Corpus, Discourse and Mental Health

Corpus and Discourse

Series Editors: Wolfgang Teubert, University of Birmingham, UK, and Michaela Mahlberg, University of Birmingham, UK

Editorial Board: Paul Baker (Lancaster), Frantisek Čermák (Prague), Susan Conrad (Portland), Dominique Maingueneau (Paris XII), Christian Mair (Freiburg), Alan Partington (Bologna), Elena Tognini-Bonelli (Siena and TWC), Ruth Wodak (Lancaster), Feng Zhiwei (Beijing).

Consisting of spoken, written or signed language, discourse always has historical, social, functional, and regional dimensions. Corpus linguistics provides the methodology to identify meaning in discourse and make it available for interpretation. The goal is to expound the differences and commonalities in the attitudes and beliefs expressed by the members of a discourse community, both contemporary and historical.

The Corpus and Discourse series features innovative corpus linguistic research into a range of discourses, it publishes key texts bridging the gap between social studies and linguistics and it showcases a wide range of applications, from language technology via the teaching of a second language to the translation of discourses. It also explores how language frames the way we perceive reality.

Corpus, Discourse and Mental Health

Daniel Hunt and Gavin Brookes

BLOOMSBURY ACADEMIC
LONDON • NEW YORK • OXFORD • NEW DELHI • SYDNEY

BLOOMSBURY ACADEMIC
Bloomsbury Publishing Plc
50 Bedford Square, London, WC1B 3DP, UK
1385 Broadway, New York, NY 10018, USA
29 Earlsfort Terrace, Dublin 2, Ireland

BLOOMSBURY, BLOOMSBURY ACADEMIC and the Diana logo are trademarks of Bloomsbury
Publishing Plc

First published in Great Britain 2020
This paperback edition published in 2021

Library of Congress Cataloging-in-Publication Data
Names: Hunt, Daniel (Linguist), author. | Brookes, Gavin (Linguist), author.
Title: Corpus, discourse and mental health / Daniel Hunt and Gavin Brookes.
Description: London; New York, NY: Bloomsbury Academic, Bloomsbury Publishing Plc, 2020. | Series:
Corpus and discourse | Includes bibliographical references and index. | Summary: "Situated at the
interface of corpus linguistics and health communication, Corpus, Discourse and Mental Health provides
insights into the linguistic practices of members of three online support communities as they describe
their experiences of living with and managing different mental health problems, including anorexia
nervosa, depression and diabulimia. In examining contemporary health communication data, the book
combines quantitative corpus linguistic methods with qualitative discourse analysis that draws upon
recent theoretical insights from critical health sociology. Using this mixed-methods approach, the analysis
identifies patterns and consistencies in the language used by people experiencing psychological distress
and their role in realising varying representations of mental illness, diagnosis and treatment. Far from
being neutral accounts of suffering and treating illness, corpus analysis illustrates that these interactions
are suffused with moral and ideological tensions sufferers seek to collectively negotiate responsibility
for the onset and treatment of recalcitrant mental health problems. Integrating corpus linguistics, critical
discourse analysis and health sociology, this book showcases the capacity of linguistic analysis for
understanding mental health discourse as well as critically exploring the potential of corpus linguistics to
offer an evidence-based approach to health communication research"–Provided by publisher.
Identifiers: LCCN 2020005657 (print) | LCCN 2020005658 (ebook) | ISBN 9781350059177 (hardback) |
ISBN 9781350059184 (ebook) | ISBN 9781350059191 (epub)
Subjects: LCSH: Mentally ill–Language. | Depressed persons–Language. | Eating disorders–Patients–
Language. | Discourse analysis. | Psycholinguistics.
Classification: LCC RC455.4.P78 H86 2020 (print) | LCC RC455.4.P78 (ebook) | DDC 616.89–dc23

LC record available at https://lccn.loc.gov/2020005657
LC ebook record available at https://lccn.loc.gov/2020005658

ISBN: HB: 978-1-3500-5917-7
PB: 978-1-3503-0200-6
ePDF: 978-1-3500-5918-4
eBook: 978-1-3500-5919-1

Series: Corpus and Discourse

Typeset by Deanta Global Publishing Services, Chennai, India

To find out more about our authors and books visit www.bloomsbury.com and
sign up for our newsletters.

For our parents

Contents

Illustrations

Figure

Tables

Content notice

This book examines the accounts of people suffering from anorexia nervosa, depression and diabulimia, a condition similar to an eating disorder developed by some people with type 1 diabetes.

It contains explicit first-hand accounts of eating disordered practices (particularly Chapters 2–4 and 6–8) and self-injurious behaviour and suicidal ideation (particularly Chapters 5 and 7–8).

Acknowledgements

Although there are only two names on its cover, this book is the product of the continued efforts and support of a far larger number of people.

First and foremost, we are grateful to the numerous online support group members – anonymous but appreciated – whose contributions are analysed in the following chapters.

We are grateful, too, to the series editors, Michaela Mahlberg and Wolfgang Teubert, and to Becky Holland and Andrew Wardell at Bloomsbury for sponsoring our proposal and for nurturing the manuscript to its fruition.

Kevin Harvey has been the quiet inspiration behind much of the research contained herein and we are especially thankful for the unflappable encouragement and unswerving intellectual guidance he has selflessly offered to each of us.

The writing of this book and everything that has entailed also owes a great deal to the unfaltering support of Svenja Adolphs, Sarah Atkins, Paul Baker, Brian Brown, Małgorzata Chałupnik, Dick Churchill, Luke Collins, Colin Gallagher, Lizzie Grove, Sam Haddow, Talia Isaacs, Joe Jackson, Lucy Jones, Olivia Knapton, Nelya Koteyko, Tony McEnery, Steven Morrison, Louise Mullany, Dave Peplow, Elena Semino and Danny Weston.

In addition, the research in this book was partially supported by the Economic and Social Research Council (ESRC) (grant number: ES/J500100/1).

Finally, much of the research presented in this book was undertaken in the School of English at the University of Nottingham and, as such, we remain indebted to Ron Carter, who died while it was being written. Although he was far too modest to ever acknowledge it, Ron represented the very best of academia; he was unceasingly generous, intellectually meticulous and wary of those who would build empires rather than bridges. In a world that seems evermore beset by complex problems, Ron's refusal to give in to the temptation of the simple, reductive explanation, his willingness to meet people halfway, and his ability to find common ground between ideas that appeared otherwise incompatible has never felt more necessary.

Mental health, discourse and corpus linguistics

1.1 Introduction

This book is about the language that people use to talk about mental distress. Focusing on the context of online support groups, the analysis presented over the forthcoming chapters examines the linguistic choices that people make when they disclose their experiences and understandings of different forms of emotional suffering. Mental distress can manifest in an extensive range of diagnosable mental disorders; the fifth and latest edition of the *Diagnostic and Statistical Manual of Mental Disorders* (*DSM 5*; American Psychiatric Association 2013), an authority on the classification of mental disorders, comprises a hefty 947 pages cataloguing 152 distinct psychiatric disorders (as well as various sub-types and unspecified disorders) (McCarron 2013). In this book we bring together two different research programmes which focus on three mental disorders in particular: (i) the eating disorder, anorexia nervosa (henceforth, anorexia); (ii) the mood disorder, depression; and (iii) an emergent, contested eating disorder known as diabulimia. While this book cannot therefore claim to be comprehensive in its coverage of mental health conditions, its focus on these particular disorders does at least provide insight into two prominent types of mental distress – mood disorders and eating disorders – as well as a currently non-diagnosable condition in diabulimia. These three disorders also enable us to account for language used in relation to conditions that are marked, respectively, by their rate of mortality (anorexia), prevalence (depression) and questions over their diagnostic legitimacy (diabulimia). Although all of these disorders are subject to contestation (explored in more depth in the next chapter), the last of these in particular brings to the fore questions over how people come to describe – or resist describing – themselves as suffering from a medical condition, how other people respond to such descriptions and how this shapes their beliefs about themselves and what they are experiencing.

In the following chapters, then, we are interested in exploring the ways in which members of online health-related support groups use language and discourse (a concept we introduce later) to represent these conditions, as well as themselves and others in relation to them, in the messages that they write. Understanding the experiences, attitudes and beliefs held about anorexia, depression and diabulimia by people who live with them is crucial to understanding the conditions themselves and to evaluating how those who suffer from them can be best treated and supported. To this end, we believe that detailed analysis of the language used by people when talking about their mental health problems offers a potent means of making sense of these experiences, attitudes and beliefs.

In this vein, a secondary aim of this book is to explore the opportunities and limitations of using corpus linguistic methods to analyse discourses of mental distress. The term *corpus linguistics* refers to a body of methods that uses specialist computer programs to study linguistic patterns in large collections of naturally occurring language data (McEnery and Wilson 2001). Corpus methods offer systematic means for pinpointing repeated and unique linguistic patterns in text and talk (Baker 2006) and hence for identifying common and more singular representations of anorexia, depression and diabulimia in this book. For example, corpus software can rapidly retrieve and present every instance of *depression* in a dataset and conduct statistical analyses based on the words that co-occur with it in order to understand how speakers typically (and atypically) talk about the condition and their relationship to it. Such affordances enable the mental health narratives of potentially thousands of individuals to be examined in ways that are not practical in purely qualitative studies. Despite the significant analytical opportunities offered by the ability to systematically analyse large amounts of data, to our knowledge there are few studies utilizing corpus techniques to examine online discussions of mental health issues (for exceptions, see Harvey 2012, 2013a; Harvey and Brown 2012; McDonald and Woodward-Kron 2016).

While our analysis places strong emphasis on the lexical and grammatical features of online support group messages, our intention in this book is not to provide a purely descriptive account of these texts. Our reasons for this are twofold: first, linguistic descriptions of computer-mediated communication are not in short supply (Baron 2000, 2008; Crystal 2001; Barton and Lee 2013). Secondly, for their participants and, we believe, the social scientist, the primary significance of these online interactions does not lie in their status as neutral language data. Rather, it lies in the rich, first-hand accounts of mental health knowledge and experience which they provide. To present a purely descriptive account of these texts would therefore disregard an opportunity to understand the subjective accounts of pernicious mental health conditions that the participants offer. This practical orientation places the present study squarely in the tradition of applied linguistics, memorably defined by Brumfit (1995: 27) as 'the theoretical and empirical investigation of real-world problems in which language is a central issue' (see also Cook 2003). To borrow Corder's (1973: 10) terms, our study 'is not a theoretical study [but] makes use of the findings of theoretical studies' to illuminate issues in the 'real world'. By its very nature, this makes applied linguistics an interdisciplinary endeavour, and the research in this book combines substantive aspects of linguistics, health sociology (Nettleton 2013) and medical humanities (Crawford et al. 2015) and orients as much to the two latter disciplines as it does to the former.

In keeping with this orientation, this book is intended for an audience drawn from a range of disciplinary backgrounds. In approaching questions about mental illness using methods from the field of linguistics, our intention is to show the value of attending closely to language even when dealing with issues more commonly associated with the disciplines of psychology and psychiatry. Likewise, attention to language can highlight the ways in which broad social changes are reproduced, negotiated and challenged at the micro level of interaction between individuals, and hence offer insights relevant to health sociologists.

We should also make it clear at this point that it is not our aim to compare or contrast the discourses associated with anorexia, depression and diabulimia, although we do flag up certain areas of similarity or difference where these are judged to support (or likewise problematize) our analytical points. Neither is it our aim to establish a general set of 'mental health discourses' that characterize online mental health support discussions. It is for this reason that we analyse online interactions related to anorexia, depression and diabulimia separately in the form of three case studies, rather than amalgamating our data and focusing primarily on the consistencies across these conditions. By first considering the data related to anorexia, depression and diabulimia discretely, we are able to examine topics that are particular to interactions around each condition – such as insulin use in relation to diabulimia – but which would have likely slipped into the analytical background had we combined the datasets together. In addition, it also enables us to consider the ways in which the representations of anorexia, depression and diabulimia that emerge during interactions in each support group are strongly related to, and best understood in relation to, the contextual norms of each forum itself.

Finally, we should also make clear that it is not our intention to identify any 'linguistic markers' of anorexia, depression, diabulimia or emotional distress more generally. Rather, we share the view of Galasiński (2008) who, writing in relation to depression, argues that the diverse ways in which people talk about emotional suffering means that it is 'quite difficult to make definitive claims as to what affect in language is supposed to look like in depression or outside it' (2008: 16–17). This is a point we will return to in Section 1.4.

In light of the interdisciplinary makeup of our intended readership, the remainder of this chapter elaborates on this general introduction with respect to the book's three central elements: (i) mental health and distress, (ii) discourse, and (iii) corpus linguistics. The next section explores the constructed and contested nature of mental health and illness, a consideration which brings us to the phenomenon of medicalization – a key concept in this book's analysis – and specifically to the processes by which some mental states come to be thought of and treated as 'normal' and others as 'abnormal' or 'deviant' and thus as requiring medical intervention. We then move on to the related topics of discourse and discourse analysis, sketching out the view of discourse we adopt in this book and the ontological assumptions this entails for our analysis. Following this, we provide a more detailed introduction to corpus linguistics as our primary methodology and approach to discourse analysis, acquainting readers with some of its key features and debates and comparing it against other approaches currently being applied in social scientific research of (mental) health language. The chapter then concludes with an overview of the remaining chapters of the book. Reflecting the diverse disciplinary perspectives from which the topic of mental health is approached in contemporary research, this book is written with a consciously interdisciplinary audience in mind. As such, we do not assume that readers have any prior knowledge of the topics of mental health and distress, discourse (analysis) or corpus linguistics.

1.2 Mental health and the medicalization of distress

An important starting point for the research in this book is our view of mental disorders as socially and discursively constituted. Epistemological debates around psychopathology have, as Pilgrim and Bentall (1999) point out, long been characterized by two polarized positions which they term 'medical naturalism' and 'social constructionism'. Medical naturalism holds that psychiatric nosology 'proceeds incrementally with a confidence that there exists a real and invariant external world of natural disease entities' (Pilgrim and Bentall 1999: 261). From this perspective, these 'natural disease entities' have been observed and studied by diagnosticians with increasing sophistication over time, rendering psychiatry's accounts of mental disorders ever more accurate – in other words, bringing them ever closer to the 'reality' of the natural disease entities they aim to describe. However, the medical naturalism position has been challenged, most notably by proponents of anti-psychiatry, an international movement inspired by the work of scholars such as Michel Foucault, Ronald David Laing, Thomas Szasz and Franco Basaglia, that is concerned with reframing the concept of 'mental health'. Exponents of this movement problematize psychiatry's explanatory and diagnostic frameworks, in many cases totally rejecting psychiatric explanations for mental distress (Szasz 1960). Some critics of psychiatry also go so far as to claim that it has yet to provide any convincing evidence of the biological 'reality' of mental illness, such as lesions or physical defects in the brain (Burstow 2015).

The second perspective, social constructionism, studies psychiatric diagnoses as 'representations of a variegated and ultimately unknowable human condition', with mental illnesses themselves viewed as 'by-product[s] of the activity of mental health professionals' (Pilgrim and Bentall 1999: 261). Influenced by the writing of Michel Foucault and Jacques Derrida, scholars and critics working in the social constructionist tradition are less concerned with studying psychopathology itself and more interested in studying how psychopathology is represented or socially constructed through different types of social practice. The social constructionist perspective has been adopted by countless discourse-based and social scientific studies of mental illnesses including, among others, anorexia (Hepworth 1999) and depression (Lewis 1996) (see Harper (1995) for a review of social constructionist research of mental health discourse).

As a means of negotiating these oppositional perspectives, Pilgrim and Bentall propose a critical realist view of mental health, which, they argue, sits somewhere in between medical naturalism and social constructionism. Associated most closely with the work of philosopher Roy Bhaskar (1975, 1979, 1990), critical realism is usefully defined by Archer and colleagues as

> a series of philosophical positions on a range of matters including ontology, causation, structure, persons, and forms of explanation. Emerging in the context of the post-positivist crises in the natural and social sciences in the 1970s and 1980s, critical realism represents a broad alliance of social theorists and researchers trying to develop a properly post-positivist social science. Critical realism situates itself as an alternative paradigm both to scientific forms of positivism concerned with regularities, regression-based variables models, and

the quest for law-like forms; and also to the strong interpretivist or postmodern turn which denied explanation in favour of interpretation, with a focus on hermeneutics and description at the cost of causation.

(Archer et al. 2016: n.p.)

When applied to the study of mental health and illness, critical realist approaches are sympathetic towards social constructionism's concern with examining psychiatric concepts of mental illness in terms of the social and historical contexts that have given rise to them but, unlike social constructionism, does not reduce psychopathology to the level of discourse alone. From a critical realist perspective, it is not reality itself but human theories of and methods for investigating reality which are understood to be socially (and discursively) constructed. These constructions are not viewed as objective but rather as 'shaped by social forces and informed by interests […] includ[ing] interests of race, class and gender as well as economic investment and linguistic, cultural and professional constraints in time and space' (Pilgrim and Bentall 1999: 262). Critical realism therefore advocates a moderate social constructionism that 'ensures a proper caution about historical and cultural relativism, without degenerating into the unending relativism and nihilism attending social constructionism' (Pilgrim and Bentall 1999: 271).

For the purpose of this book, we take a critical realist view of mental illness. We are interested in understanding how members of online communities linguistically encode their experiences of mental illness and the socially and historically contingent explanations that they draw upon when doing so. Between the poles of medical naturalism and social constructionism, critical realism is appealing because it 'respects empirical findings about the reality of misery and its multiple determinants but does not collapse into the naïve realism of medical naturalism. It accepts causal arguments but remains sensitive to the relationship between empirical methods and pre-empirical (e.g. professional) interests and social forces' (Pilgrim and Bentall 1999: 272). A further advantage of the critical realist perspective is that it allows us to sidestep the difficulties surrounding debates pertaining to the biological foundation of mental illness. Whether or not conditions like anorexia, depression and diabulimia are biological, we can be sure that they are social. They are all experienced by individuals in social contexts, and those experiences are likely to be shaped by contextual factors at the macro and micro levels and, crucially, mediated through discourse. It is this discourse that we are primarily interested in. We will expand on what this critical realist perspective on mental illness means for our view of discourse, and in turn for our analysis, later in this chapter. In the meantime, we turn our attention to the process by which forms of mental distress come to be classified and constructed as illnesses – namely, medicalization.

The concept of medicalization has been most forcefully developed by medical sociologist Peter Conrad to account for the 'process by which non-medical problems become defined and treated as medical problems, usually in terms of illnesses or disorders' (Conrad 1992: 209; Zola 1972). The remainder of this section expands upon the concept of medicalization, its emergence and influence on contemporary society, and its relevance to this book. While the majority of writing engaging with the topic of medicalization adopts a critical perspective on it and the medical institutions it supports, our intention here is not to undermine the value of the advances in medical knowledge that have led to and resulted from medicalization. Rather, we want to present research in support of three related propositions: first, that the development of medical science has occurred alongside the expansion of the medical paradigm into previously non-medical areas of life (a process of medicalization); second, that developments in health sciences are not confined to the medical clinic and its technologies; rather, and third, that the process of medicalization impels lay individuals to understand themselves in ways shaped by medical science.

Recent research on medicalization has been extensive, such that the term itself has come to refer to a number of processes occurring in different contexts. The range of activities through which medicalization can be realized is captured by Conrad's classification of it as 'defining a problem in medical terms, using medical language to describe a problem, adopting a medical framework to understand a problem, or using a medical intervention to "treat" it' (1992: 211). More recently, Rose (2007) has discussed the effects that medical developments have had on lay individuals, regarding medicalization as a process by which people come to 'describe themselves in the language of health and illness, question themselves against medical criteria of normality and pathology, [and] take themselves and their mortal existence as circumscribing their values' (2007: 700).

Inherent in both of the descriptions above is the contention that medicalization involves a reconceptualization of phenomena from a non-scientific folk paradigm into the practices and epistemology of medical science. Accordingly, Conrad (2007) asserts that society is becoming increasingly medicalized, with ever more previously natural or 'normal' aspects of social life being subsumed under disease labels and treated as medical problems. To offer an example relevant to mental health, Scott (2006) argues that shyness has undergone a process of medicalization in the form of diagnoses for social phobia, social anxiety disorder and avoidant personality disorder. Scott claims that this instance of medicalization has three main dimensions: the use of biomedical and genetic approaches to treatment, the use of cognitive-behaviour therapy and 'shyness clinics', and the so-called disciplinary regimes imposed by self-help literature on the topic. In addition to mental health issues, research has demonstrated the medicalization of a range of social phenomena as diverse as childbirth (Johanson et al. 2002), infertility (Becker and Nachtigall 1992) and hair loss (Harvey 2013b).

According to Conrad and Schneider (1980), medicalization can occur at the macro-, meso- and micro-level. As Gabe (2013) points out, '[m]acro-level actors include medical researchers and journals, governments and national organizations [,] the meso-level would include local organizations, while doctor-patient interaction concerns mainly micro-level actors' (2013: 49). The different strata at which medicalization can occur are necessarily interrelated, such that broad alterations to the political and cultural landscape refract into the types of micro-level lay interactions that are the focus of this book. While macro processes such as the market dominance of self-interested pharmaceutical companies are both worrying and eminently worthy of study, the interest of this review is to show how these changes impact upon the practices of *individuals*, both inside and outside of clinical settings.

Research into medicalization at the 'micro-level' has shown it to have far-reaching consequences for how people who are not medical experts come to conceptualize and communicate about various aspects of their very being. However, this does not mean to imply that non-experts are passive in the medicalization process. Indeed, although medicalization is driven in part by professional and institutional interests, it is important to recognize the complex roles that 'laypeople' and so-called expert patients play in promoting medicalized understandings of health and illness (Busfield 2017). Increasing internet access and the proliferation of health information websites has enabled lay individuals to adopt the roles of informed patients and health consumers who can seek out and publicize medical knowledge themselves (Barker 2008; Miah and Rich 2008).

In addition to increased exposure to medical concepts and diagnostic criteria through the internet, media and public health literature, Rose (2006) claims that recent increases in psychiatric diagnoses and rates of psychotropic drug prescription have radically altered lay individuals' self-perceptions. Rose argues that the expansion of psychiatry into conditions at the borders of normality and the ostensibly growing prevalence of psychological disorders have made both lay people and clinicians more likely to interpret behaviour in terms of psychological pathology. Democratizing medical and psychiatric knowledge, he argues,

> serves to lower the threshold at which individuals are defined, and define themselves, as suitable cases for treatment. It increases the numbers of those who enter upon a 'moral career' as a person suffering from a treatable condition, and reduces the age at which many enter upon this career.
>
> (Rose 2006: 481)

However, medicalization does not necessarily entail an uncritical acceptance of patienthood or alignment between lay individuals and medical professionals. For instance, Fox and colleagues' (2005) study of an online pro-anorexia community illustrates the proliferation of medical information among a group that remains firmly opposed to the categorization and treatment of anorexia as a medical pathology. These 'pro-anas' display a sophisticated knowledge of calorie content, body mass information, exercise regimes and weight loss pharmaceuticals, while explicitly subverting clinical accounts of anorexia and the implication that they are mentally ill. Rather than medicalization being a totalizing process, therefore, individuals who define their identities in relation to medical diagnoses can assimilate medical information into existing value systems and use biomedical knowledge while rejecting its typical therapeutic functions (Rose 2007). The medicalization of everyday life is therefore neither complete nor straightforward; although medical concepts have undoubtedly become pervasive in lay understandings of health and illness, this does not entail a blanket acceptance of a biomedical model of disease, a patient identity, or the dicta of public health messages (Fox et al. 2005; Fox and Ward 2006). Instead, lay beliefs come from a range of sources and

> do not directly correspond to those of professionals, nor are they watered-down versions of what is taught in medical schools. Lay people form their own perspectives, drawing upon a wide variety of sources not limited to scientific or proven-in-practice dimensions.
>
> (Hughner and Kleine 2004: 416)

Medical knowledge is therefore just one of many different types of resources that individuals can draw upon to understand their health and illness, and lay people typically retain a concern for non-biological features of their illness experiences, such as anxiety about the effects of illness on their social, financial and emotional well-being (Stoppard 2000; McKague and Verhoef 2003).

According to Conrad (1992), medicalization can entail both positive and negative consequences for the people affected by the particular phenomenon or embodied experience in question. He refers to these, respectively, as the 'brighter' and 'darker' sides of medicalization (Conrad 1992: 223), though, as Fox et al.'s (2005) study shows, a simple binary view of medicalization as either good or bad ignores the range of complex, partial and contingent ways in which medical discourses are taken up. Regardless, as mentioned earlier, much of the literature surrounding medicalization regards the process critically. One frequent criticism of medicalization is that it necessarily involves expanding the remit of medical pathology, which encourages lay people and professionals alike to pathologize embodied experiences according to biological models of disease. This has prompted concern that medicalization marginalizes lay conceptualizations of disease (Kleinman 1988) and isolates the causes of ill health within affected individuals rather than the social worlds they inhabit. Proponents of this argument cite as evidence the decontextualized, individualizing accounts of mental disorders provided by diagnostic manuals, including the aforementioned *DSM*, which, as O'Reilly and Lester (2016: 6) observe, are 'fundamentally developed from a biomedical perspective and have resulted in the construction of mental illness as an objective, ahistorical reality that resides within the "ill" individual' (and see Pilgrim and Bentall 1999). For example, Crowe's (2000) critique of the fourth edition of the *DSM* (APA 1994) highlighted the assumption that mental disorders are caused by universal biochemical and physiological defects residing in the individual, thereby suppressing the possibility that such disorders could be caused by responses to external events. This also has implications for treatments, with Crowe warning that an 'uncritical acceptance and utilization of this classification system excludes the possibility of more innovative research and treatment for people experiencing mental distress' (2000: 75).

As the quote from Crowe alludes, as well as curtailing non-medical explanations, medicalization can also result in responses to human suffering being delimited to those that involve clinical intervention. This is reflected in clinical practice where the primacy of models of mental illness that prioritize biological causes over social factors restricts the mandate of healthcare professionals to propose socially oriented interventions, even where these may benefit patients (McPherson and Armstrong 2009). Standardized medical models of mental illness may therefore 'imperil illness negotiation on the one hand, and curtail local healing opportunities on the other' by precluding non-medical approaches to treating illness (Lee 1995: 31).

Another consequence of medicalization postulated by its critics is that it renders individuals affected by a pathology as effectively passive, to the point that they risk becoming both over-reliant on medical interventions and uncritical of the ever-expanding jurisdiction of modern medicine (Gabe 2013: 52). The expanding authority of medical expertise is not necessarily a bad thing, particularly for people who might not feel capable of remedying their ailments on their own. However, the prospect of having other, maybe all, aspects of life dominated by medical experts is likely to be less appealing (O'Reilly and Lester 2016).

In contrast to the widespread critique of medicalization, there are also arguments that the process can bear significant clinical and symbolic benefits – what Conrad (1992: 223) refers to as medicalization's 'brighter side'. First, the increasing scope of medicalization observed by Conrad and others has at least in part resulted from advances in diagnostic tools and refinements in human understandings of the body and its ailments. These same developments have also meant that the last century has borne witness to remarkable progression in the faculties of medical science to prevent, control and even wholly eradicate disease and to sustain life far beyond humanity's previous capacities. As Conrad (2007: 147–8) puts it, '[o]n the medical side, many of us know individuals whose life has been significantly improved by psychoactive medications, who are no longer depressed, disoriented or disordered thanks to medical interventions'. As such, to define a problematic or distressing set of experiences in medical terms, as an illness, is to deem those experiences appropriate for medical attention – a process which opens up opportunities for the alleviation of the attested experiences or 'symptoms', or even a cure (Gwyn 2002; Gabe 2013).

The classification of distress as an illness, including mental illness, also has the potential to reduce some of the stigma that might be associated with certain causes of distress. This is particularly the case for conditions for which blame or moral responsibility is apportioned to sufferers (Conrad and Schneider 1980). For example, in conducting semi-structured interviews with women with a history of eating disorders, Easter (2012) found that biomedical explanatory models helped to nullify stigma associated with the belief that anorexia is a volitional condition. Similarly, during interviews with people with depression and their families, Karp (1996) observed that regarding depression as a biologically predetermined condition helped sufferers to account for their experience of uncontrollable, chronic unhappiness and enabled them to mitigate blame for their illness.

In foregrounding both its favourable and more concerning implications, the foregoing discussion remains ambivalent about how medicalization should be evaluated. As Conrad (1992) rightly asserts, demonstrating that the borders of medical pathology are expanding as a result of complex social and political processes does not mean that medicalization is inherently undesirable or, more importantly, any better or worse than alternative explanatory models of human suffering. Indeed, given the astounding capacity of contemporary medicine to alleviate disease, we may in fact have good reason to pursue medicalization (Ebrahim 2002). Similarly, just as a biomedical perspective might relegate structural and cultural factors affecting mental health to secondary concerns, any competing explanations of health, such as those provided by social and cultural theorists, will be equally partial. Put in terms of clinical practice, a professional view that privileges a patient's biological symptoms over the patient's own personal and social concerns is not inherently invalid, any more than the patient's experiences are invalidated by a biomedical description of their suffering. The difference in perspectives shows only that there is a need to understand how medical and non-medical conceptions of health are negotiated in interaction and what their implications may be for those experiencing suffering. As Rose claims, therefore, rather than simply identifying medicalization, we must also 'assess the costs and benefits of our thoroughly medical form of life – and of those that offer themselves as alternatives' (Rose 2007: 702).

Having reviewed the tensions around medicalization and medicalized accounts of mental distress, the research in this book responds to Rose's (2007) call for an investigation of the effects of medicalization. To this end, we examine communication between individuals affected by anorexia, depression and diabulimia in online support groups, a venue described as a possible 'engine of medicalisation' in contemporary society (Conrad 2005; Barker 2008). In addition to this, our analysis will also examine whether notions of morality and responsibility attend medical explanations of psychological distress. This in turn encourages a broader analytical concern with the relationships between the use of medical knowledge in talk, the negotiation of responsibility for sickness, and the construction of identities in relation to mental illness. The next section of this chapter introduces discourse and discourse analysis and outlines the particular view of discourse we adopt for our analysis.

1.3 Discourse

In analysing situated, naturally occurring linguistic patterns in people's accounts of mental illness, this book is concerned with discourse. The identification and analysis of 'discourse' has become a significant activity across the contemporary humanities and social sciences (Fairclough 2002, 2003).

Indeed, since the 1970s, the concept of discourse has been appropriated within diverse areas of intellectual inquiry, all allied by a concern with the analysis of language and text, such as linguistics, psychology, philosophy and cultural studies, to name just a few. As a result of the numerous disciplines examining spoken and written interaction within their own specific paradigms, few terms are now so freighted with meaning as the term 'discourse' itself (Mills 2005). Sunderland, for instance, observes the way in which '[d]ifferent theoretical approaches conceptualise discourse and its workings in different, though overlapping, ways' (2004: 6), while Baker (2006) describes the term 'discourse' as 'problematic, as it is used in [...] a number of inter-related yet different ways' (2006: 3).

For the purpose of this book, we wish to foreground two distinct interpretations of 'discourse' and its analysis. The first views discourse as any text 'above the sentence or above the clause' (Stubbs 1983: 1). The second, more theoretical understanding originates with Foucault, who conceives of discourse as not just groups of signs (signifying elements referring to contents or representations) but as rule-governed sets of verbal and nonverbal practices that provide systematic frameworks through which people understand, act in and communicate about the world (Foucault 1969). Foucault was interested in the power of discourses, in the plural sense, to constitute those aspects of reality with which they are concerned; that is, as Foucault himself famously states, the power of discourses to

> systematically form the objects of which they speak. Of course, discourses are composed of signs; but what they do is more than use these signs to designate things. It is this 'more' that renders them irreducible to the language (*langue*) and to speech.
>
> (Foucault 1969: 54)

The view of discourse we adopt in this book draws on both of these conceptions. The corpus linguistic techniques we use to make sense of our data facilitate analysis of language at a discourse level – as Stubbs conceptualizes it – by providing information about the frequencies of lexical and grammatical features across whole or multiple texts. Discourse in this sense is also analysed through the qualitative study of language features across sequences of support group messages. In line with the second perspective outlined above, the discourses identified at the textual level are then interpreted in terms of their power to construe the aspects of mental health and illness with which they are concerned.

In keeping with the critical realist perspective on mental illness introduced in the previous section, we opt in this study for a moderate version of Foucault's social constructionism. With this in mind, we follow Fairclough, who recommends that the distinction between moderate and extreme social constructionism be marked by the terminological distinction between 'construal' and 'construction':

> We need to distinguish 'construction' from 'construal', which social constructivists do not: we may textually construe (represent, imagine, etc.) the social world in particular ways, but whether our representations or construals have the effect of changing its construction depends upon various contextual factors – including the way social reality already is, who is constructing it, and so forth. So we can accept a moderate version of the claim that the social world is textually constructed, but not an extreme version.
>
> (Fairclough 2003: 8–9)

In this study, then, we will interpret the discourses we identify in the support group messages as 'construing' rather than 'constructing' the reality of the mental disorders with which they are concerned.

While significantly influenced by the writing of Foucault, therefore, the view of discourse we take in this book also departs from Foucault's original conception in several important respects. In addition to our more moderate view of the power of discourse to construe – rather than construct – reality, our second point of departure concerns the agency with which we interpret individual actors to engage with discourses. Echoing one of the staple principles of discursive psychology (Edwards and Potter 1992), we are sensitive to the possibility for individuals to actively invent, draw upon and challenge discourses in the ways they make sense of and understand the world they inhabit. This potential affords individuals a greater degree of agency than is implied by Foucault and more hard-line versions of social constructionism, according to which individuals are conceptualized 'only as the *outcome* of discursive and societal structures' and consequently have 'no capacity to bring about change' (Burr 2015: 27, our emphasis) – an assumption critics claim results in the 'death of the subject' (Heartfield 2002).

Finally, we regard discourses as being identifiable through the communicative (including linguistic) traces they leave in the texts in which they manifest. This departs from Foucault's original conception of discourse, which did not allude to the textual or linguistic properties of discourse but instead regarded discourses as the broader, macro-level rules that govern rather than explicitly inhabit texts, actions, behaviours and so forth. Interpreting discourses in this way allows them to be identified and examined more systematically by discourse analysts. Working in a Foucauldian tradition, Mills (2005: 15) argues that we might 'detect' a discourse by 'the systematicity of the ideas, opinions, concepts, ways of thinking and behaving which are formed within a particular context'. In a similar vein, Sunderland (2004) and Baker (2010) outline some of the possible ways in which discourses manifest in texts and which allow analysts to search for traces of discourses in a more 'systematic' and 'conscious' manner (Sunderland 2004: 36). These features include repeated lexical choices in the representation and evaluation of knowledge, individuals, ideas, beliefs and (linguistic) practices; evidence of intertextuality (i.e. one text drawing on (part of) another (Allen 2011)); and repetitive and systematic use of such linguistic features as hyperbole, euphemism, implicature, modality, agency (both grammatical and sociological), nominalization and metaphor.

Following these scholars, we conceive of discourses as ways of construing reality that are realized through different linguistic articulations. The possibility of contrasting descriptions of any phenomenon allows for reality to be construed in multiple (conflicting) ways, depending on which discourse(s) are invoked (Fairclough 2003: 124). As Burr (1995: 48) puts it, discourses 'each [have] a different story to tell about the world, a different way of representing it to the world'. To offer an example relevant to health, Cameron (2001: 15–16) observes how the concept of drugs is the object of a plethora of discourses (i.e. of criminality, recreation, medicine and spiritual enlightenment), all of which paint a different picture of what drugs are. A single discourse can be realized by consistent utterances across different times, locations and authors. Meanwhile, a single text may contribute to multiple discourses that are themselves interrelated. For example, a psychiatric research article may construe mental illness through particular descriptions of the mind and mental states, in so doing contributing to a wider discourse of psychiatric medicine that normalizes particular representations of health and illness and which itself instantiates wider discourses such as rationalism and empiricism. In this regard, texts can be viewed as containing and reiterating traces of wider social practices and forms of social organization. When a particular verbal representation is reiterated in a relatively stable and consistent manner, a discourse can become an established and accepted way of viewing the world. In this respect, Foucault's notion of discourse functions in a similar way to the historical materialist notion of ideology (Mills 2005: 27). A discourse can therefore be not just a way of representing the world during linguistic interaction but also become an epistemic resource that influences people's understanding of reality and themselves long after a specific communicative event (Willig 2000).

Although they might be drawn upon in the same text or to construe the same phenomenon, all discourses are not born equal. Instead, discourses compete with one another in the claim to dominance or to so-called truth status (Mills 2005). As Sunderland (2004: 45) puts it, discourses exist in 'constellations', for a discourse's status as dominant or marginalized relates to other, usually competing, discourses around the same topic. Returning to the issue of medicalization, one example of this is the way in which medico-scientific discourses dominate how the body and its ailments are interpreted and talked about in Western societies, while the perspectives offered by alternative medicines are generally regarded as fictitious and fraudulent (Harvey 2013a: 6–7).

Discourses and their statuses (say, as dominant or minority) not only construe aspects of the world but are also construed by it (Blommaert 2005). In this sense, discourses enter into dialectal relationships with the world; when we draw upon or invent certain discourses and exclude others, we do so in ways that are shaped by our immediate interactional and wider societal contexts. At the broader level, this means that discourses are shaped by the societies in which they take place. Meanwhile, at the local level, discourses are shaped by individuals' aims and objectives in interactions, as well as by the affordances and constraints of particular communicative media and contexts. The mental health discourses we identify in our analysis will thus be interpreted as having been shaped at the macro level by the contributors' wider social and cultural milieus and at the micro level by their interactional aims and objectives and the technological affordances of the online support group platforms on which they converse.

With this view of discourse in mind, the project of discourse analysis thus involves identifying and disentangling the various discourses that are present in a text or collection of texts or which surround a particular object or thing in the world, as well as understanding the contextual relevance of these discourses. Discourse analysis is a heterogeneous and largely qualitative methodology which has already been fruitfully applied in studies of the language of mental illness disclosure. A few recent examples include Galasiński's (and colleagues') research into the discourses surrounding men's depression and suicide (Galasiński 2008, 2013, 2017; Ziółkowska and Galasiński 2017), Knapton's (2018) study of the linguistic construction of the self in narratives of obsessive-compulsive disorder and Demjén et al.'s (2019) study of metaphorical framings of distress in lived-experience accounts of voice-hearing (for an overview of discourse analytical research of mental health, see Georgaca (2014)). In these studies (and more besides), discourse analytical approaches have enabled researchers to interrogate the constructed and culturally and historically situated nature of mental illness concepts and experiences. The approach to discourse that we take in this book combines qualitative techniques from discourse analysis with quantitative methods of corpus linguistics. What this means in practical terms will be outlined in Chapter 3. For now, we introduce corpus linguistics as our primary methodology and approach to discourse analysis.

1.4 Corpus linguistics and alternative approaches

Corpus linguistics is a collection of methods for analysing language based on large collections of naturally occurring language in-use (McEnery and Wilson 2001). Such a collection of texts is called a *corpus* (the Latin word for 'body', plural *corpora*). One of the main appeals of using large collections of data – it is not unusual for corpora to run into millions, sometimes billions, of words – is that it allows researchers to base their analyses on more substantial and representative textual evidence, thereby accounting for wider variation in the type of language or texts being analysed and ultimately producing findings that are more generalizable with respect to the particular language, social group, context or linguistic variety under study.

A corpus is not a randomly compiled collection of texts but is carefully designed to represent a particular language or variety. Corpora can comprise textual data from a range of modes (i.e. speech, writing, computer-mediated communication, gestures) and genres (e.g. spoken conversations, books, online support groups). A corpus is considered representative of the variety it is designed to represent if findings based on its contents can be generalized to that variety (Leech 1991). This issue of representativeness will therefore dictate the design of the corpus in terms of its size, the texts it contains and its balance in terms of how much each text or genre contributes to the corpus as a whole (McEnery and Hardie 2012: 8–11).

To illustrate how representativeness influences corpus design, it is useful to consider the distinction between general and specialized corpora. Where general corpora are designed to represent entire languages or varieties (usually at a single point in time), specialized corpora are designed to represent language in more specific contexts (McEnery and Wilson 2001: 5). Because they strive to represent language on a broad scale, general corpora tend to be very large in size, typically comprising thousands of texts and millions or billions of words. An example of a general corpus is the 100-million-word British National Corpus (BNC; Aston and Burnard 1998), which was compiled to represent contemporary written and spoken British English during the 1980s and 1990s. Given the practical difficulties associated with achieving representativeness on such a broad scale, large general corpora like the BNC are often designed according to sampling frames which help to ensure that they provide a balanced representation of the various genres or registers that make up the target language or variety.

Specialized corpora, on the other hand, tend to be much smaller than general corpora and usually represent a single or more restricted range of genres and registers. An example of a specialized corpus purpose-built for health communication research is the approximately one-million-word Adolescent Health Email Corpus compiled and analysed by Harvey as part of his research into the language adolescents use when seeking health advice (Harvey 2012, 2013a). However, even specialized corpora can be very large. For example, in research on patient feedback about healthcare services, Baker et al. (2019) analysed a purpose-built corpus of 228,113 patient comments (approximately 29 million words) about the UK National Health Service (NHS).

Another key feature of a corpus is that it contains naturally occurring language. In other words, corpora contain real language produced by real people in real-world contexts. The use of attested language data is a core feature of corpus study (McEnery and Gabrielatos 2006), and one that places corpus linguistics at the antipodes of the rationalist linguistics characterized by the Chomskyan tradition. In stipulating that only those discursive practices which can be intuited by the researcher are analytically relevant, Chomsky's (1957) disregard for attested data represents something of a non-starter for empirical health communication research. In contrast, an overriding emphasis on naturally occurring language rather than native speakers' verbal intuitions grounds corpus linguistics in the social sciences (Stubbs 1996) and the discipline of applied linguistics (introduced earlier), where linguists' work has a fundamental engagement with real-world concerns. The naturally occurring data used in corpus research exists prior to and regardless of its investigation by a researcher, permitting repeat analysis and the discovery of linguistic patterns not readily available to intuition (Carter 2004). The deliberate engagement with language use in contexts that are unfamiliar to the analyst is of clear relevance to the present study, where descriptions of experiences of mental illnesses would otherwise be unavailable to the researchers.

The final feature of corpora we want to address here is that the texts they contain must be stored in an electronic, machine-readable format so that they can be analysed using computers. Because they tend to be very large, it is usually not practical for corpora to be analysed by hand (at least in their entirety). Here, corpus software packages such as *WordSmith Tools* (Scott 2016) can be used by human researchers to carry out tasks which they would otherwise be unable to perform manually. These procedures, which will be introduced in more detail in Chapter 3, allow analysts to search for every occurrence of a word or combination of words, generate frequency information about linguistic phenomena of interest (e.g. words, chains of words, grammatical types), perform statistical tests on those frequencies (i.e. to measure the significance or strength of relationships between phenomena) and to present the data in ways that render it more amenable to qualitative discourse analysis (Baker 2006). The quantitative analyses are carried out automatically, removing the need for laborious manual reading and reducing the risk of researchers falling into miscalculations when confronted with overwhelming amounts data (Baker 2010). At the same time, computer assistance can be beneficial for the analysis itself, as it can render visible patterns that run counter to human intuition (McEnery et al. 2006) or which feature sparingly in one or two texts but become significant when considered as part of a larger collection of data (Stubbs 1994).

In view of their analytical benefits, the volume of research employing corpus methods has expanded rapidly in the last thirty or so years, such that it has become difficult to overstate the impact that corpus linguistics has had on the study of language. Indeed, it is no exaggeration to state, as Leech (2000: 677) does, that corpus linguistics has 'revolutionized' the ways in which we approach and now even conceptualize language. As part of this disciplinary revolution, corpus methods have been employed in increasingly 'applied' sub-disciplines of linguistics and used in combination with concepts and approaches from a range of cognate fields. The recent uptake of corpus methods by researchers working in the domain of health communication is no exception here. Indeed, Crawford et al. (2014) argue that it is unsurprising that we find corpus methods employed to analyse the language of medicine, an institution largely driven by quantitative, 'evidence-based' research. While analytically rigorous, purely qualitative studies are limited by their focus on relatively small datasets or single cases that 'can only suggest possibilities' of wider trends in health communication (Drew 2001: 267). In contrast, as Harvey (2012: 353) notes, corpora 'afford the researcher a level of analytical consistency not available to health communication research that uses small datasets'. As a consequence, following a series of studies of 373 primary care consultations by Skelton and colleagues (Skelton and Hobbs 1999a, b; Skelton et al. 2002a, b), corpus methods have proved invaluable in enabling health communication researchers to pursue lines of inquiry at the interface of healthcare research and discourse analysis. In Skelton et al.'s case, their analyses examine issues such as the role of pronouns in shared decision-making and the ways in which doctors use metaphors to present complex disease phenomena as both comprehensible and controllable. By using corpus methods, the authors are able to combine robust quantitative analysis of linguistic features diffused throughout a large dataset with a qualitative analysis that unpacks the role of these features in relation to the social, emotional and professional demands of the consultation.

Many subsequent corpus studies have been quick to capitalize on the wealth of health communication data generated through digital interactions (cf. Hunt and Churchill 2013). For instance, the aforementioned work by Harvey (2012, 2013a; Harvey et al. 2007) applies corpus methods to the analysis of a large corpus of emails submitted to an adolescent health advice website. Here, corpus techniques are vital both in offering a broad diagnostic description of the range and frequency of health concerns teenagers have and in facilitating precise descriptions of how young people understand and experience issues related to sexual health, weight and depression. More recently, synthesizing corpus linguistics with critical metaphor analysis, Demmen et al. (2015) combine data from online discussions with semi-structured interviews in order to understand the role of violence metaphors for cancer and end of life when used by patients, carers and health professionals. At 1.5 million words, their corpus is of a far larger size than could feasibly be analysed manually. However, through a corpus-assisted process of metaphor identification, the researchers are able to illustrate how the frequency of violence metaphors varies according to whether the speaker is a patient, carer or clinician, and the context in which they are communicating. Their extensive qualitative analysis of these metaphors also evinces the ways in which a speaker's choice of metaphor depends upon their role in relation to the illness, the level of formality of the communicative context, and the particular mental states they seek to express (Demmen et al. 2015: 226). When taken together, corpus-based studies of health discourse such as these demonstrate the propitious opportunities offered by computer-assisted methods for analysing health discourse in granular detail while also buttressing claims through statistical analyses of large volumes of data.

Corpus linguistics is not, however, the only method that has taken a quantitative approach to studying the language of health and illness. In particular, readers with a background in psychology or health sciences may be familiar with *Linguistic Inquiry and Word Count* (*LIWC*; Pennebaker et al. 2007), a text analysis programme originally designed to analyse narratives of emotional upheaval. The software's primary function is to assign each word in a text (or collection of texts) to one of eighty categories in a pre-set dictionary before producing an output indicating the proportion of the text corresponding to each category. As well as including grammatical features such as pronouns and prepositions, these categories are intended to indicate the psychological states of the author and their 'thinking styles' (Tausczik and Pennebaker 2010: 27). *LIWC* includes categories purported to capture words referring to positive emotions (*happy*, *good*, *love*), anxiety (*afraid*), cognitive insight (*know*, *realize*) and words that 'hint at a general social awareness', such as *talk* and *you* (Lyons et al. 2006: 255). Once measured against the *LIWC* dictionary, texts and groups of texts can then be compared in terms of the relative proportions of their constituent categories. For example, Lyons et al. (2006: 256) claim that members of online pro-anorexia communities have more 'hedonic focus' due to their significantly greater use of positive emotion words and present tense verbs when compared with members of pro-recovery anorexia networks. Pro-anorexics, they surmise, may therefore have an emotionally stabilizing thinking style.

Employing a similar approach, Al-Mosaiwi and Johnstone (2018) focus on the use of 'absolutist' words such as *always*, *totally* and *entire*, which they claim index unnuanced thinking. Comparing initial messages posted in anxiety, depression and suicidal ideation support fora against messages to several online support groups for a range of physical conditions and social problems, they identify a significantly higher use of absolutist terms in the mental health fora, particularly in the suicidal ideation support group. Absolutist terms, they conclude, therefore constitute linguistic markers of affective disorders.

These 'dictionary-based' quantitative methods are widely used and *LIWC* in particular has become an influential method for text analysis in psychology (at the time of writing, the software has over 3,700 citations). It also produces results that align with popular intuitions – and in some cases with clinical research – about different demographic and clinical groups; the finding that people with depression use more first-person pronouns (Rude et al. 2004) matches popular representations of depressed individuals as introverted and concerned with their own feelings. Likewise, the finding that increases in testosterone lead individuals to use fewer words referring to other people (Pennebaker et al. 2004) matches the gender stereotype that men are more self-regarding and less socially aware. It is also very difficult to refute the claim that there is *some* relationship between language and the mental states of speakers/writers, which is the foundation on which *LIWC*'s proponents claim to establish psychological profiles from linguistic features. However, as a methodology, *LIWC* has two related limitations that mean the outcomes of such studies offer, at best, an oversimplification of participants' language. These relate to (i) the validity of assessing psychological states through linguistic output and (ii) *LIWC*'s disregard for communicative contexts.

LIWC's viability as a method of psychological research rests upon the assumption that words used in isolation directly reflect the single psychological states or functions of their users. Yet this assumption appreciably overlooks the ways in which language is used strategically for emphatic, persuasive or genre-specific purposes. Horne and Wiggins (2009) demonstrate that new members of an online support group for people with suicidal feelings repeatedly present their circumstances in extreme terms in order to present themselves as authentically suicidal. This language, they argue, is necessary for users to be regarded as legitimate members of the online community without carrying out a suicidal threat. Linguistic features that Al-Mosaiwi and Johnstone (2018) would classify as signs of 'absolutist' thinking are therefore employed strategically as a means of validating a request for support. This is particularly important in a context where participants' continual participation in the group risks challenging their identity as someone who is genuinely suicidal: absolutist language becomes the linguistic code required to legitimize users' initial and long-term membership. Rather than identifying the language of depressed or suicidal thinking, therefore, Al-Mosaiwi and Johnstone's findings can be seen to identify the language of online support discourse in relation to depression and suicidal ideation. This is a small but important shift and one that brings into focus the social and interactional aims that participants orient to through their linguistic choices. This change in focus also entails that linguistic features cannot be transparently linked to psychological states. We would argue that it also offers a more humane representation of suicidal individuals, who are shown to be able to sensitively and strategically respond to the particular demands of the communicative context rather than being simply 'absolutist' thinkers.

Yet even if we accept that individual words *do* reflect the psychological profile of the speaker, *LIWC*'s method of categorizing words' psychological functions in isolation from each other is fraught with pitfalls. The notion that words take their meaning from their contexts of use – not least their combination with other words – is a long-standing axiom of contemporary linguistics (van Dijk 1977). However, it is not clear from the authors' description (Tausczik and Pennebaker 2010) whether many studies employing *LIWC* account for the effects of anything other than the most rudimentary word combinations. This oversight could lead to highly simplistic analytical claims: in the corpus of depression forum messages that we analyse in Chapter 5, participants collectively use the word *happy* ninety-three times compared with *sad* thirty-seven times, and *angry* thirty-two times. Using *LIWC*, we might therefore be inclined to conclude that the participants are happy two and a half times as much as they are sad. Yet even a cursory look at the forum messages themselves shows this not to be the case; participants repeatedly talk about being 'not happy' or about 'putting on a happy face' around others. Such combinations of words do not just invert the meaning of an ostensibly 'positive emotion word'; they also show that the support group members use emotion words to produce a complex array of meanings that cannot be reduced to a rudimentary 'positive' and 'negative' classification. Similarly, the implications of speakers'/writers' use of direct or reported speech, in which emotion words (and emotions) are attributed to others – 'I'm fed up of people telling me I should be happy' – are equally overlooked. In this example, the writer uses indirect speech to represent other people's injunction to 'be happy' – 'happy' is their word, not his. Yet an automated analysis can make no such fine-grained distinctions; in such an instance, 'happiness' will be attributed to the psychology of the post's author in a way that directly contradicts the contents of the text. Given the prevalence of reported speech in healthcare narratives (Hamilton 1996), this is no small oversight.

It is also not apparent if researchers using *LIWC* consider the semantic bleaching that characterizes language change, in which a word or phrase takes on a discourse marking function. For example, far from being a transparent marker of psychological anxiety, the use of *afraid* in utterances such as 'I can't help you, I'm afraid' forms part of a conventional politeness marker. In the same vein, *you know* can perform a range of discourse marking functions that do not necessarily indicate cognitive insight on the part of the speaker (Fox Tree and Schrock 2002). An analysis that fails to account for these well-attested discursive features cannot be taken as a valid examination of language in-use.

Because *LIWC*'s classification of authors' thinking styles is primarily based on the purported function of individual words, it may also overlook ways in which similar meanings can be encoded phrasally. As Galasiński (2018) observes, the 'absolutist' thinking with which Al-Mosaiwi and Johnstone (2018) are concerned could be instantiated through common phrasal constructions such as 'not on your life', 'in no way' or 'not in a million years' as well as individual words such as 'never', 'nothing' and 'all'. As a result, significant differences in the frequency of 'absolutist' language between different online groups may just reflect the methodology's insensitivity to how absolute situations are discussed by members of specific online communities.

Taken in sum, insights from discourse analytic research mean we have considerable reservations about the capacity of automated analyses like *LIWC* to accurately assess psychological traits, as well as the validity of its more general claim to identify thinking styles from linguistic features without accounting for the textual environment in which those features are embedded.

This issue is compounded by a second shortcoming of many *LIWC* studies; a decontextualized approach to discourse analysis. Pennebaker and Lay (2002) analyse transcripts of press conference responses given by Rudolph Giuliani during his time as mayor of New York from 1993 to 2001. In particular, their analysis focuses on linguistic differences during a month of personal crisis, in which Giuliani was diagnosed with cancer, withdrew from the senate race against Hilary Clinton, separated from his wife and made public his extra-marital affair. The authors note that Giuliani's press conferences during this time contained a significantly higher percentage of singular first-person pronouns relative to the periods before and after, along with a corresponding decrease in references to other people. This pattern, they contend, is indicative of high 'self-focus' and is also found in people who are depressed and socially or emotionally isolated (Pennebaker and Lay 2002: 278). Yet what's excluded from this analysis is any consideration of the questions put to Giuliani during these press meetings. Likely faced with questions specifically about his health and personal relationships, it seems wholly unsurprising that Giuliani makes greater use of *I* and *me* compared to when he discusses the city's response to 9/11. However, shorn of any such contextualized analysis, his words are interpreted as directly (and perhaps solely) indexing his psychological states. A similar issue besets a *LIWC* study by Wolf et al. (2007), who compare the language used by inpatients of an eating disorders facility against that used by members of a 'pro-recovery' online message board. The authors compare journals written by the inpatients with messages posted to the anorexia support group, claiming that differing 'cognitive styles' can be identified through significant differences in the use of past versus present tense and so-called self versus social pronouns. Yet this analysis fails to consider how use of these features might reflect broader differences in genre and audience design between personal reflective diaries and mass-participation online support groups.

Although corpus-based discourse studies employ a variety of different analytical approaches (Baker and McEnery 2015), it would be rare to find a published corpus-based discourse analysis that adopts a similarly naïve approach to context. If we are to understand accounts of mental illness as discourse rather than as a series of isolated words, we must seek to understand how salient lexical items function in their context of use, to grasp *why* particular linguistic choices are made and to appreciate the local and social implications of those choices.

In practical terms, this means complementing quantitative findings derived from corpus methods with extensive qualitative analysis that accounts – as far as possible – for the various contextual factors that influence the ways in which the participants in our data write. In our case, corpus tools provide the facility for analysing thousands of support group messages, thereby gauging a wider and more varied picture of subjective experiences and understandings of mental illness that are construed through the group members' discourse. However, automated quantitative analysis forms only one element of this approach, which is integrated with sustained qualitative interpretation of the support group messages that avoids reductive interpretations of words' meanings. In doing so, the research in this book also expands the boundaries of corpus linguistics and health communication by examining, in mental health discourse, a topic that has to-date received scant attention from corpus researchers.

Having provided this general introduction to corpus linguistics, the corpora and corpus linguistics techniques used in this book are outlined in more detail in Chapter 3. We now conclude this chapter by giving a brief overview of the remainder of this book and with a note on our terminological choices.

1.5 Overview of the book

Following this introduction, the next chapter provides a more detailed overview of the three mental health conditions considered in this book – anorexia, depression and diabulimia – in particular foregrounding the contrasting, contested perspectives held on them, including among sufferers.

Chapter 3 describes the study's data and methodology. This begins with a detailed introduction to the context of online peer-to-peer health support groups, addressing their technical affordances and utility for disclosing and discussing personal experiences of mental distress – features which we argue make them a suitable research site for our purposes. We then describe the design and compilation of the support group corpora under study, before outlining the corpus techniques we use to analyse them. This chapter also features extensive discussion of various practical and theoretical issues attending to the compilation and analysis of online linguistic data, including those to do with representing the non-standard character of computer-mediated communication, as well as the ethical considerations which underpin the collection of online accounts of distress.

The analysis is then reported across Chapters 4 to 6. Chapter 4 considers how members of an online anorexia support group discursively construe the eating disorder and their identities in relation to it, including by exploring the discourses surrounding eating, weight loss practices and the role of dietary guides in their recovery. This chapter also considers how competing accounts of anorexia, attested across separate messages posted by different users, can fulfil particular interactional goals. Chapter 5 elucidates the discourses that are used to represent depression, as well as the related topics of antidepressant medication and self-injurious behaviour. The final analytical chapter, Chapter 6, focuses on messages about diabulimia posted to online support groups for people with diabetes. As well as examining the discourses surrounding diabulimia itself, the analysis reported in this chapter also explores those contributing to the representation of the interconnected themes of insulin and diabetes, in so doing addressing diabulimia's characteristic status as a dual pathology, something which sets it apart from the other conditions analysed in this book.

Following the analysis, Chapter 7 presents a discussion of the main findings from Chapters 4 to 6, bringing together common themes emerging from the analysis of each mental condition. In particular, this chapter will consider the functions of the mental health discourses at both the micro and macro levels, in terms of enabling the users of these digital support communities to respond to and alleviate (anticipated) stigma as well as contributing towards the medicalization of mental distress both within and outside these online contexts.

Finally, Chapter 8 concludes the book by discussing the effects of the discourses identified in the preceding chapters and by considering their possible implications both for the sufferers of these conditions and the medical practitioners responsible for their care. In this chapter we also offer a series of methodological reflections on the utility of corpus methods for the study of (mental) health communication and evaluate the extent to which these approaches can meet the demand for research and practice that is both evidence-based and person-centred.

1.6 Notes on terminology

Scholars venturing into the study of mental health are presented with a freighted nomenclature with which to name (and hence construe) individuals who experience mental health problems. 'People with mental health problems' thematizes personhood over pathology, yet the lengthy post-modification is cumbersome; 'clients' reiterates and validates the uptake of commercial discourse into healthcare, a process about which we believe there are strong grounds to be sceptical; 'service users' encodes an active role, though it is not clear that all the individuals whose discourse is examined hereafter actually use healthcare services. Hence, in referring to the individuals using the online support groups under examination, we use the terms 'support group members/contributors', 'users' and 'sufferers'. We realize the last of these may appear an emotive choice. However, the ensuing analysis demonstrates that in many cases the members of the support groups we analyse do indeed consider themselves to be sufferers of the mental disorders and types of distress they are discussing.

Anorexia, depression and diabulimia

Contested conditions and online support

2.1 Introduction

Having established the aims and parameters of this study, set out our understandings of discourse and medicalization, and outlined the key features of corpus linguistic analysis, in this chapter we turn our attention to the three mental health problems with which this book is concerned: anorexia, depression and diabulimia. Each of these topics is substantial by itself, meaning that our discussion in this chapter is necessarily selective. In keeping with our foregoing arguments about the contested nature of mental illness, we aim to foreground contrasting understandings of anorexia, depression and diabulimia. As we illustrate in the following sections, these contrasts frequently arise from the different disciplinary perspectives of medical and social scientists. However, they also emerge from the diversity of experiences of sufferers themselves (which, too, can be mediated by the disciplinary perspectives of researchers who investigate and report them). In the case of diabulimia, there is a further, more fundamental debate over whether it even exists as a classifiable health condition, an issue that has important consequences for those who claim to be diabulimic.

2.2 Anorexia

Anorexia nervosa is associated with severe loss of weight and malnutrition due to lack of food intake. It has the highest mortality rate of any psychiatric disorder (Hoek 2006). Although by no means exclusively so, anorexia is typically characterized by onset during adolescence – with first diagnosis in the UK peaking between fifteen and nineteen years old (Micali et al. 2013) – and is particularly associated with adolescent girls. While the results of prevalence studies vary considerably, most estimate that between 75 per cent and 90 per cent of people affected by anorexia are women (Sweeting et al. 2015).

The *DSM 5* (APA 2013) stipulates that anorexia is characterized by weight below that which is minimally normal for an adult or expected for a child or adolescent. In addition to this physical criterion, according to *DSM 5*, individuals with anorexia are also distinguished by '[i]ntense fear of gaining weight or becoming fat, or persistent behaviour that interferes with weight gain, even though at a significantly low weight' and '[d]isturbance in the way in which one's body weight or shape is experienced, undue influence of body weight or shape on self-evaluation, or persistent lack of recognition of the seriousness of the current low body weight' (2013: 338–9). It is these psychological symptoms that distinguish anorexia from similar diagnoses such as avoidant/restrictive food intake disorder (2013: 337). Anorexia nervosa is also recognized as having two non-exclusive sub-types: restricting type, in which weight is lost through dieting, fasting and/or excessive exercise; and binge eating/purging type, in which individuals repeatedly engage in binge eating or purging through self-induced vomiting or use of laxative or diuretic substances.

Apprehension over weight gain leads people with anorexia to strictly control their diets and perceive weight loss positively, with fear of weight gain often increasing as weight is lost. Prolonged malnourishment and low weight places stress upon the body and can lead to osteoporosis and increased vulnerability to infection. In acute cases, anorexic starvation can lead to death through physical exhaustion, electrolyte imbalance, dehydration and infection (Herzog et al. 1997). People with anorexia nervosa also show an increased risk of suicide (Hoek 2006) and Steinhausen's (2002) review of 119 longitudinal studies reports a 5 per cent mortality attributable to anorexia. For those patients who do not die as a direct result of anorexia, Steinhausen reports that 46.9 per cent fully recover, 33.5 per cent have improved symptoms and 20.8 per cent have the condition chronically. Similarly, Fairburn and Harrison (2003) found that 10 to 20 per cent of patients diagnosed with anorexia go on to develop an unremitting form. Contemporary medical descriptions suggest a multifactorial aetiology for anorexia, with risk factors including genetic disposition and personality traits – such as compulsiveness and obsessionality – that may have a hereditary basis; environmental, social and familial factors; and childhood adversity such as abuse or the death of close relatives (Schmidt 2002; Strober and Johnson 2012).

While the APA's diagnostic criteria hold a preeminent position in clinical and epidemiological studies of the disease, anorexia is also the subject of extensive research across the biological, psychological and social sciences. These disciplines provide divergent accounts of anorexia that belie the simplicity of the foregoing diagnostic guidelines. The following subsections outline major themes in these perspectives, beginning with a brief history of anorexia nervosa and its contemporary treatment. We then detail contrasting critical and feminist analyses of anorexia before reviewing studies that examine sufferers' accounts of it.

2.2.1 Medical and sociocultural perspectives

The original medical formulations of anorexia nervosa were made independently by Lasègue (1873) and Gull (1868, 1874) and were based on examination of a small number of female patients. Gull emphasized that anorexia nervosa was a nervous disease with psychological causes, concluding that the cause of anorexia lies in 'hysterical' tendencies (1874: 25). Despite the ostensible neutrality of this clinical assessment, the notion of hysteria was – and still is – profoundly ideological. Attributing anorexia to the hysteria of female patients served to frame the condition as an extension of supposedly female irrationality and established the view that anorexia was a self-inflicted starvation of 'obnoxious' women (Hepworth 1999: 25). This original description conferred connotations of immorality upon anorexia that shaped social representations of anorexic patients thereafter.

Residual notions of self-infliction and irrationality that characterized nineteenth-century classifications of anorexia are still apparent in contemporary clinical descriptions. For example, Beumont describes anorexia as a 'condition of self-engendered weight loss' by individuals who are 'divorce[d] from the reality that most of us recognise' (2002: 162), while *DSM 5* states that 'individuals with anorexia nervosa frequently either lack insight into or deny the problem'(2013: 340). Self-infliction is also implied in psychiatric descriptions of anorexia, not least the previous *DSM*'s first diagnostic criteria for anorexia nervosa as a '*refusal* to maintain body weight*' (1994: 307.1, emphasis added), which defines the patient as being engaged in a conflictual relationship. Beyond these clinical descriptions, Fleming and Szmukler's (1992) study of over 350 clinical staff found that patients with an eating disorder were considered more responsible for developing their condition and less likeable than patients with schizophrenia. This mirrors more recent work by Stewart et al. (2006), who found that lay members of the public believe patients with anorexia are more to blame for the onset and maintenance of their condition than individuals with schizophrenia or asthma.

The notion that anorexia nervosa is a self-inflicted condition has important consequences for the way in which anorexia is treated therapeutically. If anorexia is perceived to be driven by the wilful choices of the individual patient, treatment will be focused on adjusting their personal psychology (Hepworth 1999). Contemporary treatment for anorexia largely reflects this model of anorexia as a psychopathology (Malson et al. 2004), with psychological interventions regarded as crucial to long-term recovery (NICE 2004). Individual psychotherapy for anorexia often draws variously on cognitive and behavioural therapies, interpersonal psychotherapy and motivational enhancement therapy, though treatment may also include family therapy that actively involves the patient's relatives in treatment (Morris and Twaddle 2007). These interventions are normally delivered in a secondary care setting on an outpatient basis, although more severe cases of anorexia – usually determined by patients' low body weight – are treated on an inpatient basis. In the UK, patients with anorexia who have a dangerously low weight and are unwilling to accept treatment may be detained as inpatients under the 1983 Mental Health Act. In-patient treatment typically includes a re-feeding programme that aims to safely increase the patient's weight, and which is carried out coercively through feeding tubes in some cases. While comparatively rare, compulsory re-feeding practices echo Gull's (1874) claims that anorexic patients display signs of insanity and that their treatment preferences can be disregarded during treatment, though this is intended to avert life-threatening physical illness.

Alongside medical, psychological and psychiatric studies, there is a large body of non-clinical literature on anorexia's social and cultural meanings. Such research frequently employs qualitative methodologies and a social constructionist epistemology. As we argued in the previous chapter, social constructionist research is particularly useful for foregrounding the way in which cultural discourses, institutions and social norms establish notions of health, illness and disease, not least those related to eating disorders. This has resulted in accounts of anorexia that stand in marked contrast to clinical studies which construe anorexia as an apolitical, individual psychopathology (Malson et al. 2004). Most notably, the fact that an individual's desire to be thinner resonates so strongly with Western cultural imperatives to pursue slenderness has been used to countermand the notion that anorexia is purely a 'self-engendered' and irrational pathology.

Giddens (1991) interprets anorexia as a consequence of developed societies. In contemporary society, he claims, manifold lifestyle choices have supplanted the traditional social roles through which individuals have historically established social identities. For example, in its moderate form, the widespread practice of dieting exemplifies the general late modern trend of bodily management through which individuals define their bodies and selves. Anorexia nervosa represents an extreme form of this reflexive identity project (Widdows 2018); a rejection of the dietary pluralism of modernity and adoption of a 'deliberate asceticism' that distinguishes the individual from others (Giddens 1991: 105). Giddens's analysis affords insight into the increased occurrence of eating disorders among women by citing the higher value placed on their physical appearance and hence their greater need for bodily regulation. Giddens also argues that weight loss and the pursuit of an anorexic identity offer women a more feasible mode of self-definition than social goals such as professional success, which remain relatively more difficult for them to achieve. This in turn accounts for the sense of self-empowerment from restrictive dieting reported in patient-based studies (Eivors et al. 2003), even while underplaying the significant feelings of distress and despair experienced by those with anorexia.

Giddens's (1991) attempt to situate anorexia nervosa in relation to social structures, and particularly those affecting women, parallels feminist readings of anorexia, which have offered trenchant criticism of medical explanations of the condition. In opposition to biomedical research, they implicate the gender inequalities that pervade industrialized Western societies as an aetiological factor in anorexia nervosa (Gimlin 1994). Feminist literature departs strikingly from medical research in its resistance to, and occasional outright rejection of, the description of anorexia as an individual pathology that distinguishes healthy and unhealthy individuals. Rather, anorexia has been reinterpreted as an acute response to cultural imperatives of bodily management experienced by all women (Orbach 1986). For example, Bordo (2003) argues that although the aetiological causes of eating disorders are indeed multifaceted, gender inequalities in Western culture play a preeminent role (2003: 52). Despite this, Bordo argues, medical models have consistently relegated cultural norms to a merely contributory role in the development of anorexia on the grounds that only a minority of individuals within developed societies develop the condition. The search for additional, non-cultural causes – such as hereditary factors – then effaces the primary role played by Western culture in the proliferation of eating disorders.

In contrast, Bordo situates anorexia in relation to cultural values that favour 'masculine' qualities of rationality and physical and mental restraint and confers associations with mental weakness and insatiability on women. This pervasive set of cultural values underscores symptomatic characteristics of anorexia nervosa including wilful suppression of appetite, a sense of security and achievement gained from bodily control and a fear of female sexual development

(Bordo 2003: 146–60). By drawing parallels between widespread values and features of anorexia, Bordo demonstrates that anorexic individuals' obsession with thinness cannot be understood wholly in terms of individual pathology. Rather, the anorexic body needs to be situated within the context of cultural values which idealize physical self-control (Malson 1998).

In this vein, the symptomatic misconception of body size and fear of weight gain in the *DSM* can be deconstructed as evidence of pervasive gender oppression. For example, women's overestimation of their own body size reflects ubiquitous media depictions of a glamorized, thin female body and, more generally, mirrors a cultural norm of feminine beauty that values a diminutive, submissive appearance (Wolf 1991; Bordo 2003: 55–7). Similarly, women's enactment of control over the size of their bodies can be regarded as symptomatic of a culture in which their physical appearance is used as an index of their social and moral worth (Rothblum 1994). A thorough response to anorexia is therefore required not just to deal with disordered eating behaviour at an individual level but also to challenge a set of cultural values that subjugates women and promotes bodily management as a virtue (Swartz 1987).

The differing accounts of anorexia outlined above usefully demonstrate two out of many possible interpretations of anorexia as a social phenomenon and a subjectively lived experience. For example, while sociocultural research consistently constructs anorexia as a means of self-control, individual studies identify distinct motivations for seeking that self-control in the first place, including – though not limited to – a crisis of self-identity (Giddens 1991); an unattainable beauty ideal and subordinate female subjectivity (Bordo 2003); and the subjugating effects of heteronormativity (McCaughey 1999). Taken together, these diverse analyses underline the lack of a single, comprehensive explanation of anorexia. Instead, as with many complex phenomena, there exist multiple explanatory models that draw variously upon a range of disciplinary perspectives to configure anorexia and the anorexic patient in different ways. These competing accounts also vary considerably in terms of what falls in- and outside of their analytical focus; just as feminist writers have argued that psychiatric research individualizes pathologies with little appreciation of sufferers' broader cultural environments, the treatment of eating disorders on the macro level of Western or late modern society can lead to generalizations that overlook considerable differences in individual experience. There is a danger that such theorizing can lead to cultural interpretations of anorexia that, while sophisticated, bear a diminishing resemblance to the accounts of individual sufferers (Berg 2002). Until recently, however, research that seeks to uncover how social discourses of feminine beauty, physical restraint and medical knowledge are negotiated interactively has been surprisingly underrepresented. As Rich avers in the introduction to her ethnographic study of an in-patient facility, there is 'a plethora of studies which explore the discourses around eating disorders. There is, however, relatively little research which addresses how young women actually manage these discourses; […] how they make sense of the various social constructions of eating disorders at an everyday level' (2006: 285). The following section addresses these qualitative studies before focusing specifically on (corpus) linguistic research into eating disorder discourse.

2.2.2 Sufferers' accounts and the 'anorexic voice'

Just as the foregoing section illustrated that anorexia remains a contested condition at a theoretical level, patient accounts of living with eating disorders reveal a similar theme of conflict experienced at a personal level. Participants in Rich's (2006) ethnography reported that their families and peers failed to understand their desire for weight loss and regarded anorexia as pathological, self-inflicted and 'deviant'; a perceived stigma that led these sufferers to seek support in alternative contexts such as online groups. These sufferers also discursively managed the social castigation of anorexia by constructing their illness in terms of the restraint and self-control attributed to esteemed social actors such as athletes. By constructing a narrative of self-empowerment, patients were able to create a positive anorexic identity that they were unwilling to relinquish, leading to conflict with their healthcare providers. Rich also argues that anorexic patients have a complex and contradictory relationship with their condition; they resist others' attempts to index their health through physiological measurements rather than subjective distress, yet remain profoundly concerned with their own body mass and calorie counting. Similarly, they engage in non-compliance behaviours during treatment and regard anorexia as personally vindicating while simultaneously being aware of the negative impact it has on their own and other people's lives.

This ambivalent experience of anorexia is echoed across other studies (Giordano 2005). On the one hand, anorexia can be experienced as a means of exerting a sense of control after a traumatic life event or transition. On the other, however, this sense of control can also lead to conflict with close relations who pathologize behaviours that people with anorexia experience as functional. In Eivors et al.'s (2003) interview study, increasing tensions with friends and family members had led participants to reinterpret their anorexia as potentially maladaptive. Nevertheless, the study participants reported feeling opposed to a pathologizing diagnosis of mental illness and experiencing a renewed sense of lost control during professional interventions that focused on managed diets. Their subsequent unilateral withdrawal from professional therapies offered the interviewees a means of reasserting control over their lives and routines. However, early drop out from treatment also left some participants with no alternative strategies for managing stressful experiences, increasing their reliance on disordered eating and leading some to adopt the identity of an 'incurable anorectic' (2003: 105).

Themes of control, conflict and resistance towards treatment pervade Malson et al.'s (2004) work with inpatients on specialist anorexia wards. Their interviewees frequently rejected professional claims that they were medically unwell, a rejection that served to undermine the legitimacy of their hospitalization. Further, the patients strongly resisted being treated solely as a case of anorexia by their attending clinicians; rather than seeing anorexia as defining their identity and behaviour (a view they largely attributed to professionals), the patients sought to present anorexia as separate from themselves (see also Malson 1998: 145). This allowed them a position from which to challenge the professionals' treatment plans as harmful to their (non-anorexic) selves, rather than this resistance being regarded as symptomatic of anorexia itself. However, at times, some recovering participants also used this 'patients are 100 per cent anorexic' view to contrast their current distance from anorexia with their previous whole-hearted adoption of an anorexic identity. Malson et al.'s work is valuable in demonstrating the fluidity of constructions of anorexia and patienthood; they illustrate that sufferers utilize different descriptions of anorexia as pathological or empowering, all-encompassing or separate from themselves, and that these constructions are used strategically to achieve interpersonal objectives through talk, such as legitimizing resistance to treatment or demonstrating personal recovery.

The ways in which individuals adopt alternative representations of anorexia to facilitate interactional goals such as treatment resistance and stigma management reflect one of the central conflicts of the condition: individuals with anorexia undertake behaviours that they know to be harmful. As Giordano (2005: 89) argues, individuals with anorexia

> are not passive recipients of mental illnesses, or mere victims of their disorder. They, instead, participate actively in the production and, to some extent, in the maintenance of symptoms.
>
> (Giordano 2005: 89)

Faced with the unacceptability of self-starvation, individuals are driven to account for behaviours that they experience as both deleterious and compelling. As noted by Hardin (2003), a discourse of psychopathology provides just such an explanation. Examining a recovery-oriented online support group of the kind introduced in the next chapter and then examined in Chapter 4, Hardin found that forum members emphasized 'anorexic thinking' over low weight as the most important criterion for being considered as an 'authentic anorexic' by others. Identifying themselves in relation to a legitimate psychiatric condition enabled the forum members to mitigate their sense of responsibility for developing the condition and for its consequences, while also distinguishing themselves from 'pro-anorexics' who see anorexia as a positive lifestyle choice and who align against medical treatment (Fox et al. 2005; Ging and Garvey 2018). However, the negative consequences of a medicalized view of anorexia are also apparent here since the forum's obligation to view anorexia through a discourse of psychopathology also entailed that members categorize themselves as fundamentally disordered (Hardin 2003: 214). Hardin also observes the potential of web users to be 'taken up' by these discourses, and new members of an online forum may be obliged to reproduce its normative discourses in order to receive acceptance from existing members (Stommel 2009; Stommel and Koole 2010). These discourses may be both empowering as a means of addressing a sense of personal shame while also divesting individuals from a sense of agency in relation to their condition.

Rather than a single, unified account of anorexia, these studies illustrate that tensions between multiple conflicting explanations of the condition are refracted at the level of the individual sufferer, who can employ a range of competing discourses to comprehend and warrant their own experiences. Although psychological and biomedical explanations of anorexia can counteract moral indictments of sufferers as '"shallow," "vain," "conceited," "selfish," or "indulgent"' (Easter 2012: 1412), these explanations may also undermine individuals' own illness narratives and lead to a fatalism in which eating disorders are considered hardwired into the individual, thereby trivializing their efforts to recover. Therefore, while they may be welcome in dismantling accusations that eating disorders are a morally culpable choice, medicalized explanations also have potentially profound implications for the identity of the sufferer and the value of their struggle towards recovery.

A collection of more recent studies suggests that, at least for some individuals, the conflict and ambivalence of anorexia is focalized through the experience of living with an anorexic 'voice' (Pugh 2016; cf. Bruch 1978). Personified as a distinct entity, individuals with anorexia describe their anorexic voice as having emerged at a point when they felt vulnerable and as offering a source of comfort and distraction from emotional distress (Tierney and Fox 2010). While initially like a supportive, guiding and ever-present parent, the anorexic voice nevertheless commands individuals to stop eating and lose weight, thereby pushing them towards characteristically anorexic behaviours. As the disease progresses, the anorexic voice is experienced as more punitive and as undermining the individual's confidence, eventually coming to dominate the individual and dictate their behaviours (Williams et al. 2016). Participants in these studies position the anorexic voice as both a comforting friend and an enemy that controls them and drives their disordered behaviours (Williams and Reid 2010). As such, even though it is distinct from the biochemical or psychological explanations of anorexia discussed earlier, the discourse of the anorexic voice also offers individuals a means to account for their condition by representing their own agency as compromised by a distinct entity. In addition, while experiences of an anorexic voice can predate contact with healthcare services (Pugh 2016), a similarly personified construction of anorexia is also apparent in professional treatment literature; Serpell et al. (1999) report asking patients to write a letter to their anorexia as their 'friend' and their 'enemy', while Lask and Hage (2013: 199) recommend that patients externalize anorexia so that it is 'conceptualised as a distinct entity'. Differing professional interventions may therefore reiterate the fundamental aspects of the anorexic voice discourse.

Overall, the picture here is one of profound difficulty for the individual with anorexia. As well as external conflict with family members and healthcare professionals, research into the 'anorexic voice' shows that recovery from anorexia is also experienced as an internal battle in which the individual must gain control over their anorexic voice and challenge the unhealthy thoughts that it generates. This is particularly challenging in cases where sufferers come to identify with their anorexic voice (Tierney and Fox 2010; Williams et al. 2016), leading to a sense of loss or incompleteness that in turn can prompt a return to disordered behaviours. As well as physical and mental healing, then, recovery also involves a search for a new, post-anorexia identity, though one that also requires the individual to see themselves as responsible for their own actions (Duncan et al. 2015).

These studies suggest that the anorexic voice is a remarkably rich, multifaceted personification that can help to explain sufferers' ambivalence towards treatment and recovery. While the experience of a tyrannical anorexic voice may have implications for professional therapies (Pugh 2016), its functional role for individuals in negotiating their personal identity and mitigating their sense of responsibility for the condition is less well addressed in foregoing research. Likewise, the role of this construction as a discursive resource deployed during interaction remains under-examined. However, as will be discussed in Chapter 4, this discourse is both salient and highly functional within the online eating disorder support group.

In addition to the thematic analyses that characterize much qualitative research on anorexia, several studies have employed discourse analytic methods to examine language data produced by individuals with anorexia. As part of a wider corpus linguistic study of adolescents' online health inquires (see Harvey 2013a), Mullany et al. (2015) observe that concerns with food and dieting permeate the health concerns of young people, with questions about weight and body shape peaking among girls at age twelve. In particular, adolescents consistently inquire into 'normal' and 'average' body weights and how they can lose weight, illustrating that from a young age children have accepted a belief in the need to regulate their bodies in order to conform to a norm, even if they remain uncertain as to what this norm actually is. These expectations of normative body size and particularly a desire to avoid being seen as overweight pervade messages that refer explicitly to 'anorexia', with adolescents constructing disordered eating through both a medical register in which anorexia is a disease and an aesthetic register focusing on the appeal of the slender body. These messages convey the profound ambivalence experienced by young people caught between the pull of compulsory slenderness and a growing concern that they may be harming themselves; as one thirteen-year-old author articulates: 'I feel stupid for wanting to look like that, because I know it's dangerous, but I want it' (Mullany et al. 2015: 220).

Outside of corpus approaches, Skårderud (2007a) draws on conceptual metaphor theory (Lakoff and Johnson 1980) to examine representations of anorexia produced by his clients when describing their experiences of the condition. The participants produced a range of metaphorical conceptualizations of food, eating and anorexia itself, testifying to a diversity of individual experiences. Common among these, however, was a tendency to conceive of mental and emotional experiences in terms of physiological ones through conceptualizations of the body as a container and food as emotions. As a result, the act of 'filling' the body through eating is experienced as filling oneself with emotions which, if overwhelming, could be removed through purging or laxative use. Likewise, the physical experience of weight and heaviness was experienced as a feeling of emotional burden. This figuration of food in terms of emotions also renders dietary restriction and weight loss as forms of emotional control. However, Skårderud (2007a, b) also argues that a central element of living with anorexia is to lose sight of the metaphorical nature of the connection between food and emotions, such that bodily restriction is experienced literally as emotional control rather than only being symbolic of it. Weight loss therefore comes to be seen as the only means of addressing difficult emotional experiences. This tendency towards concretizing emotional experiences may also go some way to explaining the prevalence of the anorexic voice noted above, in which emotions are mediated by an imaginary personified individual.

While Mullany et al. and Skårderud's respective studies illustrate how teenagers and patients with anorexia conceive of their condition, the nature of the data analysed precludes an analysis of how these beliefs may arise during and be accepted or challenged during interaction with others, not least other people with anorexia. In contrast, Knapton (2013) demonstrates the use of specific discourse metaphors in an online pro-anorexia support group. Construing anorexia as a skill and a religion enables pro-anorexia community members to represent weight loss as the successful achievement of a goal, and one that brings spiritual enlightenment based on the avoidance of 'sinful' food. Knapton argues that the representation of anorexia as a skill or religious calling does not constitute a radically new conceptualization but rather extends existing metaphors that construe conventional female beauty in terms of a skilful achievement or religion. In keeping with Bordo (2003) and Rich (2006), Knapton argues that members of the pro-anorexia community simply extend culturally available concepts of beauty and self-control to encompass anorexia, thereby establishing a value system that is in line with cultural imperatives towards thinness and which makes them resistant towards treatment and recovery. Much like Hardin (2003), Knapton foregrounds the central role played by members' discursive accounts of anorexia (and the role of metaphor within such accounts) in shaping the norms of an online community. The constructions that come to be dominant in a particular community are highly consequential for community members, since they shape individual beliefs about recovery from anorexia and decisions about whether to comply with or resist professional interventions. This will be a particular focus of Chapter 4, which illustrates the implications that the prevailing representation of anorexia has for the online community members' beliefs about medical treatment and individual responsibility. In the meantime, it will suffice to say that anorexia is the site of multiple competing discourses that offer diverging and consequential accounts of its causes, function and embodied experience. Although these experiences are normally riven by intra- and interpersonal conflicts, individual sufferers can also draw upon discursive representations of anorexia to resist stigma and feelings of responsibility as well as medical intervention. Understanding how and why these conflicting discourses are propagated and taken up during the common practice of online peer support is therefore highly necessary. This sense of conflict is also apparent in the second mental health problem that this book addresses: depression.

2.3 Depression

Despite its status as the 'common cold' of psychopathology (Seligman 1975), it is difficult to overestimate the potential severity of depression and the breadth of its effect upon the health of Western populations. Depression is the most common mental health problem and the leading cause of disability worldwide (2017) and is consistently and strongly associated with suicide across the UK and the rest of Europe, North America and Oceania (Beautrais 2000; Kessler et al. 2005; Bernal et al. 2007; Pilling et al. 2009). In addition to this tangible human loss, a Sainsbury Centre for Mental Health report (2010) estimated the annual cost of depression in the UK in 2009/10 to be £105.2 billion. This includes expenses from healthcare services and indirect economic costs such as lost productivity due to sick leave, premature death and those leaving work to care for the ill.

As with anorexia nervosa, depression is more common in women than men, with the former being twice as likely to become depressed (Stoppard 2000). Unlike eating disorders, depression is more common among individuals with a lower socioeconomic status, the unemployed and those living in poor quality housing. This demographic distribution is reflected in the multifactorial clinical model of depression which implicates both hereditary and biological characteristics which interact with negative events during childhood to render individuals vulnerable to depression. Life experiences such as job loss, bereavement, deprivation and other health problems can also lead to a debilitating level of unhappiness (Dowrick 2004). Depression also frequently presents with a range of comorbidities, especially lower back pain and heart problems, where physical and psychological problems mutually impede recovery (Dowrick 2004).

The most commonly prescribed treatments for depression are intended to address some of these different factors. In cases of major or long-standing depression, both antidepressant medication and 'talking therapies' are used to respond to depression as simultaneously a biomedical disorder characterized by neurological imbalance and a psychological problem caused by vulnerability factors (Kangas 2001). In the UK, patients frequently express a preference for talking therapies, which are typically delivered as cognitive behavioural therapy or counselling (NICE 2009). In cases of major depression, research has shown similar levels of efficacy for both antidepressant drugs and generic counselling (Chilvers et al. 2001), although concerns regarding the long-term effectiveness and suitability of drug therapies are well established (see Dowrick 2004: 80–4 for a review). In addition, systematic reviews of antidepressant trials have demonstrated a clinically negligible difference in mood improvement between antidepressant and placebos, particularly when the reviews include data from unpublished trials that may be suppressed by pharmaceutical companies (Kirsch et al. 2008).

Although many people may recover from a period of depression with or without professional treatments, experiences of debilitating unhappiness are often chronic or recurrent. For individuals admitted to psychiatric units, longitudinal studies report recovery for between 24 per cent and 40 per cent of patients (Piccinelli and Wilkinson 1994; Surtees and Barkley 1994). In a large, twenty-five-year study, Brodaty et al. (2001) report a symptom recurrence rate of 84 per cent and readmission of 58 per cent of former inpatients, with symptoms improving in 27 per cent of patients over a fifteen- to twenty-five-year period, remaining the same in 55 per cent, and deteriorating in 18 per cent of cases. These studies demonstrate that major depression remains a frequently intractable condition that dominates the lives of sufferers and resists sophisticated psychiatric and pharmacological interventions.

Aside from feelings of profound sadness, the experience of depression can vary considerably between sufferers. This variation is captured by *DSM 5*'s diagnostic criteria for major depressive episode:

- depressed mood most of the day, nearly every day, as indicated by either subjective report (e.g. feels sad, empty, hopeless) or observation made by others (e.g. appears tearful);
- markedly diminished interest or pleasure in all, or almost all, activities most of the day, nearly every day (as indicated by either subjective account or observation);
- significant weight loss when not dieting or weight gain (e.g. a change of more than 5 per cent of body weight in a month), or decrease or increase in appetite nearly every day;
- insomnia or hypersomnia nearly every day;
- psychomotor agitation or retardation nearly every day (observable by others, not merely subjective feelings of restlessness or being slowed down);

- fatigue or loss of energy nearly every day;
- feelings of worthlessness or excessive or inappropriate guilt (which may be delusional) nearly every day (not merely self-reproach or guilt about being sick);
- diminished ability to think or concentrate, or indecisiveness, nearly every day (either by subjective account or as observed by others);
- recurrent thoughts of death (not just fear of dying), recurrent suicidal ideation without a specific plan or a suicide attempt or a specific plan for committing suicide.

(APA 2013: 160–1)

For a diagnosis of a major depressive episode to be made, individuals must present with five or more of these symptoms, including depressed mood and/or lost interest in activities, in a period of two weeks or more. The symptoms should also significantly impair a person's ability to function in their daily life.

These diagnostic criteria have often acted as a point of departure for trenchant criticisms of the concept of clinical depression. The following sections shall consider arguments against this medical formulation and the problems it generates when employed for diagnosis and treatment. Section 2.3.2 then details qualitative and discourse analytic studies of depression narratives that further problematize conventional diagnostic and treatment measures.

2.3.1 Problematizing the diagnosis of depression

The value of the diagnostic category of depression is its identification of psychopathology that transcends subjective accounts of unhappiness (McPherson and Armstrong 2009; Stoppard 2000). As such, a diagnosis of clinical depression is intended to distinguish depressed individuals from those who experience a normal, non-pathological unhappiness and from people who suffer from other mental pathologies (Dowrick 2004). However, the seventy different possible combinations of the *DSM* symptoms reproduced above mean that individuals who do not share a single symptom can be positively diagnosed as sharing the same underlying pathology (Pilgrim and Bentall 1999). An individual can also experience a number of symptoms yet remain within the parameters of medical normalcy, while those with sub-clinical symptomatology may experience significant personal impairment (Dowrick 2009a).

Looking beyond the *DSM*, there is continuing theoretical disagreement over the definitive criteria for clinical depression (Pilgrim and Bentall 1999).

Whereas the *DSM* affords primacy to depressed mood and anhedonia (a lost sense of pleasure), Beck et al. (1979) state that depression's defining feature is a negative view of the self and the future, and Willner (1985) claims there is no essential symptom for depression at all. Depressive symptoms also overlap with several other conditions such as adjustment and anxiety disorders. Debate continues over whether these conditions should remain separate or be regarded as different presentations of a shared underlying problem, as well as whether depression should be divided into several sub-types (Dowrick 2004). In light of these enduring arguments, Pilgrim and Bentall conclude that there is 'no consistent transcultural, transhistorical agreement about minimal necessary and sufficient pathognomic criteria' for diagnosing depression (1999: 263), and further that there are no definitive divisions between various mental disorders and between mental disorder and normality. Therefore, despite the *DSM*'s position as the international standard of mental illness diagnosis, its concept of depression is as much a product of professional and institutional trends as it is an objective description of a mental health condition (Bentall 2003).

As Galasiński (2008) argues, the objectivity of the *DSM* is further undermined by the vagaries that beset the language of the diagnostic criteria presented above. Alongside a series of vague quantifiers ('most of the day', 'nearly every day', 'almost all'), it is unclear how a reader (and a diagnosing clinician, for that matter) should distinguish between diminished and 'markedly diminished' interest, since if lost interest has been noticed, it must have been marked by something. Assessing whether a patient feels 'excessive or inappropriate guilt' will depend upon the doctor's subjective judgements about the gravity of any wrongdoing and the perceived extent of the patient's role in it. Similarly, accurately determining whether the patient is indecisive requires the doctor to understand the patient's perceptions of the magnitude of a decision and its consequences (Galasiński 2008). This information will be difficult to ascertain and, at the very least, subject to value-laden judgement by the clinician. Consequently, far from being clear-cut descriptions, both the ambiguities of the diagnostic criteria and the need for their interpretation in relation to each patient introduce manifold opportunities for interpretive license on the part of the diagnosing clinician.

The lack of objective diagnostic criteria means that for borderline cases, 'no subjective checklist of a patient's history and complaints can infallibly separate clinical syndromes that qualify as disorders from human discomfort of a lesser intensity' (Chodoff 2002: 628). However, when faced with such a dilemma, the diagnosis of depression offers general practitioners an effective way to respond to patients' distress and reduce a large and heterogeneous set of experiences into a single label with an available treatment protocol (Chew-Graham et al. 2002; Dowrick 2009b). The strategic use of diagnosis for simplifying patients' complicated personal and social problems represents an example of the medicalization of unhappiness that might otherwise be interpreted as a non-pathological reaction to adverse personal circumstances (Burroughs et al. 2006). Such diagnosis may bring the patient relief through professional recognition of previously confounding distress. At the same time, diagnosis may well catalyse an individual's entrance into treatments that can radically alter their lives and personal identity (Karp 1996). While these arguments are derived from research in primary care settings, they apply equally to the types of online support groups introduced in the next chapter, in which diagnoses performed by lay peers provide members with a means of validating the experiences of new users who join seeking explanations for their distress. Just like health professionals, lay diagnosis provides a means for online peers to respond sympathetically to others who narrate feelings of despair, regardless of how well such narratives match diagnostic criteria. We return to the uses and potentials of online peer support later in the chapter.

2.3.2 Personal experiences of depression

Whether diagnosed by a clinician, a peer or not diagnosed at all, the experience of depression has profound effects on the individual and their self-identity. These effects are extensively attested in a growing body of qualitative social science research investigating subjective experiences of depression. While these qualitative studies do not uniformly oppose the medical treatment of depression, they do emphasize that illness narratives such as those analysed in Chapter 5 'provide meaning, context, and perspective for the patient's predicament' and can be used in shaping therapeutic interventions (Dowrick 2004: 194). Indeed, these studies fundamentally endorse individual sufferers' accounts as a source of valid information on depression and critique quantitative studies for homogenizing complex longitudinal experiences into quantifiable variables that are predetermined by researchers (Stoppard 2000).

A preeminent theme across these qualitative studies is the feeling of isolation engendered by depression, with sufferers frequently describing both intractable feelings of social discomfort and a simultaneous longing for interpersonal connection (Karp 1996; Kangas 2001). As noted above in relation to professional diagnosis, research participants also report a fear of revealing their constant unhappiness to others, as well as persistent difficulties in articulating their feelings, leading to strained personal relationships and a sense of frustration that increases their social withdrawal and subsequent depression (Epstein et al. 2010; Harvey 2012). These communicative difficulties also go some way to explaining the popularity of online support groups for individuals with depression, who may well feel less anxious about articulating feelings of depression to people who, by dint of the context, are likely to have had similar experiences themselves. In addition, alongside the support and advice available through electronic support groups, the very process of electronic communication may alleviate the sense of isolation that pervades many people's experience of depression (Ziebland and Wyke 2012).

In comparison with clinical explanations of depression's aetiology, lay accounts frequently foreground a relationship between depression and situational and social factors. In interviews with South Asian immigrants in America, Karasz (2005) found that 85 per cent of explanations of the cause of depression implicated situational factors, particularly ongoing problems with a spouse or in-laws. These respondents also offered the markedly non-medical explanation that depression could be caused by 'thinking too much' (2005: 1630) and many did not see depression as a disease unless it led to physical illness. By contrast, when describing situational factors, Karasz's middle-class white interviewees were more likely to cite specific life events such as bereavement, divorce or miscarriage that could precipitate a depressive reaction (similar findings are reported by Lewis (1995) and Cornford et al. (2007)). Karasz's respondents also displayed a more granular understanding of depression that differentiated between a reactive depression identified as an indirect object – 'depressed by something' – and depression used substantively – 'it's depression' (2005: 1629). When discussing depression as a distinct phenomenon, respondents were more likely to provide a complex explanation that demonstrated the influence of medical knowledge. Three quarters of white American respondents mentioned possible biological causes of depression and utilized psychodynamic concepts of emotional triggers and childhood trauma, but also offered twice as many explanations that identified social problems.

These and other studies testify to the hybridity of lay individuals' explanations of depression, which not only foreground harmful life events, failed relationships, social structures and unemployment but also draw on psychodynamic theories and biomedical notions of neurotransmitter disruption and genetic predisposition (Rogers and Pilgrim 1997; Kangas 2001; Ridge and Ziebland 2006; Wittink et al. 2008). In doing so, this past research complicates any binary between 'lay' and 'professional' models of depression, as supposedly 'lay' accounts integrate folk and scientific discourses in complex and sometimes contradictory ways (Kangas 2001: 89) and attribute depression to factors both internal and external to the individual. Their variety notwithstanding, these non-professional accounts share a common theme of locating depression outside of the individual's control. That is, whether the cause of unhappiness is attributed to social or biological factors or to childhood or relationship traumas, explanations of depression consistently displace culpability from the individual sufferer. As such, these accounts of depression also signal sufferers' need to 'patch up the moral rupture presented by illness' (Kangas 2001: 77) and justify depression to those who do not otherwise comprehend it. Indeed, across, all the qualitative literature we have encountered, the most consistent feature of depression narratives is that narrators construct depression in such a way as to legitimize the condition in order to avert its perceived stigma. For Karp (1996), neutralizing stigma and constructing depression as beyond individual control is a necessary aspect of living with chronic depression, particularly when feelings of abject unhappiness persist in the absence of situational or social problems. As noted in Chapter 1, in interviewing people with long-term depression, Karp found that a medical model of biological predisposition offered a compelling explanation for the feeling that depression was beyond their control. Positive experiences with antidepressant medication validated this explanation and encouraged participants' long-term gravitation towards a medicalized understanding of depression.

Existing linguistic research into depression narratives has helped to provide a more granular picture of the ways in which sufferers can take up, resist and embellish existing discourses of depression. Examining a corpus of messages submitted to a teenage health website between 2004 and 2005, Harvey (2012) notes that adolescents are readily able to attribute depression to themselves, reaching for this label to explain otherwise inexplicable enduring distress. In this way, the teenagers construct depression as a pathology that defies their own dispositions towards happiness. The website users also distinguish between the condition of having 'depression' and the state of being 'depressed'; while the former is represented as a psychological aberration, the latter is a reactive state recurrently related to situational factors such as difficulties with friendships or parental relationships. In both cases, however, the adolescents' messages serve to legitimize their online help-seeking by providing evidence for their emotional turmoil as well as by emphasizing their powerless over the causes of their unhappiness.

A comparable finding is noted in Galasiński's (2008) extensive study of men's narratives of depression. Based on fine-grained analysis of the grammatical choices made by men describing their experiences of depression, Galasiński observes that participants consistently represent the condition as separate from themselves and as able to act independently of their control. For example, one participant states that depression 'takes away the possibility of logical thinking, of assessment of situations', while another says that depression 'did contribute significantly to the break-up of my other relationships' (2008: 46). In each example, depression is presented as acting of its own volition but also as only affecting the speaker indirectly, either via a contribution to relationship breakdown or by affecting a generic 'thinking'. By presenting themselves as neither in control of nor controlled *by* depression, Galasiński argues, the interviewees are able to maintain a sense in which their identity remains unblemished by an illness associated with dependence and emotionality.

Beyond grammatical choices, sufferers may also opt for metaphorical representations of depression that maintain a sense of their own agency (Semino 2008). By representing depression as an external space through constructions such as 'I went through a phase of depression' or by speaking of 'coming out of' depression (Semino 2008: 180–2), sufferers separate themselves from depression's onset and are able to conceptualize themselves as actively moving themselves out of the condition. In contrast, Semino (2008: 185) also observes that an opposing metaphor is used by a clinical psychologist, who describes sufferers as 'thinking in very black and white terms' and 'magnify[ing] anything awful that happens to them'. By drawing on a conventional metaphorical relationship between seeing and thinking, the psychologist implicates the sufferer's own thinking in perpetuating their depressed state (see also McMullen 1999; Thomas-MacLean and Stoppard 2004; Charteris-Black 2012). Taken in sum, these studies highlight discursive choices at the level of lexis and grammar (between 'being' depressed and 'having' an active depression) and metaphor that offer contrasting representations of the condition and the moral culpability of the sufferer. In parallel with Karasz (2005), Harvey's (2012) work also illustrates the way that lay individuals combine accounts of 'feeling depressed' due to external, non-medical circumstances and the internal psychological malfunction denoted by 'having depression'. As the analysis in Chapter 5 reveals, this choice between *depressed* and *depression* is central to contrasting representations of the condition and the sufferer.

Despite this overlap between lay and biomedical descriptions, sufferers are ambivalent towards a model of depression as a medical disease. While allowing individuals to avoid blame for depression (Schreiber and Hartrick 2002), capitulating to a biochemical explanation also cues the adoption of a passive patient identity and acceptance of professional pharmacological interventions (Lewis 1995). Similarly, Epstein et al.'s participants claimed that describing depression as a chemical imbalance reduced personal stigmas but also 'neglected the uniquely personal aspects of the depression experience and devalued behavioural or psychological treatment options' (2010: 960). It is hard not to see parallels between these findings and the research into anorexia discussed earlier. In both cases, medical discourses offer a way out of illness stigma while also presenting a challenge to individuals' own experiences and explanations of suffering. In both instances, even while seeking to account for the difficulties engendered by their conditions, individuals may still seek to resist a passive patient identity by advocating personal responsibility, stoicism and emotional stability rather than dependence on healthcare. These individual coping strategies can enable sufferers to maintain a sense of agency and empowerment even when uncontrollable factors lie at the heart of their aetiological models of illness (Cornford et al. 2007).

The above research highlights a number of interrelated conflicts anchored to the clinical model of depression and the embodied experience of being depressed itself. At a conceptual level, depression remains subject to internecine debates regarding its defining symptoms and distinction from other psychiatric conditions. Disagreement over the nature of depression is also borne out in lay accounts that emphasize the role of immediate situational and social factors in emotional suffering while also drawing on biomedical models of depression in order to mediate perceived responsibility for illness. Nevertheless, completely accepting a biomedical model is believed to negatively affect a sufferer's self-identity and sense of agency and many resist the victim identity that a disease model entails. Living with depression can also be characterized by conflictual interpersonal relationships and uncertainty over how best to cope with psychological distress; while individuals may be desperate for emotional support, belief in the value of emotional self-reliance and fear of social encounters can also lead to anxiety towards admitting distress to healthcare professionals. Against this background of competing tensions, the potential of online peer support groups as a venue in which sufferers can seek to understand their experiences becomes clear (a consideration that we will return to in more depth in the next chapter). The analysis offered in Chapter 5 aims to describe the patterns that underlie how members of one such group articulate their experiences and to illuminate how they collectively navigate the discursive quandaries of what depression is, how it can best be treated and how to understand the individual's role in its onset and alleviation.

2.4 Diabulimia

The final mental health problem explored in this book, diabulimia, is an eating disorder in which individuals with type 1 diabetes, who are insulin dependent, restrict their insulin in order to shed calories and control their body weight. Diabulimia is a contested disorder insofar as, unlike the other mental health conditions examined in this book, it is not recognized as a legitimate mental disorder by medical authorities and, by extension, medical practitioners. Indeed, the term *diabulimia* is not an official diagnostic label, meaning that it is not possible for anyone to receive an official diabulimia diagnosis from a medical practitioner. Rather, it is a term invented and used by sufferers, mainly in online contexts, for the purposes of exchanging experiences, advice and social support with others. Instead of viewing it as a disease, medical authorities tend to conceive of diabulimia as an inappropriate compensatory behaviour and sign of non-adherence to prescribed diabetes management regimen (Mathieu 2008).

Despite campaigns from those affected by it, diabulimia was not recognized as a disease in *DSM 5*, which instead offers the following categories under which diabulimia might be classified: 'inappropriate compensatory purging behaviour', 'misuse of medications for weight loss', 'bulimia nervosa' and 'other specified feeding and eating disorders' (OSFED). However, activists and some researchers have argued that these labels are problematic, as they fail to capture diabulimia's central dual diagnostic component – that is, that people with diabulimia necessarily have pre-existing diabetes. As Sharma points out,

> [u]nfortunately, the presence of Type 1 diabetes only appends a much deeper level of psychopathology – lending patients a higher probability of developing disordered eating than their normal peers. This is one reason why it is so crucial that 'diabulimia' be resolved from other 'inappropriate compensatory behaviours' and general symptoms of eating disorders. It involves a completely discrete demographic with markedly different psychological baselines, an exclusive method of weight control, and even distinct impetuses.
>
> (Sharma 2013: 19)

Some researchers have also advocated a distinction be drawn between disorders that involve the withholding of insulin and those which involve the restriction of other types of medication (Shaw and Favazza 2010). Meanwhile, the use of the *DSM* labels *bulimia nervosa* and *OSFED* to describe diabulimia can be criticized on the basis that they risk conflating diabulimia, on both a linguistic and conceptual level, with other eating disorders, potentially obscuring the nuances between them and implying that their attendant experiences, symptoms and prognoses are the same.

The naming, or lexicalization (Jones 2013), of diseases and other health-related phenomena has long captured the interest of scholars researching at the interface of language and health (Crookshank 1923; Cassell 1976; Fleischman 1999, 2001), and indeed forms an important element of our own analysis in this book. Underlying such discussions is the understanding of the body and its ailments as cultural, medical and linguistic constructs. From such a view, the names and labels attributed to diseases are assumed to have implications for the ways that both experts and non-experts alike understand, communicate about and ultimately attempt to remedy them (Warner 1976; Fleischman 2001: 490). The foregoing discussion of the naming of diabulimia itself raises several important considerations concerning who does (and should) ultimately determine the name of a disease. Jammal (1988) argues that this matter sits within the remit of the lexicographer, while Fleischman (2001) proposes that diagnostic names and labels should result from specialist consensus. Jammal's view, though only posited in the late 1980s, might seem somewhat dated and out-of-touch to those aligning with the broadly poststructuralist view of health and illness as socially constituted phenomena (Brown 1995). At the same time, although Fleischman's (2001) position most likely reflects the ways in which diagnostic labels do in reality come into being, it paints a rather disempowering picture from the perspective of those experiencing the health phenomenon in question, affording limited scope for them in terms of shaping how that issue is talked about and understood (Conrad and Barker 2010). We agree with Fleischman (2001) that official names for health-related phenomena typically emerge as the product of specialist discussions and academic inquiry. However, we also believe that this process should endeavour to account for the ways in which the disease or health problem in question is labelled and described by non-experts, particularly those who have first-hand, lived experience of it.

In the absence of a ubiquitously accepted label, in the last couple of decades a plethora of names and umbrella terms for diabulimia have emerged from the research literature on this topic. In addition to the term *diabulimia* itself, the origins of which will be explored in more detail later in this section, these include *insulin abuse* (Schuler et al. 1989), *insulin misuse* (Bryden et al. 1999), *insulin omission* (Affenito and Adams 2001), *insulin resistance* (Riddle 2002), *insulin manipulation* (Battaglia et al. 2006), and *deliberate insulin omission/underdosing* (Shaw and Favazza 2010). Another umbrella term under which diabulimia might be categorized is *Eating Disorder in Diabetes Mellitus Type 1/2*

(ED-DMT1/2). This label was proposed by an international group of clinicians at a conference in Minnesota, USA, in September 2008. Despite receiving some degree of clinician approval, this term is still open to the criticism that it fails to distinguish diabulimia from other, non-insulin-omitting eating disorders experienced by people with diabetes and has, as far as we have observed, failed to gain any significant traction among either experts or non-experts.

Although the term *diabulimia* has yet to gain clinical approval, it has afforded the phenomenon of deliberate insulin restriction with a discursive presence in online spaces as well as in some contemporary research (Ruth-Sahd et al. 2009). This point is supported by Sharma (2013: 14), who argues that the word *diabulimia* 'grants patients a discrete nomenclature to identify with', before going on to argue that,'[p]utting a label on a pathology is a powerful preliminary step towards support manoeuvres and treatment approaches'. Moreover, in the UK, the term *diabulimia* has begun to enter public discourse through popular media and served as something of a 'catalyst of [...] awareness' in recent years (Sharma 2013: 12). For example, in 2017 the BBC aired a documentary titled 'Diabulimia: The World's Most Dangerous Eating Disorder'. In the same year, the BBC also published a news story with the headline, 'The suicide note that told Megan's diabulimia story', centred on a twenty-seven-year-old woman who attempted to commit suicide and cited her diabulimia and the lack of support as the cause in her suicide note (http://www.bbc.co.uk/newsbeat/article/40888659/the-suicide-note-that-told-megans-diabulimia-story). Since this time, national newspapers such as *The Guardian*, *i*, *Daily Mail* and *Daily Telegraph* have also published stories about diabulimia, usually focusing on individual cases as a way of introducing the condition to the general public.

For the purposes of this study, the apparent traction that the term *diabulimia* has gained among sufferers in online communities, as well as in more general public discourse through popular media, attest to its suitability for examining the discourses that surround this emerging health phenomenon in the context of online support groups. However, like the other disease labels discussed above, it is important to acknowledge that even the term *diabulimia* has met with some opposition, mostly from practitioners but also from some researchers. Weinger and Beverly (2010: 451), for example, observe how some practitioners have opposed the use of this term due to its perceived associations with sensationalistic media reporting. Others have taken issue with the word *diabulimia* on grounds of semantic inaccuracy; for example, Colton and colleagues (2009: 138) avoid using the term because they argue that it implies what is, for them, a false distinction between eating disorders experienced by people with diabetes and those experienced by people who do not have diabetes. Likewise, although she uses the label diabulimia in her own work, Sharma (2013) acknowledges that the inclusion of the word 'bulimia' (as in dia*bulimia*) – intended to signal the purging of sugar from the body before it is used – might inaccurately imply that sufferers of diabulimia induce vomiting, akin to bulimia. These objections aside, for now *diabulimia* remains the most widely accepted term, particularly among sufferers communicating about the condition online. As our term of choice, we will now briefly consider *diabulimia*'s linguistic complexion and etymology.

Diabulimia is a portmanteau word constructed by means of contamination – that is, the word-building process by which two existing words are combined in both form and meaning to formulate a new word (Das 1984: 263). In the case of diabulimia, the words *diabetes* and *bulimia* are fused together, broadly to convey the use of insulin manipulation as a purging tool to lose weight. As Sharma (2013: 8) observes, '[o]riginally coined to convey the purging characteristic of bulimia nervosa, "diabulimia" stripped to its starkest definition is the "use" of diabetes […] to eliminate unwanted calories or weight.' *Diabulimia* was therefore likely constructed via contamination for descriptive purposes. However, another theorized function of contamination as a method of word construction, and one which might also be applicable in the case of diabulimia, is euphemistic circumlocution – that is, the use of an innocuous word or phrase to talk about a taboo or sensitive topic (Lavrova 2010). This strategy might be particularly relevant regarding health concerns that people may feel embarrassed or ashamed to disclose in candid and explicit terms, as it grants them the opportunity to seek out and communicate with similar others more implicitly for the sake of exchanging advice and support. On the linguistic obscuration of diseases via euphemistic circumlocution, Lavrova writes,

> the designation is appropriate for being cryptic and euphemistic: it camouflages the disease, its treatment and enables the patients to freely communicate with each other without feeling the curious or condescending gazes of others. […] The structural model of contamination seems to be an adequate way of camouflaging some painful notions and meanings.
>
> (Lavrova 2010: 227)

As a term constructed via contamination, then, *diabulimia* might offer people who deliberately restrict their insulin a code word for communicating about their illness with a particular circumscribed group and in a way that backgrounds the (potentially dangerous) act of insulin restriction itself, perhaps to spare feelings of embarrassment or to evade anticipated negative evaluation from others.

Despite its relatively brief history, the precise origin of the term *diabulimia* is difficult to trace and, much like the condition itself, subject to contest and debate. Brink claims to have coined the term in 1987 (Brink 1997), yet others claim that the term was created by sufferers and their family members (Ruth-Sahd et al. 2009). Whatever the case may be, the term is widely accepted to have entered the 'blogosphere' in the early 2000s, where its popularity among sufferers and other non-expert groups grew exponentially via blogs, support groups and other online media. As Sharma (2013: 14) puts it, '[t]he era of both the social networking website and the blogosphere witnessed the true emergence of diabulimia into both the private as well as public consciousness'. Given that the focus of our study is online support groups, the label *diabulimia* should therefore provide a suitable starting point for exploring the discourse around this phenomenon online.

At this point, it is important for us to acknowledge that our use of the term *diabulimia* in this book could be interpreted as a signal that we perceive the health phenomenon that it denotes to be a discrete disease, rather than a mere complication of diabetes. While it is not the aim of this book to judge or argue for or against diabulimia's pathological legitimacy (for neither author possesses the expertise necessary to contribute to such a debate), our analysis in Chapter 6 will demonstrate that the majority of the contributors to the discussions about diabulimia in our data did indeed communicate about it using decidedly medicalizing language. In other words, the support group members communicated about and thus potentially conceived of diabulimia as a disease. We will return to the topic of diabulimia's clinical status later in the book, as part of the discussion which follows our analysis. In what remains of this section, we will review existing research on this topic.

2.4.1 Clinical and epidemiological studies of diabulimia

Likely as a consequence of its contested status, diabulimia has received scant attention from researchers in both the medical and social sciences. Indeed, Darbar and Mokha (2008: 32) rightly remark on the 'extremely limited' availability of research into diabulimia, while Hughes (2010: 11) comments on the 'scant' literature dedicated to the topic. Of the limited number of studies that *have* set out to explore this issue, the majority has adopted a decidedly positivist perspective (Thorne 1997), setting out to describe diabulimia's prevalence and its biological consequences. However, due to its contested status, establishing firm prevalence figures is more challenging for diabulimia compared to other mental health conditions, meaning that we do not know exactly how many people are currently affected by it. This notwithstanding, research suggests that diabulimia is likely to constitute a significant health concern among people with type 1 diabetes, with Goebel-Fabbri et al. (2008) estimating that as many as 30 per cent of people with insulin-dependent diabetes have intentionally restricted their insulin to control their body weight at some point in their lives. Furthermore, Shaban (2013: 104) describes the practice of deliberate insulin restriction as 'the most favoured means of weight control in people with type 1 diabetes'. Consistent with the epidemiological trends reported for other mental disorders, including anorexia and depression, diabulimia is understood to affect women more than men, with estimates suggesting that around 40 per cent of women with type 1 diabetes take less insulin to lose weight, while the figure is closer to 10 per cent for men (Colton et al. 2009; Hasken et al. 2010; Shih 2011; Callum and Lewis 2014).

By restricting their insulin, people with diabulimia are placed at increased risk of a range of serious and potentially fatal complications. These include diabetic neuropathy, kidney disease, diabetic retinopathy and ketoacidosis, as well as heightened susceptibility to heart attack and stroke (Rydall et al. 1997; Mathieu 2008; Shaban 2013). Studies into the long-term effects of diabulimia suggest that, when compared with non-insulin-restricting controls, the risk of death from diabetes complications increases more than threefold for diabetics who deliberately restrict their insulin (Goebel-Fabbri et al. 2008). Moreover, compared to those who take requisite amounts of insulin, the lifespan of individuals with diabulimia is estimated to be reducible by as much as thirteen years (Shih 2011: 25). Diabulimia is therefore a dangerous practice with potentially fatal outcomes, and it is in view of these outcomes that Zabka (2011: e221) characterizes it as 'a flirtatious relationship with toxicity and fatality'.

2.4.2 Sufferers' experiences of diabulimia

The foregoing studies of diabulimia have provided tentative epidemiological data and serve to highlight the biological impact that it can have on sufferers' bodies. However, this research does not reveal anything about diabulimia from the perspectives of those suffering from it. The small number of studies that have set out to elucidate lived experiences of diabulimia have done so rather tentatively, usually as an aside, and mostly without recourse to empirical data representing the perspectives of individuals with first-hand experience of it. Instead, research has focused on interviews with practitioners (Mathieu 2008) or on anecdotes and sufferer accounts invented by researchers (Sharma 2013). Consequently, the voices of non-experts, including people with first-hand knowledge and experience of diabulimia, have generally been elided from the research picture.

One exception to this trend is a recent study carried out by Hastings et al. (2016) that explored the role of relationships and associated identities in recovery from diabulimia. These researchers conducted five online focus groups with thirteen members of an online support group. Thematic analysis of the focus group transcripts showed that individuals who have recovered from diabulimia are likely to be well placed to provide psychological support to sufferers and are thus able to play a positive role in supporting others' recovery. However, these relationships could also be harmful if the online groups' norms were not carefully managed. This study thus highlights the power of online support group membership to aid recovery but also serves to flag up the influence of group norms in these settings. We will return to these features of online support groups more generally in the next chapter.

Aside from Hastings et al.'s study, which focused specifically on the role of support groups and relationships in the context of recovery, in empirical terms, we still know very little (if anything) about individuals' subjective experiences and understandings of diabulimia (Balfe 2007; Goebel-Fabbri et al. 2008; Powers et al. 2012). Moreover, while Hastings et al.'s analysis revealed themes around recovery in diabulimia, its focus on content rather than linguistic form means that the linguistic choices that sufferers make in representing their knowledge and experiences of this health issue remain unexplored. This gap in knowledge, along with the general lack of research on diabulimia more broadly, is not just a cause for academic curiosity but could also constitute a significant obstacle to effective clinical intervention. For instance, Sharma (2013: 14) describes how diabulimia has 'mystified' practitioners who lack awareness of its seriousness, as well as the ways and extent to which it impacts upon the lives of sufferers. Consequently, both scholars and healthcare practitioners alike have urged research that elucidates sufferers' subjective perspectives on diabulimia (Hasken et al. 2010; Weinger and Beverly 2010; Shih 2011). By exploring the discourses on which people draw to talk about and represent their experiences and understandings of diabulimia in the context of online support groups, the analysis reported in Chapter 6 can be viewed as responding to such calls. Although that section of our analysis focuses primarily on the discourses surrounding diabulimia specifically, the findings emerging from that chapter will also contribute insight into how these discourses are shaped by those surrounding the related themes of diabetes and insulin. In the next section we conclude this chapter by providing a more detailed introduction to the context under study: online support groups.

2.5 Chapter conclusion

While encompassing research into three distinct conditions, this chapter has consistently illustrated the contrasting and disputed understandings of anorexia, depression and diabulimia. Given their greater public and academic recognition, these debates are more well developed in relation to anorexia and depression and rather less-so in relation to diabulimia. Nevertheless, there are some consistencies across the existing research into each condition. Most obviously, qualitative studies of sufferers' accounts of these conditions reveal experiences of profound distress and personal conflict that in turn drive sufferers both to try to make sense of their illness and to seek support from others. In providing narratives of their illnesses, sufferers consistently employ representations that legitimize their experiences as genuine suffering and seek to explain how their distress has come about. Even in the case of diabulimia, where sufferers' experiences remain notably understudied, this legitimizing tendency is revealed by the label for the condition that sufferers have adopted, which gestures towards medical terminology. Indeed, perhaps inevitably, medical discourse has a significant place in lay accounts of all three of these conditions. In the case of anorexia and depression, participants in qualitative studies have been shown to challenge the perceived stigma of their illnesses by conceiving of them as a form of biological malfunction. However, these medicalizing explanations have a double edge for sufferers, serving to place their illness beyond the limits of both their moral responsibility and their attempts to situate it within their own personal, social and cultural circumstances.

Although the negotiation of stigma, agency and responsibility in relation mental illness has been a recurrent motif of foregoing qualitative studies, there has been comparatively little examination of the details of the language used by sufferers in these negotiations. At best, linguistic research into anorexia, depression and diabulimia is nascent, particularly in relation to online communication. This is somewhat surprising, given that the techno-psychological features of online support (outlined in the following chapter) mean they are apt venues for the candid discussion of experiences of mental illness. With a few exceptions (Harvey 2013a; Hunt and Harvey 2015; Mullany et al. 2015; McDonald and Woodward-Kron 2016; Brookes 2018), linguistic research into online mental health communication has also taken a micro-analytical approach to discourse analysis. While offering insightful and effective examinations of the experiences of those suffering from psychological distress, in addition to the interactional dynamics of online fora, such studies are unable to harness the large volumes of data available online. Here, then, is where the present study seeks to intervene by attending closely to the linguistic characteristics of sufferers' discussions of anorexia, depression and diabulimia in large online fora and by employing the unique perspective afforded by corpus linguistic methods to do so. The nature of this online context and the data and the methods that we use to analyse it are presented in the next chapter.

Corpora and methods of analysis

3.1 Introduction

In this book we adopt a corpus-based approach to analysing mental health discourses in online support group interactions. This methodological chapter describes both the nature of online health support and the particular sets of data we have gathered, as well as the corpus-based discourse analysis approach through which we have examined them. We begin by introducing the context of our data, online health support groups, considering their implications both for people who use them and researchers who study them. While there are ongoing debates about the values and dangers of peer-to-peer health support online, we are also concerned with exploring how the technical features of online support groups make them well suited to discussing and debating personal experiences of mental illness. As a consequence, our interest also lies in understanding online support groups as contexts with their own norms and shared beliefs about illness that are discursively produced, negotiated and contested. It is in this contested territory, in which mental health conditions are the subject of multiple conflicting academic and lay discourses, that our own study is positioned.

Following this, we outline the corpora of online support group interactions that are analysed in this book, including describing their design, construction and attendant ethical considerations, before outlining the specific corpus linguistic techniques that facilitate our analysis of anorexia, depression and diabulimia discourses in these contexts. The chapter then concludes with a review of the main strengths and limitations, as we see them, of our data and methodological approach.

3.2 Online fora and mental health support groups

An internet forum (plural *fora*) is an online, computer-mediated communicative platform which offers its users the chance to interact with large numbers of (usually) unknown others for the purposes of sharing ideas, telling stories and seeking and providing support about a range of topics (Claridge 2007). Fora are typically dedicated to specific topics or themes, the nature of which can vary widely on a forum-to-forum basis and can include, for example, sports, film, music, current events (Largier 2002) and, since the early 1990s in particular, health (Collot and Belmore 1996). Like many other forms of computer-mediated communication (CMC), the popularity of internet fora grew exponentially during the 1990s due to the increased availability of domestic computers (Thomas and Wyatt 1999). In fact, the number of active fora on the internet is so great that it lays beyond estimation (Crystal 2001). The content of internet fora is generated by users in one of two ways: either by creating a thread (a series of chronologically ordered messages or posts relating to a specific topic that have been contributed by numerous users) or by posting a message to an existing thread that has been created either by another user or by a forum moderator (Antaki et al. 2005). Messages tend to be primarily linguistic in content, although most fora are also capable of hosting non-linguistic content too, meaning that some messages are multimodal and contain, for example, emoticons, emojis, images, embedded videos, Graphic Interchange Format files (GIFs) and other audio/visual elements.

Internet fora constitute an accessible and popular avenue for health-related disclosure and advice-seeking, affording individuals the unique opportunity to interact with and read about the feelings and experiences of large numbers of similar others from whom they can receive social support, advice and even validation with regard to their health-related experiences (Coulson et al. 2007). Joinson refers to this phenomenon as 'the benefit of being in the same boat' (2003: 151), and particularizes these benefits to those seeking health-related support in internet fora and other online communities thus:

> [m]isery loves company for a number of psychological reasons, the key being social comparison. Social comparison is a process of comparing ourselves with others. In general, we can compare ourselves with those doing better than ourselves (upward social comparison) or those doing worse (downward social comparison). Within a self-help context, the two forms of comparison serve two independent functions: downward social comparisons may improve a person's mood and self-esteem by showing that there are others worse off [...], while upward comparisons may provide a guide for actions.
>
> (Joinson 2003: 151)

Indeed, in their review of social and health science literature on the topic of e-health, Ziebland and Wyke (2012) characterize the desire and benefits of sharing and accessing peers' stories of health and illness as one of the key features of e-health when they write, '[t]he value of first-person accounts, the appeal and memorability of stories, and the need to make contact with peers all strongly suggest that reading and hearing others' accounts of personal experiences of health and illness will remain a key feature of e-health' (2012: 242). Accordingly, Fox and Duggan's (2013) study found that one in four American internet users had watched or read about someone else's experience of illness online in the last twelve months.

The benefit of having access to the disclosure of experiences of similar others is likely to be particularly attractive to individuals experiencing health concerns that are routinely subjected to social stigma (Stommel 2009), including forms of mental distress (Sartorius 2007), where sufferers might be less inclined to seek face-to-face support from practitioners and even friends and relatives for fear of negative judgement or social sanction (White and Dorman 2001). Online fora also offer significant practical benefits, such as providing their users with the opportunity to overcome spatial, temporal and other accessibility barriers that might otherwise impede them from seeking advice and interacting with similar others (Salem et al. 1997).

Despite their benefits, health fora have also been the focus of numerous criticisms. One such criticism concerns the questionable credibility of the information they contain, particularly on peer-led platforms, whose typical users are unlikely to have received any formal medical training (ten Have 2002). Indeed, it is possible for health forum contributors who have little to no knowledge or experience of a particular health issue to nevertheless publish information about it, including that which is inaccurate or misleading. Moreover, even when contributors do have relevant knowledge or experience, another challenge of user-generated health information is that users can present their opinions as facts (Coulson and Knibb 2007). It is difficult to ascertain how much of the information contained in online fora is factually misleading, though it seems probable, given the vast numbers of members and contributions that they typically host, that most health-related fora will contain at least some factually misleading information. However, many fora operate with moderator-led measures and mechanisms which monitor user-generated content in an effort to prevent the circulation of offensive or unscrupulous material. While in some cases this may involve users' contributions being amended or deleted altogether, in other cases users may correct or 'pull up' others, should their contributions be deemed factually misleading or otherwise unhelpful.

Another potentially negative characteristic of many health fora relates to the contribution of scaremongering and negative information which might frighten other users (Sandaunet 2008a). In a study carried out by Broom and Tovey (2008), a group of cancer patients self-reported that they were actually more worried by negative medical statistics and scaremongering in internet fora than they were by misleading information circulated on such platforms. Health professionals have expressed similar concerns over the potential for online communication to legitimize damaging health practices. In the case of mental health, these concerns have focused in particular on online networks related to self-harm and suicide and to pro-eating disorders, in which anorexia and bulimia are presented as legitimate dietary and lifestyle practices. By proliferating representations of health behaviours and mental illness that, broadly speaking, run counter to medical orthodoxy, these online spaces are claimed to legitimize practices that involve harming the body and which dissuade individuals from pursuing professional treatment and recovery. Indeed, it is because such online networks produce content that contradicts psychiatric views about self-harm, suicide and eating disorders that they are considered dangerous (Baker and Fortune 2008). Space limitations mean it is not feasible to provide a thorough discussion of pro-self-harm and pro-eating disorder communities here. However, we concur with Baker and Fortune's (2008) perspective that a more nuanced response to purportedly dangerous online communities would involve seeking to understand the discourses circulating within them and the value they have for their users, and hence why some sufferers may opt to participate in online networks either in addition to or instead of conventional psychiatric care.

Perhaps the main reason that online fora constitute such popular avenues for (mental) health-related disclosure and social support is that they provide conditions for more open and less inhibited expression. Relevant here is the concept of the 'online disinhibition effect'; a theory developed by Suler (2004) to account for the less inhibited nature of individuals' communication and behaviours online compared against offline, face-to-face contexts. Suler argues that when interacting in anonymous computer-mediated contexts, people tend to 'loosen up, feel less restrained, and express their selves more openly' (2004: 321). Accordingly, the disinhibiting effect of CMC is brought about by six characteristics of communication in this context: anonymity, invisibility, asynchronicity, solipsistic introjection (imagining others' reactions), dissociative imagination (being able to imagine that other interactants are not real people) and the minimization of authority. Although Suler argues that these factors work simultaneously and co-operatively, he also acknowledges that the 'lion's share' of this effect is created by three of these factors (2004: 322): (i) anonymity, (ii) invisibility and (iii) asynchronicity. We will now consider each of these factors in turn.

According to Suler (2004), dissociative anonymity is the main contributory factor underlying the disinhibited nature of online communication. In the context of CMC, anonymity involves either the complete concealment of one's identity or the presentation of one's identity to others in an altered way that either conceals intimate aspects of the self or completely betrays one's offline identity altogether. The anonymous nature of some online communication allows users to dissociate themselves from both their online behaviours and the offline behaviours that they describe and disclose online. Thus, Harvey (2013a: 22) offers the analogy of users' donning a 'protective cloak of anonymity' when communicating online, which allows them to 'express the way they truly feel and think'. Researchers propose that the anonymity of online environments can facilitate feelings of equality, potentially making contributors feel more at-ease to express information of a personal and sensitive nature (Attard and Coulson 2012). The opportunity for anonymity is particularly attractive to individuals who wish to disclose potentially face-threatening and stigmatizing health-related concerns. For example, Grohol (1998) notes how individuals experiencing mental health issues are able to talk more openly and freely about their experiences in anonymous online environments because they can do so without anticipating negative judgement and evaluation, as might be the case (or at least as might be perceived to be the case) in non-anonymous contexts.

The concept of invisibility in CMC is not too dissimilar to that of anonymity. Despite the increasingly multimodal character of CMC, hastened further by the emergence and growing convenience of multimodal media (such as video call applications), significant swathes of online communication remain text-driven, with interlocutors typically unable to see one another (Goddard and Geesin 2011; Barton and Lee 2013). Typed exchanges are frequently only accompanied by user profile pictures, or images or videos incorporated into the body of the message itself, none of which need actually depict the users themselves. It has been argued by scholars researching CMC that the invisibility afforded by platforms such as internet fora lends bravery to interlocutors, allowing them to talk about potentially face-threatening issues in an open and candid way (Joinson 2001; Suler 2004; Goddard and Geesin 2011). Invisibility also grants forum users the means to contribute to, or simply to visit and read, discussions about topics that they would never openly discuss in visible communicative contexts (e.g. a face-to-face conversation with a medical practitioner) for fear of prejudice and negative evaluation. Furthermore, the double-blindness of online peer-to-peer support fora means that even if a user is negatively evaluated by other users on the basis of a forum contribution, unless that negative evaluation is expressed in a typed message, the impression of accommodation and acceptance is created by default (Joinson 2003). Another effect of invisibility is that interlocutors can communicate unhindered by the fear that they will be negatively prejudged or stereotyped on the basis of their ethnicity, sex or any other aspect of their identity that might be evident in their physical appearance. As Harvey argues, 'invisibility produces a reduced sense of public awareness and, with this, a propensity for increased self-disclosure [...] users of email do not have to concern their selves with how they look or sound when they send a message' (2008: 38).

Finally, communication can be considered asynchronous if it does not require the simultaneous participation of all interlocutors. Asynchronicity contributes to the online disinhibition effect in as much as it does not require interlocutors to deal with others' reactions and responses immediately. Suler (2004) contends that the 'light' temporal demands placed on interlocutors in asynchronous, compared to synchronous, communicative contexts means that greater amounts of time and thought may be committed to the creation of their contributions (i.e. forum messages), the result being that the interlocutor's 'train of thought may progress more surely and rapidly towards deeper expressions of disinhibition that sidestep social norms' (Harvey 2008: 39; see also Wright and Bell 2003; Malik and Coulson 2008). Suler (2004) also proposes that the relaxation of these social norms in asynchronous communicative contexts can be particularly appealing to people who wish to disclose potentially embarrassing or face-threatening concerns (particularly in relation to their (mental) health), since they are comforted by having the option to depart from or leave behind the communicative situation at any point of discomfort or embarrassment (Suler 2004: 323).

In light of the foregoing discussion, the communicative context of internet fora provides a platform on which people with mental health concerns can make sensitive self-disclosures and share their personal difficulties with a level of candour that would be unlikely in more inhibiting offline settings, such as face-to-face interactions (Barak 2007). Moreover, these factors might facilitate less inhibited personal disclosure in the internet fora examined in this book, and so conceivably offer a data source that is more reflective of these individuals' naturalistic discursive routines compared to data collected in environments in which the researcher is present and visible, such as interviews and focus groups (Joinson 1999).

A significant body of linguistic research into online support groups has focused on how users linguistically formulate advice-requesting and advice-giving messages (see Stommel and Lamerichs (2014) for a review). These studies have shown that requests for advice in online support groups are often not straightforward. For example, in a study of messages posted to online support groups for people with bipolar disorder, Vayreda and Antaki (2009) reported that first postings were frequently framed not as specific requests for advice but rather as more generally worded requests for help. Stommel and Lamerichs (2014) suggest that the indirectness of requests for advice in these contexts could be linked to participants' need to present themselves as competent (despite requesting advice), as well as to limit the possibility of receiving potentially undesirable responses from other members. In terms of advice-giving, many studies have focused on the need for support group members to establish their knowledge and credibility as advice-givers. One way in which group members can establish their credibility is by giving advice in the format of a comparable story or narrative, with the resolution acting as an implied piece of advice to the requester (Veen et al. 2010). So, the requesting and giving of advice can be both more and less direct in the context of online support groups, with the chosen format and level of directness likely intertwined with users' need to construct positive online identities while also attending to the group's norms and (implicit) conditions for membership.

Narrowing our focus to linguistic studies of online mental health support groups specifically, a key area of focus in this body of work has been the way in which contributors to support groups establish legitimacy with respect to their membership of specific online communities. An early example of such a study is Lamerichs's (2003) investigation of the discourse emergent from an online support group for people with depression. Her analysis revealed how the support group contributors went to great lengths to present themselves as being 'truly depressed', for example by embedding into their narratives precise details as to when and where their depression started, thereby situating their suffering within both time and space, and by displaying and accounting for their experiences (see also: Lamerichs and te Molder 2003; Sneijder and te Molder 2004). Another important finding from Lamerichs's study was the requirement that support group members attend to concerns surrounding blame and accountability in relation to their illness at the same time as having to manage the authenticity of their own and others' illness-related identities – a theme mirrored by Hardin's (2003) observation of the need for contributors to online anorexia support groups to perform the identity of 'authentic anorexic' mentioned in the previous chapter.

The theme of legitimacy also emerged in Horne and Wiggins's (2009) analysis of two online support groups for people with suicidal thoughts. Using methods from discursive psychology (Edwards and Potter 1992), their analysis showed how group members displayed their being 'authentically suicidal' through four practices: narrative formatting, going 'beyond depression', displaying rationality, and not explicitly asking for help (see also: Smithson et al. 2011). Like Lamerichs's work, their analysis also revealed how multiple posts could 'work up' the identity of the suicidal users being psychologically 'on the edge' of life and death. However, unlike in Lamerichs's study, the contributors to the support groups they analysed did not present themselves as being sufficiently competent in dealing with their problems. They concluded that the support group they analysed worked in part 'as a site for suicidal identities to be tested out, authenticated and validated by individuals' (Horne and Wiggins 2009: 170).

Another study which addresses issues to do with authenticity in online mental health-related support groups was carried out by Stommel and Koole (2010), who combined methods from conversation analysis and membership categorization analysis (Sacks 1992) to examine contributions to an online support group for people experiencing eating disorders. Their analysis showed how new members' interactions with existing members were shaped by their desire to display their legitimacy for membership of the group. Thus, they argue that the group operates as a Community of Practice (Lave and Wenger 1991), with membership to it organized through joint participation in certain writing practices; namely, those which allow the members to show that they subscribe to normative requirements of group membership, primarily in terms of displaying the acknowledgement that they are ill. In the case they focus on, this includes members relinquishing the pro-anorexia 'membership category'. Since the new member they analysed was not ready to subscribe to this norm, the threshold for support-seeking was heightened in that group. In this regard, even while the respective participants display contrasting attitudes towards anorexia, Stommel and Koole's study reflects Knapton's (2013) examination of online pro-anorexia communities, which illustrated a normative conception of anorexia as a pseudo-religious and aesthetic practice, and which served to demarcate legitimate contributions to those communities.

Expectations based on existing interactions in an online community and an individual member's status within it can therefore play a role in the ways in which support group members linguistically frame their messages, as well as the discourses on which they draw to construe their understandings and experiences of the health conditions they are communicating about. Such considerations are worth bearing in mind for the present study, as they are likely to influence the discourses on which individuals draw in their messages about anorexia, depression and diabulimia. In short, this means that health fora are not simply repositories of monadic individual narratives. Rather, individual forum posts must be understood as contributions to online communities that have established norms and expectations for communicating about illness (what Wenger (1998) refers to as 'interactional repertoires'). In some cases, these norms are codified through overt 'forum rules' and explicit moderation practices, while in others they are implicit in the ways in which their members express themselves (and the ways in which they do not) and how their messages are structured. In this way, forum members' contributions and the responses they receive can themselves be seen to orient to the collective norms of a forum, such as by reinforcing a forum's norms by reiterating its prevailing view of an illness. In seeking to understand the discourses of mental illness expressed by sufferers, the analysis in Chapters 4–6 of this book will seek to situate participants' messages against the contexts of the fora in which they are posted. As will become clear over the course of the forthcoming sections, the corpus linguistic approach that we use to interrogate the data is particularly well suited to evincing the interactional repertoires of online communities instantiated in the form of repeated linguistic signatures. For now, we turn our attention to the corpora assembled for the analysis in this book.

3.3 Corpora

The analysis presented over the forthcoming chapters is based upon three specialized, purpose-built corpora which, respectively, represent interactions within online support groups offering information and supportive communities for individuals experiencing anorexia, depression and diabulimia. To help to preserve the contributors' anonymity, we shall refer to these support groups and their corresponding corpora using the fictitious monikers, *anorexia.net*, *depression.net* and *diabulimia.net*. In the ensuing section, we describe the design and development of each of these corpora. As will become clear over the course of the section, while there is a large degree of overlap in terms of the steps taken in the construction of each of these datasets, in some respects they differ.

3.3.1 Corpus design and compilation: Sampling, size and representativeness

Peer support for anorexia and depression is highly accessible online, with both conditions the focus of extensive networks that span mainstream social networking sites such as Facebook, general health websites such as *WebMD.com* and condition-specific websites that include discussion boards. The data for all three corpora came from websites dedicated to peer support for living with and – in the case of depression and anorexia – recovering from the conditions. Support fora for anorexia and depression were identified through Google searches for 'anorexia forum' and 'depression forum', respectively. The identification of support groups for diabulimia, however, proved to be more challenging as we were not able to identify a support group with a specific diabulimia focus at the point of corpus construction (and indeed at the time of writing) – testament, perhaps, to both the general lack of awareness about this condition as well as to its contested medical status. We therefore decided to include diabulimia-related messages from online support groups for people with diabetes, which were identified through a search engine query using the terms 'diabetes forum' and 'diabetes message board'. This decision reflects the co-morbidity that underlies diabulimia, since those suffering with it will also have a prior diabetes diagnosis. We could have focused on interactions around diabulimia in mental health or eating disorder support groups. However, to do so would be to impose an interpretation of diabulimia as a mental disorder (or eating disorder specifically) at the point of data collection, whereas sourcing data from a diabetes support group allows for such disease conceptions and self-identifications to arise from the data more naturally.

For each condition, we narrowed the list of candidate support groups from the first 100 search engine results by keeping only those websites which were English-speaking, hosted peer-to-peer (as opposed to practitioner-led) interactions, not affiliated to a healthcare provider or charity (whose content is typically monitored by practitioners and specialists) and which met our ethical criteria (see Section 3.3.3 below). This reduced the number of websites to one each for depression and anorexia and three for diabetes. Where the anorexia and depression corpora consisted of interactions from just one support group each, as will become clear later in this section, the small number of diabulimia-related threads within these diabetes support groups required messages to be sampled from all three websites in order to compile a dataset sizeable enough for corpus analysis. Nevertheless, we will refer to these websites collectively using the term *diabulimia.net*.

Once the websites were identified, the next step involved sampling messages for inclusion in the corpora. Each website hosts asynchronous bulletin boards to which users can read and contribute and which cover a range of topics. Within these boards, individual messages are organized into sequential threads which are started by users, with each post therefore either contributing to an existing, ongoing thread, or beginning a new thread under a different subject. Each website's message board is large and has a highly active membership. At the point of corpus compilation, *depression.net* contained over 40,000 individual messages authored by nearly 900 registered members, *anorexia.net* has several thousand registered members and supports a repository of over a million messages, and the websites making up *diabulimia.net* collectively have just over half a million members and over 4 million messages. This significant volume of data is a clear testimony to the popularity of seeking support for (mental) health problems through the internet and the attendant need to understand this context more fully.

The discussion of geographical locations in messages and the details accompanying users' posts indicate that members of each forum reside in numerous countries across the world but predominantly in the English-speaking contexts of the United Kingdom, United States, Canada and Australia. Based on members' usernames and textual clues such as descriptions of themselves as daughters or mothers, we surmise that the vast majority of *anorexia.net* users are female, while the membership of *depression.net* and *diabulimia.net* is more balanced in terms of gender.

In keeping with a number of other online health community studies (Winzelberg 1997; Barker 2008), the online communities have identifiable cores of frequent posters, as well as peripheral members and new users. Among the core membership, much discussion serves the function of providing ongoing support for emotional troubles, advice on relationship, job and family issues and of seeking advice regarding experiences with healthcare providers. New members may of course move from the periphery to become core members over time or may post in a more episodic manner.

As with many web communities, posting members of all the support groups under study are obliged to adhere to explicit forum rules reached through a link displayed prominently in the forum interfaces themselves. These include generic 'netiquette' principles, such as not posting deliberately provocative or inflammatory remarks and not disclosing addresses or phone numbers. The guideline pages of each website expressly state that their support groups are designed to facilitate discussion and are not intended as a substitute for professional medical care. In addition, *depression.net*'s rules proscribe posts that detail methods of suicide on the grounds that forum users are likely to find these upsetting. Similarly, *anorexia.net* prohibits discussion of suicidal ideation as well as a number of eating disorder-specific rules. These prohibit the use of numbers in posts relating to body mass index, weight, calorific intake and frequencies of self-induced vomiting on the basis that other users find specific discussion of such issues intensifies their own anorexic compulsions. *Anorexia.net* also explicitly proscribes posts that present anorexia positively or which encourage others to restrict their own diet. From reviewing other web fora, it is apparent that such guidelines are common to a number of other depression and anorexia websites. In the case of *anorexia.net*, its rules also clearly establish it as a 'pro-recovery' site that promotes recovery and support for anorexia as an illness. The site authors thus explicitly situate *anorexia.net* in opposition to the types of 'pro-anorexia' or 'pro-ana' websites studied by Fox et al. (2005) and Knapton (2013), among others. By contrast, given that that their focus is on a chronic disease in diabetes rather than a disordered practice, the fora making up the *diabulimia.net* data do not contain such explicit warnings to users. On each website, the rules for posting are enforced by forum moderators who edit users' messages – for example, by replacing numbers with asterisks – or occasionally delete entire posts.

The guidelines for using these websites inexorably affect the communication which takes place in their respective fora and hence the discourses of mental health which we are likely to find there. Forum users on *depression.net* may be reluctant to seek help for some aspects of suicidal thinking and so either not communicate these or use a different website to do so. Similarly, those wishing to discuss anorexia as a lifestyle choice rather than a serious illness will be prevented from doing so on *anorexia.net*.

All three websites support several 'modules'; that is, parts of the forum in which topic-specific messages can be posted. For example, *anorexia.net* contains separate modules for posting messages on anorexia, bulimia and compulsive overeating as well as modules for discussing sexuality, literature and films. While many if not all of these modules are likely to contain some messages relevant to understanding sufferers' experiences of each condition, messages were only taken from those modules explicitly labelled 'Depression' on *depression.net* and 'Anorexia' on *anorexia.net* in order to ensure the respective corpus content was consistently focused around discussion of these conditions. Because the diabetes websites did not contain modules on the specific topic of diabulimia, for this corpus we had to sample specific threads on this topic. Specifically, threads were sampled if the term diabu* (with the asterisk acting as a wildcard to include the terms *diabulimia* and *diabulimic*) occurred in the thread title once and/or throughout the body of the thread at least three times. This ensured that the content of the sampled threads was sufficiently 'about' (Hutchins 1978) the topic of diabulimia, rather than merely containing a mention in passing.

The corpora analysed in this book were sampled at different points in time. A time-based sampling method is the favoured choice among electronic discourse researchers (Herring 2004), allowing the content of the online corpora to be determined by the interests and preferences of the respective forum users during those time frames. The *anorexia.net* corpus contains messages to all new threads and all existing threads that had posts added to them during a four-month period (December 2009 to April 2010), providing a total of 1,074 posts and 155,600 words across 71 threads. Due to the website's smaller membership, the same sampling method applied to *depression.net*'s forum resulted in a much smaller corpus and messages from this site were therefore sampled across a longer time span of eighteen months in order to construct a corpus with a comparable level of representativeness (discussed on pages 73–74). This gave a corpus of a similar size to the anorexia data (see Table 3.1). Due to the comparative scarcity of diabulimia interactions, for the *diabulimia.net* corpus we employed a more opportunistic approach, gathering all qualifying threads (see criteria mentioned earlier) from the three constituent websites at the point of data collection (2014), with the earliest post occurring in 2007.

We should note at this point that for all three corpora, forum threads were included in their entirety. For the purpose of this study, we view each thread as constituting a 'text', with their asynchronous and sequential structure meaning that posts are frequently written in response to one or several previous contributions. Sampling only individual posts would have meant divorcing them from the messages to which they were responding and from those which were subsequently written in response. Even at the point of data collection these 'texts' are not necessarily 'complete', in the sense that users can continue to add posts to threads for as long as they remain active, which could be months and even years after they have been sampled for corpus inclusion. Table 3.1 profiles the number of threads, posts and words per corpus.

Each post was accompanied by a substantial amount of textual data that provides details about its author and the time and date of its posting. This

Table 3.1 Profile of the Corpora[1]

	Anorexia.net	*Depression.net*	*Diabulimia.net*[2]
Total threads sampled	71	150	81
Total posts	1,063	1,709	1,072
Mean posts per thread	14.97	11.39	13.23
Total words	155,619	169,412	119,982
Mean words per post	146.40	99.13	111.92

peripheral data is ancillary to the discussion of the mental health phenomena in question and would appreciably affect frequency, keyword and collocation calculations for each corpus. Consequently, only the substantive content of each message was used to compile these corpora, though the peripheral data could be recovered by viewing the original web pages when necessary.

Even by the standards of specialized corpora, the datasets analysed in this book are relatively small (Flowerdew 2004). While Sinclair (1991, 2004) avers that the larger the corpus the better, having a corpus that can supply thousands of concordance lines for every query does not guarantee that all these concordances will be investigated. In such cases, the volume of data would defy the time (and patience) needed by a single researcher to exhaustively investigate the corpus (McEnery et al. 2006). In contrast, Flowerdew (2004) and McEnery (2006) demonstrate that smaller corpora enable a level of detailed qualitative analysis that would be impractical on a larger corpus. This point is echoed by Harvey, who observes that

> [s]pecialised corpora, [...] given their size and composition, their essential manageability, are often subjected to qualitative-based analyses. The close examination of concordance lines with recourse to the linguistic co-text afforded by qualitative approaches, for example, provides a rich source of data to complement more quantitative-based studies. [...] Indeed, a characteristic feature of many specialised corpora studies [...] is their use of both quantitative and qualitative data.
>
> (Harvey 2013a: 75)

Harvey's assertion is of particular relevance to corpus-based studies of health-related communication, which typically examine language produced by a certain clinical population or within a particular clinical context, and so construct specialized corpora to represent this specific variety of communication (Crawford et al. 2014). In this vein, Adolphs et al. (2004) studied the interactional strategies employed in the context of telemedicine by examining a corpus of NHS Direct recordings that amounted to approximately 62,000 words, and Harvey et al. (2007) examined the key topics and linguistic features of adolescent health-related communication emergent from a 400,000-word corpus of messages sent to an adolescent health advice website. Similarly, in their analysis of cancer metaphors, Demmen et al. (2015) compared three specialized corpora of online cancer fora communication comprised of interactions between health professionals, patients and carers, which were approximately 500,000 words, 253,000 words and 500,000 words in size, respectively.

As well as being well suited to studies of health(care) communication, in the context of the present study, smaller corpora are arguably more conducive to the type of fine-grained qualitative analysis that is necessary for identifying the specific discourses on which people draw to make sense of and communicate about health. Such qualitative analysis is especially valuable for scrutinizing *how* these discourses are invoked and the ways in which they might be corroborated, elaborated or challenged by other interlocutors, at which point we can also draw upon insights from other health-related social science disciplines. Despite their limited word counts, then, the corpora analysed in this book provide apposite datasets with which to increase our understanding of the discourses surrounding anorexia, depression and diabulimia in online support groups.

Notwithstanding their usefulness for close, qualitative discourse analysis, the small size of the corpora analysed in this book nevertheless raises questions around their representativeness. Biber (1993: 243) defines representativeness as 'the extent to which a sample includes the full range of variability in a population'. The extent to which a corpus can be described as being representative thus depends upon the extent to which the findings issuing from it can be generalized to the wider language or variety that it is designed to represent (Hunston 2002). Representative corpus design is typically achieved by sampling data based on non-linguistic criteria – spoken and written modes and multiple genres, geographical regions, speaker genders and speech communities – to achieve adequate coverage of all relevant variability in the target language or variety (Biber 1993). To confidently measure the representativeness of a corpus, we therefore need to be cognisant of the consistency of the total number of texts making up the target variety – what Titscher et al. (2000: 33) refer to as the 'universe of possible texts' from which we have extracted samples for our corpus. However, attempts to compile representative corpora from anonymous online communication are hampered by the absence of speakers' demographic details (King 2009) and because the full extent of language available on the internet is impossible to ascertain (Mautner 2005; Claridge 2007). Similarly, although the listed membership of each online support group offers one measurement of the potential audience of a post, when using corpora compiled from online support groups it can be challenging to ascertain how representative a post's reception may be in terms of how widely a post is read and by whom.

In the absence of such contextual information, we adopted a measure of lexical representativeness based on corpus-internal linguistic criteria. Lexical representativeness can be measured by the degree of 'closure' (McEnery and Wilson 2001: 166) or 'saturation' (Belica 1996: 61–74) achieved in a corpus.

Saturation for a linguistic feature of a variety occurs when that particular feature appears to be finite or at least subject to limited variation after a certain point. Lexical saturation is typically measured by dividing the corpus into equally sized segments (in terms of number of tokens) and then tracking the number of new types that are introduced into the corpus with the inclusion of each segment. Once the addition of a segment yields a similar number of new lexical items (or better still, fewer), and thus lexical growth plateaus or dips, then 'saturation point' is judged to have been reached (see also: Teubert 1999). However, in this study we take a slightly different approach; since our analysis is based on keyness, we judged the lexical representativeness of our corpora in terms of the saturation of keywords.

Lexical representativeness of the *anorexia.net* corpus was assessed by adding a fortnight's worth of forum messages to the corpus at a time and generating a keyword list (under the conditions described in Section 3.4.1). When the incremental keyword list stabilized – that is, when adding another fortnight's worth of messages made negligible difference to the resulting keywords – the corpus was judged to be lexically representative of the forum communication. The same method for the *depression.net* messages resulted in a comparably sized corpus, though one that encompassed a larger number of message threads. Although the scarcity of possible diabulimia data precluded the possibility of collecting more messages for the *diabulimia.net* corpus (at the time of original corpus compilation), we nevertheless ran this same procedure on this corpus by dividing it into six segments of approximately 20,000 words. As with the anorexia and depression corpora, the keywords stabilized before the inclusion of the sixth and final segment, indicating that lexical representativeness had also been reached within the threads sampled.

Having explored the issue of representativeness, it is important for us to acknowledge at this point that the corpora analysed in this book contain posts written by a mixture of support group users who do and do not have direct experience of the mental health conditions in focus. Moreover, we are also aware of the possibility for contributors to falsely present as either having or not having such experience, in the latter case to avoid anticipated negative responses and in the former case to provide so-called disguised presentations (Holmes et al. 1997: 80), for example to seek advice on behalf of another. For the purpose of this analysis, we have little choice but to take the contributors' claims at face value. However, this feature of the data does not undermine our analysis to any significant extent, as the discourses that circulate in these environments contribute towards the broader construal of the mental health conditions regardless of whether or not the person typing them out actually had direct experience of the condition in question.

3.3.2 Typos, non-standard spelling and multimodality: Capturing and representing computer-mediated discourse

Aside from the challenges surrounding their representativeness, corpora derived from online communication present a number of issues for corpus linguistic approaches. Ringlstetter et al. (2006) outline numerous classes of orthographic inconsistency that regularly occur in online, web-based registers and which include, *inter alia*, typographical errors and non-standard spellings (Barton and Lee 2013). This issue is of particular relevance to sites of online peer-to-peer health-related communication, in which non-experts routinely draw upon morphologically complex medical and technical jargon in their interactions (Barker 2008). The result is a potentially 'dirty' corpus which, while containing much usable data, is also likely to be replete with orthographic variations (Kilgarriff and Grefenstette 2003: 342). Leaving these alternative spellings unaddressed has the potential to skew automated word counts operationalized in corpus procedures like frequency, keyness and collocation (introduced later in this chapter), which constitute points of analytical departure in the each of our analysis chapters.[3] To offer an illustrative example, the *depression.net* corpus contains sixteen instances of *counsellor*, but also four instances of *counselor*, two instances of *councillor*, one instance each of *counceller*, *counciler*, *council/er*, *councillor* and three uses of *counsellors*. An analyst considering the frequency of only the most common spelling, *counsellor*, would therefore overlook 38 per cent of the total references to this professional role. This contingency necessitated the manual survey of frequency lists for each corpus to identify spelling variations that could be combined and treated as the same word in subsequent calculations. Manual standardization of spellings was conducted as thoroughly as possible in order derive more accurate frequency data so that calculations based on word frequency were not skewed by variations of orthographically complex words such as *counsellor* and *dietician*. In addition, we manually standardized spellings in the original data in the case of words that were the focus of collocation analysis. For example, we standardized the US variant *behaviors* to *behaviours* in the original corpus files in order to ensure that collocation analysis identified the collocates of this word, regardless of its orthographic presentation.[4]

Another challenge arising from this type of data is that the forum posts under study can involve use of what Herring and Dainas (2017) refer to as 'graphicons', including emoticons, emoji, stickers, GIFs, images and videos (see also: Collins 2019: 82–7). These rebuses are an attested feature of online communication designed to emulate prosodic and physical indices of emotional states and interpersonal relations in spoken discourse (Wright and Bell 2003; Dresner and Herring 2010). Such elements are removed from our forum data once it is rendered into a text-only format. While we could have replaced graphicons with a series of tags to indicate their type and presence, the graphicons evident in our corpora seem to perform a largely supplementary function to the linguistic exchange of information in the fora, often repeating visually what is explicit in the adjacent text rather than conveying new information (Claridge 2007). Moreover, the present investigation is primarily concerned with discursive constructions of anorexia, depression and diabulimia rather than the negotiation of interpersonal relationships online, for which an analysis of graphicon use would be more germane. While presenting a potentially rich resource for the study of computer-mediated pragmatics, these features therefore fall outside of the remit of the present study, where their inclusion would require an amount of work that is arguably not commensurate with the types of analytical insight they would provide for our purposes.

The websites from which the forum posts were sampled utilize relatively simple interfaces compared to those seen in contemporary Web 2.0 websites, and their overwhelmingly text-based formats make the interactions well suited to compilation as text corpora. One aspect in which the websites vary is whether or not they contain hyperlinks. *Anorexia.net* prohibits users from posting hyperlinks to external webpages. While links are permitted on *depression.net* and *diabulimia.net*, they are relatively infrequent in both, appearing a total of four times in the threads sampled from *depression.net* and thirty-six times in the *diabulimia.net* data. In the depression messages, these links lead to the website of the seasonal affective disorder association, an online shop for nightlights, a Wikipedia page on psychoanalysis and a webpage on keeping guinea pigs. In the diabulimia data the hyperlinks connect users to other threads within the discussion boards, other diabetes support websites, diabetes-related Facebook groups and YouTube videos, news articles on diabulimia and diet and calorie-counting websites. Mautner (2005) suggests that the presence of hyperlinks disrupts the linearity of the texts which web users encounter, since readers can pursue any number of hyperlinks before returning to the original webpage. This poses the question of whether the storage of hyperlink-rich webpages in linear text files accurately reflects how those texts are encountered by their original users. However, the comparably minimal presence of hyperlinks in our corpora encourages users to read message threads in a relatively linear fashion. While it may be that forum users are simultaneously browsing multiple message threads or websites through different windows, evidence of these browsing behaviours cannot be obtained from the forum interfaces. Instead, the composition of the corpora directly reproduces the manner in which each website organizes users' contributions into threads of sequential messages.

3.3.3 Ethics and online linguistic research

The collation of corpora from messages to online mental health fora necessitates a consideration of the ethics of online research, and particularly research involving the analysis of communication around sensitive topics. In the case of the present study, the process of data collection took place before the publication of more recent papers on internet research ethics (Markham and Buchanan 2015, for instance) and the European Union's 2018 General Data Protection Regulation (see Collins 2019 for a discussion). As a result, reflecting on the study's ethical position involves a dual consideration of both the steps that were taken at the time of data collection and the different perspective offered by more recent ethical guidelines and greater public awareness of how online data is used.

Guidance on ethical decision-making for online research has recognized that blanket policies that seek to account for all forms of internet study will quickly unravel in the face of the manifold different forms of online communication and the myriad contexts in which it takes place (Markham and Buchanan 2012). Instead, they recommend a process-driven approach to ethical decision-making, in which ethical assessments are made on a case-by-case basis at each stage of a study (identifying a potential research field, accessing the site, gathering data, publishing results, etc.) and undergirded by a commitment to fundamental research regulations such as the Declaration of Helsinki (World Medical Association 2013). Within our own discipline, the British Association for Applied Linguistics' (BAAL) recommendations (2016) for research practice stress the importance of respecting participants' sensitivities, their rights to privacy and autonomy, and the need to avoid exposing participants to harm.

Given the diversity of online research and the multiple ways in which online communication can be conceived, making ethical decisions in relation to these factors often necessitates the negotiation of seemingly contradictory positions. For example, the blurred distinction between private and public communication on the web is perhaps the most long-standing and recurrent tension in online research. From a technical perspective, many online contexts – and particularly websites whose content is predominantly user-generated – are freely accessible to the public, with their content comparable to a publicly authored digital book (Frankel and Siang 1999). From this perspective, web users have opted to communicate in a public setting and their data can be used for research purposes without their notification or consent. However, even while technically public, web users may nevertheless perceive their interactions as at least partially private and can suffer harm when information that they perceived to be private is published in different contexts (Frankel and Siang 1999). As a result, recent studies have employed Nissenbaum's (2010) model of 'contextual integrity' in order to understand the norms and expectations held by web users regarding the use and flows of their information in specific online contexts. For instance, Mackenzie (2017) describes a shift from regarding the *Mumsnet Talk* forum as an essentially public environment to recognizing that its users held some expectations of privacy since they seldom anticipated that their interactions would be viewed by a general public. This shift also accompanied a change in the extent of the ethical obligations required of the researcher, most notably the increased need to contact research participants to gain informed consent prior to subjecting their messages to linguistic analysis. Mackenzie writes that the change in her perspective arose as a result of her moving from a position as a passive observer of the forum to adopting the role of an 'observer-as-participant' who held a personal affinity for the forum and its community. Mackenzie also writes that her self-positioning as a member of the *Mumsnet* community as well as her political views and role as a mother facilitated her attempts to broker access to the forum and its participants and to secure consent to analyse their interactions. Subsequent discussions held with *Mumsnet* users further sensitized Mackenzie to the informational norms of *Mumsnet*, or at least those perceived by the participants with whom she interacted.

While Mackenzie (2017) provides a clear illustration of how to achieve contextual integrity that is attuned to ethnographic methods of online research, it is unclear how such an approach would function in the present study. As Collins (2019: 35) notes, identifying the discourse norms of an online community through direct contact with its participants is more difficult for corpus linguists who seek to collect a range of texts across multiple websites 'and for whom it is not feasible to ascertain the perceptions of all of the participants, across a range of platforms and contexts'. It would, for instance, be disingenuous of either of us to act as participant observers in the online fora – neither of us have diabulimia, for example – and the diversity of participants in the fora included in this study would make it difficult to leverage access on the basis of similarities in social identities between ourselves and the fora participants. As a result, some other means of determining the obligations on the researcher are required.

Rather than adopting an ethnographic approach, Giaxoglou (2017), following Page et al. (2014), offers a means of determining the level of risk that a study's choice of data and methods poses to participants. Giaxoglou's matrix is based on four binary oppositions: (i) large scale 'big' data versus small-scale data obtained through observation, interviews and surveys; (ii) quantitative versus qualitative analytical methods; (iii) the use of sites with in-built settings for controlling access to content, such as Facebook versus sites with no privacy settings; and (iv) a focus on texts and discourse patterns versus a focus on people and their lives. A study involving more 'high-risk' characteristics (the latter in each pair) should necessitate greater precaution on the part of the researcher. Again, however, corpus studies may not fit neatly into these dimensions; while some of the findings presented in the following chapters are determined from quantitative analysis of large amounts of data, there is also extensive qualitative analysis that is intended to explicate the relationship between forum contributors' representations of mental illness and the online communities in which they are posting. Similarly, while we are concerned with texts and patterns of discourse, we also draw data from sites that have varying privacy settings for their users. At best, we could argue that this study presents a medium level of risk for participants, though it is unclear quite what precisely is at risk for participants and what actions the researcher should take in this situation.

More tangible information can be gleaned from the characteristics of the sites from which our corpora are compiled. Specifically, we have collated data from websites that do not require registration or permission to access; what Sveningsson Elm (2009) would call 'public environments' rather than semi-public, semi-private or private environments. In addition, each forum contained a visually prominent set of user guidelines that emphasized both the public nature of the forum and/ or the breadth of people that may read users' contributions. These guidelines did not prohibit research from taking place on the forum, and one forum contained a number of threads explicitly seeking participants for offline research. In addition, each forum also had between several hundreds and tens of thousands of members, with these high numbers arguably correlating with contributors' perceptions that their messages will have a wide-ranging audience (Eysenbach and Till 2001). All of the fora also have facilities that enable users to communicate with greater privacy, such as direct messaging, specific password-protected sub-fora and personal 'diaries' to which members grant access to other individual users. As a result, by examining interactions that take place in the websites' open discussion boards, we have collated data from contexts where participants have opted to communicate in the most public of several options (though admittedly the privacy/publicity of their messages is unlikely to be the participants' sole consideration in this decision). The range of more or less public venues on each forum should in turn heighten participants' awareness of the public nature of posts in the open discussion board. Giaxoglou (2017) also recommends analysing online contributors' discourse in order to understand their orientation to the online context as one that is private or public. In our own case, contributors' messages were typically orienting to a wider audience as indicated through their adoption of plural first-person pronouns to speak on behalf of the forum and the addressing of initial posts in a thread to 'anyone' or 'everyone', though the request for advice on illness-related issues also suggested a more limited intended audience.

While features of the websites may encourage contributors to perceive their messages as being published in a public domain, the publication of extracts from the fora will nevertheless open users' contributions to an audience that is highly unlikely to have been imagined by the users themselves (Baym and boyd 2012). In addition, anorexia, depression and diabulimia are clearly personal and sensitive subjects whose discussion opens sufferers to social stigma. This vulnerability in turn requires that the study should be undertaken with a due sense of responsibility to the forum users.

In order to respect forum contributors' privacy, we have used pseudonyms for the fora and removed all identifying information from the data quoted in subsequent chapters, including contributors' pseudonyms. More importantly, where possible, we have sought to collate our corpora from fora that are not indexed on search engines so that online profiles cannot be identified from the quotations that we reproduce. These measures should help to minimize threats to contributors' anonymity and privacy.

Responding to contributors' right to autonomy – and particularly their control over how their online interactions are used – through informed consent is more contentious. On a practical level, gaining consent from the thousands of contributors whose messages make up the three corpora would be largely unfeasible, regardless of whether it was undertaken prior to or after data was sampled (Collins 2019); contributors may log-in infrequently, may have ceased using the forum altogether or may simply not respond to researchers' consent requests.[5] The resulting patchwork of data would be too threadbare to fully represent the interactions in each forum or to realize the potential of corpus methods for contributing to the understanding of online mental health discourse.

However, letting practical implications drive ethical decisions would be putting the cart before the horse. More important is the need to weigh the consideration of obtaining informed consent against the implications of doing so (Elgesem 2015). The current BAAL (2016) research guidelines emphasize the obligation to mitigate disruption to participants' lives and environment. In this case, we were mindful that the participants' online environment constitutes an important source of social and emotional support and that this should remain undisturbed by the research process. We believed that imposing on the fora to request informed consent from a large number of contributors would risk disrupting the fora and undermining their primary role as supportive, recovery-oriented communities, thereby affecting the research participants and wider forum communities in a negative way (Nosek et al. 2002). We perceived this risk to be greater than the potential harm that covert research would pose to contributors.

Existing publications provide a clear precedent for our position on consent, with both recent corpus (Seale et al. 2010; Demmen et al. 2015) and non-corpus (Giaxoglou 2017) studies analysing health-related or sensitive data without participants' informed consent. Nevertheless, we are conscious that our position is a debatable one, especially in the light of recent public concerns over the (ab) use of web users' data such as Facebook's Cambridge Analytica scandal. Indeed, negotiating the ethical issues of online corpus linguistic research can feel like choosing between a series of variously dissatisfying options. Nevertheless, the position above represented an attempt to respect the participants' privacy and the equilibrium of their online environment while also minimizing their risk of harm, which represent cornerstones of ethical research conduct.

3.4 Methods of analysis

Having introduced the corpora that we have compiled for the purpose of this study, we now outline the corpus-based approach to discourse analysis that we use to analyse them. Since corpus linguistics offers a range of analytical techniques, there is no 'standard' set of procedures for a corpus study (Baker et al. 2008: 274). However, the analysis presented over the course of the next three chapters is based upon three established analytical perspectives on corpus data: keyword analysis, collocate extraction and manual analysis of concordance lines, each of which was conducted using version 7 of *WordSmith Tools* (Scott 2016). We will now introduce each of these analytical procedures in turn, describing how they assisted us in the identification and examination of mental health discourses and outlining, where relevant, our choices regarding parameters, statistical measures and cut-offs.

3.4.1 Keywords

Keywords are words which occur with an unusually high frequency in the corpus we are analysing when compared against another corpus. The corpus that we compare our dataset against to obtain keywords is referred to as the 'reference' corpus. Words are deemed to be keywords by the computer based on statistical comparisons of word frequency lists for each corpus, with the frequency of each word in the analysis corpus compared against its equivalent in the reference corpus. If a word is very much more frequent in our corpus compared to the reference corpus, and the frequency difference is judged to be significant (according to a user-determined statistical measure), that word will be flagged as a keyword by the computer. The choices of reference corpus and statistical measure are therefore important here, as both shape the keyword output. When selecting a reference corpus, we usually want one that is at least similar in size to, but preferably larger than, the target corpus and which belongs to broadly the same genre and register as the texts in our corpus, so that our keywords will flag up what is lexically distinctive about the language in our corpus, including the 'aboutness' of the texts in contains (Hutchins 1978; Scott 1996), rather than merely reflecting features of the genre or register to which they belong (Baker 2006).

The concept of keywords precedes the relatively recent, mechanical conception outlined above which is most familiar to corpus linguists. Firth (1957: 10), for example, discussed focal or pivotal words, while Williams (1983) later coined the term 'keywords' to describe those words deemed to encapsulate meanings of some significance to a particular cultural and historical moment. In contrast to these conceptions, the computational method of generating keywords is not based on subjective judgements about what is significant but allows for potentially any word to be a keyword, provided it occurs frequently enough in the corpus under analysis compared to the reference corpus.[6] Indeed, the corpus linguistic generation of keywords is arguably more sophisticated than these earlier approaches, since it can reduce, or at least delay, the influence of the researcher's *a priori* biases in the selection of keywords for analysis (Baker 2010). We will revisit the strengths and limitations of computer-assisted corpus linguistic analysis compared to manual discourse analysis towards the end of this chapter.

The keywords procedure is used as an inductive measure in this study, providing a 'way in' to our corpora by identifying the most characteristic language and themes in the support group messages. To generate keywords for the support group corpora introduced in the previous section, we compared the word frequency information for each against the word list for the spoken component of the updated version of the British National Corpus (henceforth: Spoken BNC2014; Love et al. 2017). This corpus comprises approximately 11 million words of casual spoken conversations which took place in British English across the United Kingdom between 2012 and 2016 (inclusive). As a corpus of conversational spoken British English, the Spoken BNC2014 might not at first appear to be well suited for generating keywords from a corpus comprising posts to online mental health support groups. Indeed, ideally we would compare our corpora against a reference corpus which represents multiparty, web-based interactions, such as a more general corpus of forum interactions on a range of topics. However, such a corpus is not, to our knowledge, available at the time of writing. Therefore, we were left with the choice of either constructing our own general corpus of forum posts or relying on existing general corpora. Due to practical considerations, we opted for the latter.

Computer-mediated language has conventionally been characterized as a hybrid register which combines elements of spoken and written language (Baron 2000; Crystal 2011). In view of this, we initially generated keywords for our corpora by comparing each against the wordlist for the original British National Corpus, including both its spoken and written components. While this comparison provided a lot of keywords for each corpus, including content-rich words indicative of the 'aboutness' of each corpus's constituent texts, it also less helpfully prioritized keywords that were suggestive of the support groups' less formal and interactional register, such as contractions, vague language and spoken discourse markers. Although such elements would be useful for the study of register features, they are less helpful in the identification of mental health discourses. In contrast, although comparing our corpora against the Spoken BNC2014 gave fewer keywords overall, this comparison did filter out the markers of register while retaining keywords that were more indicative of the 'aboutness' of our data and the mental health discourses it contains. Moreover, this comparison also yielded new keywords that were more promising for the purpose of identifying discourses, such as *family* in the anorexia and diabulimia corpora, *support* in the depression and diabulimia corpora and *since* in all three. With this in mind, we proceeded using the Spoken BNC2014 as our reference corpus.

Corpus analytical software packages, *WordSmith Tools* included, offer a number of statistical tests which measure either effect size or statistical significance. Effect size metrics indicate the strength of an observed difference or relationship, while measures of statistical significance indicate the level of confidence the researcher can have that a difference or relationship is dependable and not merely the result of a sampling error (Gabrielatos 2018). In other words, effect size indicates strength, while statistical significance indicates confidence. For generating keywords, it is recommended to combine metrics of effect size and statistical significance to make the results more robust.

In this book, we generated keywords using log ratio (Hardie 2014). This measure combines the log-likelihood test of statistical significance (Dunning 1993) with a measure of effect size, which quantifies the strength of the difference between the observed frequencies, independent of the sample size. Log-likelihood is a hypothesis-testing measure that assigns to each word in the corpus a score which reflects the likelihood that the word is key when the corpus is compared against the reference corpus. The higher the log-likelihood score, the greater confidence the analyst can have that a given word is a keyword. Different cut-offs can be applied, but a log-likelihood score of 3.84 indicates a confidence level of 95 per cent (standard in social sciences (McEnery 2006)), while a score of 6.63 indicates a confidence level of 99 per cent. In this study, we stipulated that keywords should have a log-likelihood score of 15.13, indicating a confidence level of 99.99 per cent (in other words, the chance of a keyword resulting from a sampling error is 0.01 per cent). Each statistically significant keyword is then assigned a log ratio score based on the size of the observed difference between the relative frequencies in our corpora and the Spoken BNC2014, with bigger differences producing higher scores. This measure therefore uses log-likelihood as a cut-off to ensure that keywords are significant but has the advantage that it also allows us to rank those keywords according to how unusually high, or 'marked', their frequency is. Since log ratio privileges low-frequency keywords, we also stipulated that keywords had to occur across a minimum of 5 per cent of the forum posts in the corpus. As well as adding a frequency threshold for keyness (since a word used in 5 per cent of 1,000 messages must occur at least fifty times, for example), this added measure also helped to ensure that keywords were reflective of recurrent discourses across the support groups under study and not simply the repeated use of a word in one or two messages.

We decided to keep our three corpora separate for our analysis, including for generating keywords, as this helped to maintain our focus on what is linguistically characteristic about the discussions of each condition, rather than looking to identify a general 'mental health' discourse. To have amalgamated our corpora would have risked overlooking such nuances, in turn rendering the analysis less useful to readers who have specific interests in one or more of the particular conditions.

Once obtained, the keywords for each corpus are then grouped into thematic and semantic categories. This step in the analysis resembles, somewhat, the thematic coding of keywords operationalized in previous corpus studies of discourse (Baker 2004; Baker et al. 2013), including in health-related contexts (Seale et al. 2006; Charteris-Black and Seale 2010; Harvey 2013a), and essentially involved assigning keywords to categories based on manual analysis of them in their original contexts using concordancing (introduced later). This constitutes an interpretive and subjective step in our analytical procedure (Baker 2010: 107–8) and can be contrasted, in this sense at least, with the automated grouping of words by semantic tagging software (e.g. the USAS tagger; Rayson 2008), used, for example, by Demmen et al. (2015) to identify metaphorical patterns in their corpora of conversations about cancer.

A key consideration pertaining to the application of a semantic tagger such as USAS to analyse specialized corpora such as ours relates to the generality of its constituent categories, which are not always particularly enlightening where specialized corpora are concerned. For example, the USAS tagger would assign many of the high-ranking keywords across our corpora to the categories B1 (Anatomy and physiology), B2 (Health and disease) and B3 (Medicines and medical treatment). While such a categorization could provide a useful thematic entry point for a study of a corpus comprising texts centred on a range of topics, they are decidedly less useful for our study of online health interactions and do not tell us much that we do not already know about or expect of them. Moreover, on a practical level the non-standard spelling evident in much CMC, and so across our corpora, can pose problems for such automated taggers which struggle to reconcile such orthographic presentations with their intended spellings and meanings. This is also problematic for the categorization of alternative forms of orthographic representation, such as acronyms and abbreviations which abound in CMC, as well as for relatively 'standard' spellings of non-standard terminology, including not least the word *diabulimia* and its associated forms.

The appeal of manual keyword grouping, then, is that it retains the replicability and statistical validation of computational keyword identification, but augments this with the interpretative sensitivity of the human analyst's perspective. The result in this case is the development of keyword categories which are more responsive to the nature of the context under study and which correspond more closely to the study's particular aims, all the while answering to broader appeals for triangulating the interpretation of statistically validated corpus evidence with human intuition (McEnery and Wilson 2001: 11). The manual grouping of keywords therefore provides a series of analytical entry points through which to examine the mental health discourses permeating the forum posts across each of our corpora. However, to examine what those discourses are, and how and why they are drawn upon in these contexts, we need to follow them up in more fine-grained fashion through collocation and concordance analyses.

3.4.2 Collocation

Collocation refers to the association between words based on patterns of co-occurrence. In corpus linguistics research, collocation is calculated using a word association measure that tells us how often two or more words occur within close proximity of one another in the corpus, and whether this association is notable as a sizeable effect (i.e. that the words have a measurably strong preference to occur together as opposed to being randomly associated). Following Firth's (1957: 6) dictum that 'you shall know a word by the company it keeps', corpus linguists have long sought to learn about words' meanings and patterns of use by examining them in terms of the words with which they tend to co-occur, or 'collocate'.

Indeed, corpus-enabled analysis of collocational patterns can provide a valuable perspective on the discursive structures that surround a word or phrase of interest. For example, Stubbs argues that the consistent co-articulation of particular lexical items around node words indicates 'the associations and connotations they have, and therefore the assumptions which they embody' (1996: 172). In short, the meaning of a node's collocates influences the meaning of the node itself. Louw (1993, 2000) refers to this dispersion of meaning as 'semantic prosody' – semantic associations established through the co-occurrence of collocates (see also Stubbs (2001) on 'discourse prosody'). Louw (1993) notes that the primary function of semantic prosody is to express the attitude of the writer or speaker, with prosodies coalescing into positive or negative inflections of a node's meaning. Similarly, Morley and Partington observe that analysis of semantic prosody offers the analyst 'insight into the opinions and beliefs of the text producer' (2009: 140). Drawing on Sinclair (2003, 2004), Hunston (2007) expands upon Louw's claims by arguing that prosodies established through consistent collocation can convey more granular semantic information than just positive or negative attitudes. Prosody, Hunston argues, indicates not only the broad attitudes of speakers towards a node word, but also the semantic and conceptual associations it carries. Baker (2006) also highlights the ideological nature of collocation, claiming that collocation indicates that 'two concepts have been linked in the minds of people and have been used again and again' (2006: 114).

In light of this analytic potential, collocation analysis has come to play a central role in the identification of discourses in texts and the development of linguistic theory more generally (Sinclair 2004; Stubbs 2011). Concordant with Baker (2006; Baker et al. 2008), we argue that recurrent collocations constitute textual traces of discourses because they establish particular, partial representations of phenomena that are normalized through their constant articulation. Given its utility for identifying frequently co-occurring words and broader formulations, the collocation tool is therefore ideally suited to provide an account of such 'systematic' language use that might signal the presence of discourses in corpus data (Baker 2006). As an aspect of textual representation, collocation can also be the site of ideological contest in which differences 'between socially, ideologically, or historically distinct discourses often crystallize in different semantic prosodies of key lexical items' (Koller and Mautner 2004: 223; Orpin 2005). Discursive struggles over meaning and resistance to dominant discourses can thus be traced systematically to alternative collocational patterns in texts.

The use of collocation analysis also provides a rejoinder to Wooffitt's (2005) accusation that discourse analyses (and particularly critical discourse analyses) present only inexplicit means of identifying discourses. Echoing Foucault's assertion that discourses systematically form the objects of speech, Mills suggests that discourses can be 'detected because of the systematicity of the ideas, opinions, concepts, ways of thinking and behaving which are formed within a particular context' (2005: 15). As with Foucault, systematicity is central to Mills's definition: discourses can be identified in texts as consistent, systematic choices in the linguistic representation of particular phenomena. By identifying frequently co-occurring words, collocation analysis objectively highlights just such systematic linguistic representations – that is, discourses – in texts (Baker 2006). The provision of corpus frequency information also allows discourses to be quantified in order to adduce dominant and minority discourses in terms of their respective collocation frequencies across a corpus (Baker et al. 2008). In this respect, corpus-based discourse analysis offers a systematic and transparent method for the identification and classification of discourses instantiated across corpora in the form of collocations and semantic prosodies (Baker et al. 2008). As a result, collocation analysis is utilized extensively in the following chapters to identify frequent and less frequent patterns in the representations of anorexia, depression and diabulimia.

Switching our focus to more practical considerations, like generating keywords, the process of obtaining collocates requires a series of decisions be made, for instance regarding the collocational span, choice of statistic and use of a minimum frequency threshold, all of which will ultimately shape the amount and type of words that are flagged as collocates by the computer. Beginning with the collocational span, this refers to the number of words to the left and/or to the right of the search word within which we want to search for candidate collocates. Tighter spans will produce fewer collocates which occur within closer proximity to the node, while wider spans will give more collocates, some of which might not occur in such close proximity to our search word. For this study, we decided to use a span of five words to the left and right of our given search word (otherwise expressed as L5>R5). This is a fairly standard collocational window in corpus linguistic research, as it is generally judged to provide a 'good balance between identifying words that actually do have a relationship with each other (longer spans can throw up unrelated cases) and [gives] enough words to analyse (shorter spans result in fewer collocates)' (Baker et al. 2013: 36). We imposed a minimum frequency threshold of five, which meant that a word had to co-occur within the aforementioned span of our a given search word at least five times throughout the corpus to be considered a candidate collocate.

Candidate collocates were then ranked using the cubed version of the Mutual Information statistic (MI^3). Mutual Information (MI) determines collocation strength by comparing the observed frequency of each collocational pairing against what would be 'expected' based on the relative frequency of each word and the overall size of the corpus. The difference between the observed and expected frequency of co-occurrence is then converted into a score (MI score) which indicates the strength of collocation, with higher scores assigned to stronger collocations (Gablasova et al. 2017). We selected the cubed version of MI for the present study because, in contrast to traditional MI, which tends to emphasize exclusive and unusual word combinations involving low-frequency words (Evert 2008), MI^3 favours collocates which have a higher frequency of co-occurrence and so tend to be 'more established in the discourse' (Brezina et al. 2015: 160). This means that MI^3 is not only useful for corpus-based discourse analysis, but also offers the practical advantage that it helps to control for the presence of typos and non-standard spellings (both of which are common in CMC) by pushing them down the list in favour of more frequent collocates.

For the purposes of the present study, then, collocation helps to take us beyond the solitary linguistic item displayed in keyword lists, offering a logical 'next step' following this inductive procedure. However, even collocation provides only a narrow glimpse at the discourses that can inhere in the use of a keyword. To fully apprehend how keywords and their collocates contribute to discourses, we have to explore them more qualitatively in their wider textual contexts through the prism of concordance.

3.4.3 Concordance

Concordancing essentially provides a way of viewing corpus data that allows us to examine every occurrence of a user-determined word or phrase in context, facilitating close inspection of recurrent patterns of use. To provide an example of what a concordance output typically looks like, Figure 3.1 shows a sample of concordance lines of the word *anorexia*, taken from the *anorexia.net* corpus.

With our node running down the centre of the screen, and a few words of context displayed on either side, the concordance view offers a useful means for spotting patterns that might be less obvious during more linear, left-to-right readings of the data (Sinclair 2003). Concordance lines are displayed in the order in which they occur in the corpus. However, they can also be sorted, for example, alphabetically according to the word either directly preceding or directly following the node, which can be useful for spotting recurring patterns. For a more contextualized view of the data, we can also access each original text (i.e. each forum post) in its entirety, as well as those posts that occur before and after it in that particular thread. Although one of the main advantages of concordance lines is that they provide a view of the textual context surrounding a particular word or phrase, their span can still be relatively narrow relative to the size of the text from which they originate. Context is, as Baker and McEnery (2005: 223) remind us, 'still paramount' in corpus analysis, just as it is in discourse analysis. Thus, it was usually beneficial (and often necessary) for our analysis to go beyond the prism of concordance and explore entire messages, and threads of messages, to explicate the mental health discourses that were signalled by the use of keywords and collocational patterns.

Throughout the foregoing section, we have described the specific corpus procedures that we use to identify and examine the discourses surrounding anorexia, depression and diabulimia in our corpora of support group interactions. Specifically, we combine the above corpus techniques in an approach that involves first engaging with the corpora quantitatively using the about it during or after meals. I told a good friend of mine that I am trying to recover from **anorexia**/bulimia and she said, 'im bulimic/overeater. I told another friend and she told me

I have no rational explanation for this. and experts even say this is a behavioral trait of **anorexia**. At first I thought I was doing it so I'd have some good food ideas for after recovery

allow myself my "alloted" foods and no more than that. Whenever I am stuck in the cycle of **anorexia** I become very obsessed with anything to do with food I dream about food. I look

how else to help yourself, but counselling with the right person - who is hip to the fact that **anorexia** is not age-limited - is a good place to start. Take good care. believe you are

) Others think that's too stigmatizing and limiting. I do believe that you can live well with **anorexia**. That's what I want. With people I love and trust in my life. With the ability to let go.

way to live. Your self-denial and strictness does sound anorexic, and lots of folks view **anorexia** as an addiction. like alcoholism. from which you get to be in recovery all your life

) I live with depression. PTSD, low-self esteem, and body image distortion. And good ol' **anorexia**. which was dormant until my world fell apart in late ***********. when I

. You could be ME!! I have no idea how old you are - I'm sixty-one - and almost died of **anorexia** a few times in my late teens. twenties. and thirties. Then. I seemed to get better.

for someone who has had anorexia and anorexia symptoms for a long time. I had acute **anorexia** in high school over two decades ago. I've been of normal weight for a long time

it's extremely difficult to find diagnostic criteria for someone who has had anorexia and **anorexia** symptoms for a long time. I had acute anorexia in high school over two decades

. because it's extremely difficult to find diagnostic criteria for someone who has had **anorexia** and anorexia symptoms for a long time. I had acute anorexia in high school over

me how bad it was because at times I will forget. I never got married because of my **anorexia**. I lost my teeth (wear dentures now.) It takes me away from God. I can't love or

Hi! This a to look at **anorexia** as what it is - something evil. Whenever you are tempted to see it as a friend.

I cried so much) and someone really heard me. that need to restrict lessened. For me. the **anorexia** was in part a way of validating the fact that I was hurting so much inside. I felt

I would cause my family if I died. was unbearable. Plus spiritually. I knew that dying from **anorexia** was not God's will. I also have seen in IP the power of denial. There were so

reasons for wanting it to go away. A couple years back I was in the middle of a relapse into **anorexia** and I had a realization. the further entrenched I got in my behaviors the stricter my

voice" by stating that one needs to be nourished before therapy can be very productive with **anorexia**. I could be countered by someone else on here who says that I'm full of poop by

. It is not me. Its not me pulling tubes out. Its the anorexia. The real me wants to be free. **Anorexia** is an enemy that speaks to me. Your brain can get so malnourished that u can

are. and cannot think. I am not in commtrol. It is not me. Its not me pulling tubes out. Its the **anorexia**. The real me wants to be free. Anorexia is an enemy that speaks to me. Your brain

Okay so I have been 'flirting' with **anorexia** and starving myself for the past couple of months. I can't take what I have done to

this sheepshly...His reply. very kindly. "I know. and the blood work I've been doing is for **anorexia**. and I can make all the appointments." Why do I tell you this exchange? Because

and I was one of the best. truth is my 'success' was fuelled for almost twenty years by **anorexia** and all the misconceptions about my own power it brought. I'm a physical and

to look into) Throw out your laxatives....big Read up on the medical complications of **anorexia**. Really read them and tell yourself that these things will happen to you. For me.

to begin to be responsible for this as I now have the skills to regain part of my life from **anorexia**. I'm not sure if she was clear about the meaning of her messages. however. and

No reputable. caring. professional counselor would tell someone with an ED. especially **anorexia** that it is okay to cut out foods and that they would only see them when they lose

not a failure at your anorexia you are a success at beating the physical symptoms of your **anorexia**. and you HAVE to keep thinking of it like that or you'll just end up where you

and that means that we are all "supposed to die of anorexia". you are not a failure at your **anorexia**. you are a success at beating the physical symptoms of your anorexia. and you

my obligation to restrict again. i'm anorexic i'm not supposed to eat! i'm supposed to die of **anorexia**. at least that's what my ed tells me. i feel i'm not a good anorexic because i'm

I was twenty. I thought that was what I wanted. I am very. very glad I am still here. I hate **anorexia**. I also love it, or I wouldn't still be actively ill. I hate what it has done to you - a

a unique case in that I am male but also ADD so I don't fit into any of the "boxes" here. Male **Anorexia** Nervosa is almost unheard of here. and especially someone my age. At least

. and a couples therapist. I just find it hard to keep up with my meal plan each day. The **anorexia** voices are strong in my head and at times I feel like I just can't say no. I don't

willing to give you the support you need. Best of luck! don't use it as an excuse to revert to **anorexia**. u'll just feel more sorry for urself if u end up where u were again. I do have an

I just got out of the hospital for IP treatment for my **anorexia**. I am struggling today with restricting and following my meal plan. I feel like the

Figure 3.1 Sample of concordance lines of *anorexia* from the *anorexia.net* corpus.

keywords procedure to identify statistically salient words and themes in the support group messages. Following this, we use collocation to develop a sense of the wider linguistic patterns within which our keywords of interest tend to occur, before finally examining those keywords and collocational patterns more qualitatively to identify recurring mental health discourses with the help of the concordance technique. Although the description above suggests a largely linear movement from keyword analysis to collocation to concordancing, in practice the process of analysis is considerably more variable and involves a consistent movement between these different analytical lenses and between different sections of the data. We would argue that this more iterative approach is more common than the polished descriptions in the methodology sections of some corpus studies would suggest and, furthermore, that it is one that enhances the researcher's immersion in the data itself. Crucially, our approach rests on the interaction between computational (and statistical) measures and human-led, more theory-sensitive interpretation of the data. At this latter stage, we draw on theories and findings relating to mental health from linguistics and other social science disciplines to make sense of the linguistic features that we identify, as well as the discourses we relate them to. Having provided a practical overview of our methodology, in the final section of this chapter we provide a brief review of the corpus-based approach to discourse analysis adopted in this study, highlighting what we perceive to be its major benefits, but also challenges and even limitations.

3.5 Methodological strengths and limitations

The foregoing discussion indicates that the methodological benefits of using corpora in the analysis of discourse are both manifold and reciprocal. From the perspective of carrying out discourse analysis, one of the main attractions of corpus methods is that the computer programs they involve facilitate the interrogation of large volumes of language data that would likely be too great to analyse using purely manual approaches. Indeed, the datasets analysed in this book, though relatively small by corpus linguistics standards, would still be at the very least impractical to analyse by hand. Moreover, by basing insights on larger collections of forum data, as opposed to a handful of interviews for example, the analysis presented over the course of the coming chapters is able to shed light on a likely wider range of mental health discourses, drawn upon by a far greater number of participants. Relatedly, with recourse to large corpora and corpus techniques, our analysis can also better account for such discourses' 'incremental effect' (Baker 2006: 13) in the context of the support groups; that is, the potential for discourses to be subtly established through linguistic patterns that might feature sparingly in one or two forum posts, but which become more significant when considered as part of a wider collection of posts across the support group.

Although frequency-based techniques privilege recurrent and so-called dominant discourses (van Dijk 2008), corpus methods can also be useful for revealing 'minority' discourses that are likely to be less pervasive and which might run contrary to or challenge directly more 'dominant' discourses, ideas or beliefs around mental health. While restricting our analysis to a single or small number of texts runs the risk of over-representing (and thus over-reporting) the status of 'minority' discourses (O'Halloran and Coffin 2004), the examination of larger and more representative corpora can help to produce analyses that are more sensitive to the relative statuses of discourses and how they interact with one another within and across texts (Baker and McEnery 2015). With the option of studying and comparing multiple discourses around anorexia, depression and diabulimia, then, the corpus approach arguably provides a more solid evidence base on which to assess the relative statuses of such discourses in the context of the online support groups represented in our data.

Because they afford researchers the opportunity to analyse large volumes of authentic language data, it has been argued that corpus methods are well suited to the commitment to more objective and empirical approaches to sizeable datasets within the domain of evidence-based health communication research (Adolphs et al. 2004; Brown et al. 2006; Crawford and Brown 2010; Crawford et al. 2014). Evidence-based interventions are those practices which have a basis of 'consistent "scientific evidence" to demonstrate improvements in client outcomes' (Kiyimba 2016: 47–48; Drake et al. 2001). Carter (2013: xiv) argues that as a series of approaches based on examining large amounts of authentic language data, corpus methods are able to provide the kind of substantial quantitative evidence that is accepted within the scientific, evidence-based world of medicine. This consideration is particularly apt in the context of research into mental health, given that the emphasis of therapeutic practice is increasingly placed on evidence-based intervention (Brown and Lloyd 2001). According to O'Reilly and Lester (2016: 10), this drive in evidence-based practice is 'especially important for the field of psychiatry, whereby there is ambiguity regarding the aetiology of conditions and many interventions are based on experience and intuition' (see also: Hopton 2006).

Because they are guided by more objective criteria, such as statistically significant keywords and collocations, corpus-based approaches to discourse analysis can help to allay the influence of our cognitive and social biases on the research process (Baker 2006). This increased objectivity is supported by corpus linguistics' commitment to methodological transparency, which is underpinned by two guiding principles: (i) no systematic bias in the selection of texts included in the corpus (i.e. do not exclude a text because it does not fit a pre-existing argument or theory) and (ii) total accountability (all data gathered must be accounted for) (McEnery and Hardie 2012). Combined, these principles of methodological transparency can help analysts to overcome the methodological criticisms levelled at more traditional forms of (critical) discourse analysis. These arguments have been most stridently articulated by Widdowson (2002, 2004), who asserts that conventional critical discourse analyses are biased by researchers' existing ideological commitments. This political stance, he avers, encourages the pre-analytical conclusion that traces of powerful, subjugating discourses are linguistically encoded within texts. This leads researchers into analysing both those texts and those textual features that suggest such discourses are present, while simultaneously suppressing evidence for contrasting readings. In short, (critical) discourse analyses are claimed to involve the partial selection of linguistic features that are themselves interpreted in a partial fashion, leading to social critiques that have been extrapolated from small amounts of textual data, 'cherry-picked' to support the researcher's own preconceived argument (Toolan 2002; Widdowson 2004). In contrast, by working with a large corpus of data that has been compiled according to transparent criteria and by using more objective computational methods to identify linguistic features for closer scrutiny, corpus linguistics can provide a riposte to the claim that discourse analyses selectively examine only those texts and linguistic features which the analyst preconceives to be relevant.

Nevertheless, although corpus techniques can help to reduce the influence of researcher bias, it is important to acknowledge that this cannot be removed completely from the research process. As the previous sections of this chapter demonstrate, the human user of corpus linguistic techniques is necessarily required to make numerous methodological decisions over the course of a study – including those pertaining to corpus selection/construction and choice of analytical techniques, statistical measures and thresholds – all of which will shape the corpus outputs. Moreover, those outputs, delivered in the form of keywords and collocates, for example, do not provide ends in and of themselves. Computers alone cannot provide explanations for the linguistic patterns in a corpus; it is up to the researcher to interpret the significance of such patterns and explain why they occur. This issue seems to be particularly acute in the case of corpus-aided analyses of discourse, as Jones points out:

> being able to detect 'Discourses' through the computer analysis of corpora requires the creative combination of multiple analytical procedures, and it also necessarily involves a large amount of interpretive work by the analyst. Corpus-assisted discourse analysis is not a science, it is an art, and perhaps the biggest danger of employing it is that the analyst comes to see it as somehow more 'scientific' than the close analysis of texts just because computers and quantification are involved. The computer analysis of corpora does not provide discourse analysts with answers. Rather, it provides them with additional information to make their educated guesses even more educated and their theory building more evidence based.
>
> (Jones 2012: 33–4)

Thus, although corpus linguistics provides explicit procedures for conducting replicable linguistic inquiry, it does not preclude politically motivated interpretation, and its findings remain vulnerable to accusations of analytical bias. Further, human influence is also likely to play a role in the selection of which words and patterns are analysed; the use of keyword and collocation analyses entails that only some lexical items and pairings are isolated for investigation, even though 'every word in a corpus contributes to the discourse' (Teubert 2005: 3). With this in mind, the extent to which the adoption of corpus techniques truly overcomes Widdowson's (2004) accusation of analytical 'cherry-picking' in discourse analysis is debatable at best. Yet, while Widdowson's argument is robust, it is surely also defeatist in its outlook. It is, for instance, difficult to imagine any form of linguistic inquiry that would satisfy Widdowson's criteria for impartiality, since even analysis of short texts will be non-exhaustive and necessarily prioritize some linguistic features over others. The ensuing examination of online mental health disclosures is no exception to this, and the investigation of linguistic features not addressed in the subsequent chapters may indeed augment our findings.

Discounting all analyses on Widdowson's grounds of partiality also neglects the fact that much can be learnt even from partial analysis. Rather than objective, dispassionate analysis, corpus-based discourse analysis offers transparent and replicable analytical procedures, automated processes for identifying salient textual features and quantitative information with which to triangulate qualitative interpretations across large datasets. While ultimately dependent on human interpretation, these methodological processes allow corpus linguists to interrogate large amounts of data and 'arrive at general conclusions in an adequate and convincing way without having to understand them as objective' (Blommaert et al. 2001: 6). This quality constitutes an advantage for any qualitative social science research and makes corpus linguistics a strong methodological foundation for the present study.

By this point, readers might be forgiven for thinking that only discourse analysis stands to benefit from its combination with corpus linguistic methods. However, in reality, both approaches are enhanced by their methodological synthesis, as the introduction of qualitative discourse analysis can bring with it a more theory-sensitive and contextually robust view of the social reality that is captured by and reflected in the corpus. This is important, as greater awareness of the social conditions under which discourses are produced is vital in explaining why discourses are present, as well as for interpreting their contextually embedded functions (Fairclough 1989: 25). It is for this reason that Mautner (2009: 33) argues that although it views language as a social phenomenon, it is through its specific application to a theory-informed method of discourse analysis that corpus linguistics' social concern is foregrounded particularly well. This is a key consideration when debating mental health, as despite the predominance of quantitative evidence, for example in the form of data arising from randomized controlled trials, scholars in the social sciences, and particularly those writing from social constructionist positions, argue increasingly in favour of the value of qualitative evidence for understanding lived experiences of mental distress, as well as for foregrounding the voices of people affected by forms of it. As Lester and O'Reilly argue,

> [m]ental distress has typically been examined from a biomedical or biopsychosocial perspective with quantitative evidence (especially, randomised controlled trials) being favoured. Over the last few decades there has been a growth and greater acceptance of qualitative methods and an increasing emphasis on applied qualitative research, which has been useful in the field of mental health. […] [T]here is a growing acceptance that qualitative approaches offer a great deal for understanding the complexities of mental distress. More specifically, qualitative methodologies, such as conversation and discourse analysis […], have the added benefit of involving a close examination of the realities of individuals diagnosed with mental health conditions and the many interactions that surround their everyday lives.
>
> (Lester and O'Reilly 2016: 23)

By allowing us to move beyond quantitative and aggregate-level data, then, the use of qualitative discourse analysis in the present study can provide richer, deeper insights into the discourses that permeate our corpora of support group interactions, all the while bringing to the fore the voices and perspectives of the individuals disclosing their experiences and understandings of mental health and distress.

Anorexia online

Pro-recovery in the ED community

4.1 Introduction

This chapter considers the linguistic signatures emerging from the *anorexia.net* corpus. In keeping with the rationale set out in the opening chapters, the aim of the analysis in this chapter and those that follow is neither to provide a formal description of the participants' discourse nor to remotely diagnose the nature and extent of the participants' mental health problems. Rather, our intention is to harness flexible corpus methods to illuminate participants' experiences of mental illness without making the analysis subservient to particular linguistic categories or diagnostic criteria. This entails going beyond the simple identification of those frequent lexical items, collocations and grammatical structures that populate the corpora by examining how different speakers use these linguistic signatures to convey their understanding of anorexia, depression and diabulimia, represent themselves as sufferers, and provide accounts of treatment. To this end, this chapter focuses particularly on how the users of *anorexia.net* construe anorexia and its relation to their own self-identities, how they represent their relationship to food and involvement in weight loss practices, and how they view recovery. It is, however, important to situate these representations in the interactional context of the *anorexia.net* forum itself. As such, the final section of this chapter focuses on the discussions across multiple messages and the ways in which competing accounts of anorexia are used by the forum participants to perform interactional goals.

4.2 Establishing themes for analysis

This analysis begins with keywords. A list of keywords derived from the *anorexia. net* corpus provides myriad avenues for possible investigation. While a keyword list presents an objective representation of the most characteristic words in a corpus, how best to approach these keywords and how best to proceed thereafter are decisions that should reflect the aims of the research. A straightforward approach is to use the ranked list as the point of analytical departure, beginning with the highest-ranked keyword on the basis of its statistical salience in the whole corpus, and then proceeding stepwise down the list. However, doing sufficient analytical justice to even a small portion of the total keywords (of which there are, in this instance, ninety) would require more word space than this chapter – and indeed book – would permit.

As a result, corpus-based discourse analyses often group keywords together in order to manage the vast investigative possibilities offered by the keyword list (Baker 2006; Jaworska and Kinloch 2018). The keywords could, for instance, be categorized solely according to linguistic categories to examine, for example, the relative frequency of reflexive pronouns (*yourself*, *myself*) or mental processes (*guess, think, feel*). However, such an approach would likely err towards the formal analysis described above, offering a comprehensive illustration of the textual characteristics of the forum discourse at the expense of duly relating these features to the lives of individuals suffering from anorexia. Our motivation to provide insights into sufferers' experiences of anorexia as well as the linguistic particularities with which such experiences are disclosed necessitates a different approach to the keyword data. This involves recognizing that the keywords are of course not just language data but also the linguistic traces of real individuals reflecting on lived experiences of anorexia and responding to others' accounts of their own experiences.

Accordingly, the majority of the keywords are organized here into thematic categories specific to the experience of anorexia (Table 4.1). These emergent discursive domains represent central areas of meaning that characterize the forum users' discussions of anorexia, offering both a feasible avenue into the corpus (Seale et al. 2006) while also prioritizing topics that the forum participants themselves are discussing. As well as reflecting the forum's discussion of disordered eating, a minority of the keywords are also revealing of stylistic features of mediated advice-giving genres, resulting in categories comprised of hedging devices and words that constitute formulaic expressions of empathy and positive regard, such as 'good luck' and 'keep posting' used at the beginning and end of posts in online support groups (Locher 2013; Pounds et al. 2018). Finally, there is a category containing a selection of high-frequency, multifunctional grammatical words that typify the forum when compared against the Spoken BNC2014.

Table 4.1 Key Thematic and Lexical Categories and Associated Keywords of the *anorexia.net* Corpus, Ranked by Log Ratio (Frequencies in Brackets)

Thematic/lexical category	Associated keywords
Anorexia and illness	*anorexia* (77), *ED* (623), *disorder* (103), *illness* (99), *weight* (265), *issues* (69), *body* (184), *health* (67), *sick* (72), *life* (264), *part* (132), *sense* (64)
Disordered behaviours	*restricting* (71), *behaviours* (123), *thoughts* (145), *scale* (116), *control* (159), *self* (117), *myself* (390), *voice* (115), *telling* (89)
Food and eating	*eating* (367), *meal* (79), *plan* (91), *food* (256), *eat* (352)
Recovery	*recovery* (277), *gain* (64), *treatment* (121), *support* (210), *healthy* (109), *myself* (390), *step* (74), *help* (355), *ways* (66), *deal* (82), *life* (264), *better* (287), *huge* (66), *normal* (72), *change* (108), *able* (154), *honest* (71), *taking* (84), *trying* (178)
Feelings and emotional responses	*ok* (85), *feelings* (145), *fear* (74), *alone* (111), *self* (117), *feeling* (189), *trust* (68), *feel* (667), *glad* (70), *felt* (145), *scared* (72), *feels* (72), *hard* (294), *better* (287), *makes* (125), *hate* (78)
Forum-related	*thread* (93), *post* (142), *luck* (68), *hope* (156), *thanks* (102), *totally* (68), *keep* (259), *anyone* (91), *honest* (71), *today* (148), *understand* (105), *sense* (64), *head* (80)
Healthcare and health professionals	*therapy* (69), *treatment* (121), *doctor* (98), *T* (249), *care* (122), *team* (76), *seeing* (60), *N* (68), *talk* (129)
Hedging	*may* (151), *seem* (60)
Other grammatical	*etc* (97), *am* (1,067), *others* (119), *myself* (390), *its* (148), *yourself* (205), *without* (127), *also* (266), *since* (93), *my* (2,007), *me* (1,465), *sometimes* (125)

Viewed in isolation, many of these keywords do not readily lend themselves to a specific thematic category. *Makes* and *seeing*, for instance, are high-frequency polysemous verbs that are not obviously bound to particular health-related topics. All keywords were therefore viewed in a concordance to identify and refine the category (or categories) to which they belong. In the case of *makes*, collocations of the form *makes me*+[emotion] and *makes me feel*+[emotion] indicated its consistent use by the forum members when disclosing disclosures of the effects of external events on their emotions; in 72 per cent of instances, *seeing* is used to refer to contact with healthcare professionals. These keywords were therefore assigned to the 'Emotions and feelings' and 'Healthcare and health professionals' categories, respectively. Given the multiple denotations of many words and the overlap in the thematic categories, a neat division of all the keywords into mutually exclusive groups is not possible, and several keywords in Table 4.1 appear in more than one category.

Rather than representing flaws in the categorization process, words that span multiple themes offer some preliminary insights into the forum users' representations of their experiences. For example, *self* is used to refer to a range of deleterious and self-injurious practices in which participants report engaging as well as ostensibly more optimistic discussions of 'self esteem' and 'self confidence'. The keyword *honest* appears both in recurrent recommendations for forum members to 'be honest' with healthcare professionals and in the discourse marker 'to be honest' that prefaces evaluative statements. As a result, it appears in both the 'Recovery' category and the group of 'forum related' keywords. Similarly, *myself* collocates with a range of reflexive processes described by the forum contributors but appears most frequently in the phrases *weigh myself* and *make myself* (do something to recover), and hence appears in the 'Disordered behaviours', 'Recovery' and 'Other grammatical' categories. The use of abbreviations such as *T, N* and, less frequently, *pdoc* to refer to specific healthcare professionals (therapist, nutritionist and psychiatrist, respectively) is common on *anorexia.net* and constitutes part of a forum-specific jargon; their meanings appear to be resolved by the forum members from the abbreviation without requiring the orthographically standard form.

These ambiguous keywords aside, the keyword list indicates the discussion of anorexia in terms of weight, food and behavioural characteristics but also in relation to a range of negative emotions, social relations and medical interventions. There are also some surprising absences from the keyword table. In particular, it is noticeable that the word *fat* does not emerge as key from the keyword analysis. While *fat* is used sixty-four times in the corpus – comparable, in terms of raw frequency, to *gain, seeing* and *huge* – it features in only 4.52 per cent of the sampled messages. Despite the fear of becoming fat being a central diagnostic criterion for anorexia (APA 2013), therefore, *fat* constitutes a relatively peripheral aspect of the forum users' discussions of their experiences, especially when compared with *weight*, which features in 16.56 per cent of posts.

The following analysis focuses on keywords related to the first four categories shown in Table 4.1. It begins by examining the ways in which the forum contributors lexicalize anorexia in order to understand how they construe the condition and their relation to it. Thereafter, it considers the ways in which forum participants discuss their eating disordered behaviours, their discussions of eating and the ways in which they refer to dietary meal plans in relation to recovery. In each of these sections, the analysis begins by considering keywords in terms of frequency before moving to consider collocational patterns and their associated meanings in the forum messages. The final analysis section (4.6) takes a more concertedly qualitative approach by considering the ways in which contrasting representations of anorexia function as discursive resources for conducting various facets of online peer support.

4.3 Lexicalizing anorexia

The keywords also highlight that the forum members employ various lexical choices for referring to anorexia itself. Relative to *anorexia* (*log ratio* = 10.00), the lower keyness value for *ED* (*log ratio* = 8.59) is somewhat misleading given that it has a different meaning in the forum – an abbreviation of 'eating disorder' – than its homograph's use as a man's name in the BNC2014. However, *ED* is by far the most frequently used term for referring to anorexia, occurring 623 times in the corpus and across 86 per cent of the sampled threads. In terms of frequency, *ED* is followed distantly by *eating disorder* (seventy-nine occurrences), *anorexia* (seventy-seven occurrences) and *disorder* unmodified by *eating* (fifteen occurrences). Two other abbreviations, *AN* and *ana*, were used to refer to anorexia four times and once, respectively. Given that the corpus data is compiled exclusively from an anorexia forum, the comparatively low frequency of *anorexia* is somewhat surprising. The forum users' clear preference for the shortened form, *ED*, could simply be regarded as typical of the abbreviation of common lexis that characterizes electronic communication (Baron 1998). However, this interpretation overlooks the fact that the forum users also adopt a form denoting the superordinate term 'eating disorder' despite posting messages in a forum module intended specifically for the discussion of anorexia and not bulimia, compulsive overeating or eating disorders more generally. It is also notable that there are no such equivalent abbreviations used for depression and diabulimia in the corpora analysed in Chapters 5 and 6. Consequently, although the available labels for referring to anorexia have some denotational equivalence, it would be ill-considered to presume each label therefore communicates the same meaning (Fleischman 1999). For example, the forum participants' use of a hypernym in place of the more specific *AN* or *ana* orients to anorexia as part of a general category common to all the website users, even though clinical literature indicates clear differences between the various eating disorders (WHO 1992; APA 2013). As with the use of *T*, *N* and *pdoc*, the absence of clarification when the abbreviation *ED* is used in the forum also implies that its members are able to resolve its meaning without difficulty. That is, users have sufficient communal understanding of the meaning of *ED* that they do not need to write 'eating disorder' or 'anorexia' in full.

The preferential use of a noun form, *ED*, to nominalize anorexia also renders incongruous certain articulations of the relationship between the individual writers and their anorexia. For example, verb phrases which posit an attributive relationship between speaker and condition such as 'I'm ED' or 'I'm ED'd' are harder to parse compared with 'I'm anorexic' and remain entirely absent from the corpus. As shall be elaborated below, the avoidance of constructions that directly equate forum users with anorexia is typical in the *anorexia.net* corpus and is sustained through various consistent linguistic choices.

Collocation analysis offers an effective basis through which to understand how forum contributors represent anorexia and different aspects of illness experiences. As Harvey argues, grammatical choices made when discussing diseases 'are important, since preference for a certain form encodes a particular version of events which, in turn, will have consequences for how experiences are constructed and understood' (2012: 361; Fleischman 1999). Indeed, analysing grammatical collocates of *ED* is especially revealing in the *anorexia.net* corpus and, as such, we initially consider them in isolation from lexical collocates before illustrating how its lexical collocates play a complementary and reinforcing role in encoding a particular relationship between sufferer and anorexia.

Collocation analysis using a L5 > R5 word collocational span indicates that *ED* occurs most frequently with *the*. While this is unsurprising given that *the* is the fourth most frequent word in the corpus, *the* is also the strongest collocate of *ED* ($n = 310$, $MI^3 = 20.91$). Indeed, the two words even have a relatively strong association when using the standard mutual information measure ($MI = 4.35$), a calculation that penalizes high-frequency combinations such as those involving function words. *The* occurs overwhelmingly in an L1 position to form *the ED* ($n = 200$). This bigram accounts for 32 per cent of instances of *ED* with 78 per cent of instances of *the ED* constituting a noun phrase for referring to anorexia, rather than forming part of a longer noun phrase such as *the ED ward* or *the ED voice* (see below). The next strongest collocate of *ED*, *an* ($MI^3 = 18.95$), forms the bigram *an ED* on eighty-four occasions, while *my ED* is used sixty-one times in the corpus to refer to anorexia. These frequencies indicate a clear preference for referring to anorexia as *the ED* or *an ED*, using determiners that do not encode grammatical possession and which construe anorexia as a singular, countable entity. As the most frequent determiner+*ED* construction, *the ED* is the generic form used by the forum participants to refer to their condition. Representative examples of this collocation are presented in the paragraph that follows. Except where noted, in these examples and those extracts provided hereafter, data is reproduced with its original spellings and with relevant keywords and collocates highlighted in bold. Square brackets are used to indicate our amendments of the data for clarity and very occasionally for brevity.

1. I know I need it [a nutritionist appointment] because **the ED** always convinces me that I am having plenty ... even though clearly that isn't the case.
2. I feel that most people are really scared of high fat food and it's just another way of **the ED** telling me that I don't have a problem since I eat chocolate (my biggest weakness)....
3. but it went against everything **the ED** tells me. I felt like I was gross and lazy. I didn't think I could stand it and **the ED** was telling me how much I would have to compensate today by not eating much and by walking a lot.
4. I have been doing much better the past few days and **the ED** is getting scared. I reached out for support from my parents when I needed it before and after meals and made it through.
5. But I know that I have to trust my team and those around me rather than **the ED**.
6. But then I get guilt later that I'm a failure even at **the ED**, or when the scale is off by ****-**** pounds!

These examples provide an initial snapshot of the diverse concerns that the forum contributors communicate in the anorexia forum. These include a need for appointments with and trust in healthcare professionals (extracts 1 and 5), discussion of particular foods (ex. 2), engaging in exercise perceived to compensate for eating (ex. 3), entreating parents for help with eating (ex. 4) and the relationship between weight and self-esteem (ex. 6). Throughout these examples, the authors' use of the definite article when nominalizing anorexia aptly reflects their knowledge of a condition with which they have a long-standing familiarity. Nevertheless, it would be possible to substitute *my ED* for *the ED* in each of the above extracts without changing their overall propositional meaning or syntactic structure; each excerpt refers to a singular condition associated with the writer, yet each author refrains from grammatically encoding possession of their eating disorder. Where use of a possessive determiner at least indicates a relationship of ownership between anorexia and the writer, the definite article elides this relationship, leaving it as one of neither identity nor possession. In addition to indicating the authors' familiarity with anorexia, therefore, recurrent use of a definite article in place of a possessive determiner serves to dissociate these sufferers from their condition and objectifies their own anorexia as a discrete entity that exists apart from themselves (Malson et al. 2004). Moreover, the forum members consistently personify this objectified *ED* by attributing to it verbal and emotional processes characteristic of people; *the ED* is variously described as 'convincing' and 'telling' the sufferer things, as well as 'getting scared'.

Although it is striking in its use and frequency throughout the corpus, this grammatical objectification and personification of an illness is by no means unique to the *anorexia.net* support community. On three separate threads on *anorexia.net*, members refer to self-help books by Schaefer (2004, 2009) that personify anorexia from the outset. For example, in the introduction to *Goodbye Ed, Hello Me*, Schaefer writes that she 'learned to think of it [anorexia] as a distinct being with unique thoughts and a personality separate from my own' (2009: 1). Similarly, in a chapter subtitled 'Separating from Ed', Schaefer writes that 'If I could just keep my weight low enough, Ed said that I could be in complete control of my life' (2004: 3). Texts by psychiatric professionals provide comparable examples. Freeman's CBT-based self-help book, *Overcoming Anorexia Nervosa*, for instance, contains personified representations of anorexia including, *inter alia*, 'As the illness takes hold, it seems to squeeze out the ability to think' (2002: 30) and 'it is your AN that has taken over the reins and is controlling you' (2002: 93). Similarly, as noted in Chapter 2, Serpell et al. (1999) describe a therapeutic exercise in which patient with anorexia are encouraged to think about their condition as an external friend and then an enemy. The personification of anorexia as a distinct speaking and acting agent clearly resembles the forum users' messages, with posts to *anorexia.net* displaying intertextual parallels with therapeutic practices that also construe a verbal separation between sufferer and eating disorder and attribute agency to anorexia itself.

More generally, the depiction of diseases as definite, objectified entities is an attested and long-standing characteristic of medical discourse (Nijhof 1998; Warner 1976). Cassell argues that 'the prevailing philosophy of disease that underlies modern medicine [which] sees diseases as objects' (1976: 143), and that this is reflected in the language used by professionals and lay people alike. For example, patients suffering from physical illness frequently refer to their disease or affected body parts as distinct objects using 'it' or 'the'. In grammatically objectifying medical conditions, patients enact a separation from them, indicating that their sense of self cannot be equated with their disease (Mintz 1992). Examples such as extracts 1 to 5, in which the forum users refer to *the ED* rather than *my ED*, provide evidence that this linguistic disconnection features prominently in the forum posts, and hence that the forum members align themselves with a medical discourse of psychopathology. However, Cassell also claims that less physically discrete conditions such as diabetes are seldom objectified and that patients' concept of mental illness are not objectifying at all; 'it would be odd', he argues, 'to hear someone speak of "*the* depression" when speaking about his own depression' (1976: 145). Nevertheless, just such a construction abounds on *anorexia.net* as the forum members reify anorexia through their choice of determiner. The repeated personification of anorexia as 'the ED' therefore represents an extreme version of the medical discourse of diseases as distinct objects in which the condition is construed not only as separate from the individual, but also as being able to perform actions independently. Indeed, as demonstrated below, the use of the objectifying definite article when lexicalizing anorexia is the most frequent among a number of linguistic strategies through which the forum users extricate themselves from the phenomena denoted by *ED*.

This objectification is particularly lucid when members use the same bigram to refer to other individuals' conditions and to anorexia in general:

7. Remember that that pain is the reality of **the ed** and not about recovery. Turning pain into self harm in whatever form is no answer.
8. WHY do we feel this way about ourselves, other than that **the ED** is making us feel this way?
9. this thread is fro myself and anyone else who would like to join to finaly let go off **the ed** by realisin the things we get from it are not woth it and that we have so many other qualities to us that we need to celebrate and remember.
10. I realize now that that was **the ED** talking and ED LIES!!!

These extracts illustrate that the forum participants not only refer to their own condition as an object but also construe the multiple personal conditions of every forum user as the same single entity. For example, the plural pronouns 'we', 'ourselves' and 'us' in extract 8 clearly signify reference to the forum members as a group, yet the author also refers to a singular 'the ED' that is 'making [them] feel this way'. Similarly, extract 9 not only contains three references to plural 'we' but also uses a 'the ed' and an anaphoric 'it' to represent anorexia as a singular condition that affects numerous individuals. Such verbal choices naturalize anorexia by presenting it as an objective phenomenon that exists separately from the group members themselves, even while they refer to its subjective effects upon them (Fleischman 1999). According to Nijhof (1998) and Wenger (1998), this process of linguistic naturalization also serves a social function by solidifying important aspects of social reality and discursively assigning them the status of natural, objective phenomena. This social function in turn helps to explain the predominance of *the ED* on *anorexia.net*; rather than multiple, subjective experiences of anorexia, using 'the ED' allows the forum members to present anorexia as an independent object that all the community members share in common. In lieu of shared personal histories, geographical spaces or offline networks, this representation of anorexia provides a means of expressing shared experience with other forum members and hence a discursive foundation upon which the online community and its interactions are based.

In contrast to *the ED*, instances of *my ED* ($n = 71$) emphasize the idiosyncratic nature of anorexia and are far less frequent in the *anorexia.net* corpus, accounting for only 11.4 per cent of L1 collocates of *ED* in the corpus and appearing in 5.49 per cent of the sampled posts. In keeping with Koller and Mautner's (2004) claim that different representations of phenomena coalesce around alternative collocation patterns, examples of *my ED* indicate that it is used in a different verbal context to *the ED*:

11. I have been recovering from **my ed** for about a year now. When I did have **my ed**, I used to be the SAME exact way! I used to make sure everyone around me ate, but I never did.

12. During the many years I had **my ED** I ate very little, but what I did eat was alot of candy, sweets, etc.

13. I really don't want **my ED** back but am torn because I always think I was happier when I was thinner.

14. I have been honest with my caregivers (I was already receiving services for trauma) about **my ED** from the beginning, and it has brought nothing but good. I encourage you to give T all the information and honesty you can.

15. My friend doesnt know about **my ED**, and im having a hard time telling her. Hopefully Ill be able to attend the party still, Ill have to get my Ts opinion.

16. I am doing some work with my therapist at the moment to look at how I can accept that **my ED** will always be a 'part' of me rather than having this ideal that I will be 'cured' and free. We are going to do a piece of work to help me to gain a bit of weight (which I am terrified of) and to work on accepting me for me ED and all - as it is part of me afterall.

Compared with *the ED*, the instances of *my ED* above illustrate the preference for this bigram among forum members who report either having recovered from anorexia or being in the latter stages of professional treatment and recovery. This is indicated by the use of spatial deixis – 'I really don't want my ED back' (ex. 13) – and the use of past-tense verbs forms – 'When I did have my ed', 'During the many years I had my ED' (ex. 11 and 12) – to signal past experience of anorexia. Similarly, extract 14 illustrates the use of present perfect tense – 'I have been honest with my caregivers' – which functions to signal that her positive experience of treatment is relevant to her advice-giving in the present (Crystal 1995). Such reference to recovery or foregoing experience of treatment frequently prefaces the provision of advice to another forum member. As such, we see *my ED* occurring when forum members are describing their experiences of recovery as a means of representing themselves as legitimate advice givers in an online context where authority may not otherwise be apparent (Potter 1996; Morrow 2006).

The use of *my ED* by those in recovery creates an interesting contrast to instances of *the ED*. While the possessive determiner makes explicit the speakers' association with their condition, the wider messages in which this collocation is situated frequently involve expressions of temporal and psychological distance from anorexia. Instances of *my ED* that encode possession of anorexia by those currently suffering from it, such as extract 15, constitute 39 per cent of instances of *my ED* and represent a minority discourse on the forum (Baker 2006). There appears, therefore, to be a trade-off between temporal distance from anorexia and the degree of grammatical possession which the community members convey towards it; forum members using *the ED* describe immediate and ongoing struggles with an eating disorder that is distanced from them grammatically. Conversely, forum users who represent themselves as recovered or in remission from anorexia are more likely to construe it as something they have possessed – *my ED*. In accordance with this, present tense existential clauses such as 'I'm anorexic', which collapse the relationship between speaker and condition to one of identity, occur only twice in the entire corpus. Example 16 illustrates that this is a distinction to which the forum users themselves are indeed sensitive, with the author claiming that part of her ongoing psychological treatment involves accepting anorexia as a part of her identity.

Having considered the grammatical collocates of *ED*, the analysis that follows focuses on its lexical collocates and draws upon Orpin's (2005) 'semantic profiling' approach, in which a node word's meanings and associations are evinced from its strongest lexical collocates. Table 4.2 presents the twenty strongest lexical collocates of *ED*.

These lexical collocates reinforce much of the picture of *ED* evinced in the foregoing discussion; contributors repeatedly state that anorexia 'makes' them do certain things and those who are experiencing relief from the condition talk

Table 4.2 Top Twenty Lexical Collocates of *ED*,
Ranked by MI³

Rank	Collocate	Frequency	MI³
1	*voice*	43	17.40
2	*OCD*	24	15.91
3	*tells*	10	13.68
4	*back*	24	13.57
5	*about*	36	13.13
6	*talking*	12	12.89
7	*without*	15	12.70
8	*telling*	14	12.59
9	*voices*	8	12.57
10	*life*	19	12.18
11	*go*	19	12.17
12	*unit*	5	12.12
13	*group*	8	12.01
14	*really*	22	12.00
15	*now*	19	11.91
16	*thoughts*	13	11.89
17	*makes*	12	11.75
18	*things*	18	11.73
19	*part*	12	11.67
20	*specialist*	5	11.61

about 'go[ing] back' to it, seemingly construing anorexia as a former romantic partner. Even more noticeable, however, is that five of the strongest twenty collocates of *ED* – as well as the weaker collocates *saying* (*MI³* = 11.29) and *says* (*MI³* = 9.64) – refer to speech acts or voices (*voice, tells, telling, talking, voices*). These collocations signal that verbal processes are a consistent feature of how anorexia is represented on *anorexia.net*. Concordances of these collocates and their related lemmas reveal a usage not dissimilar to *the ED*, in which verbal and material processes associated with human agents are attributed to the disorder itself (see also ex. 1–3 and 10 above):

17. We all have a ME and an ED. Sometimes the ED **voice talks** and sometimes the REAL **voice talks**. Your you **voice** is **telling** the ED that you can have bread and eat normally and it's okay to eat and gain some needed weight.

18. Now the goal is to not let my emotions dictate my eating this weekend because, as I have written before, Saturdays are often the hardest day for me and therefore the day when the ED **voice** screams 'RESTRICT' and 'EXERCISE' the most.

19. There was one line in my friend's email reply that sounded just like what the ED **voices** yell at me - 'Please don't do this to the ministry.'
20. I now have to combat the ED **voices telling** me 'I had a good week, so I am all done now.' Ovbiously that isn't the case but it is very convincing.
21. the ed **voice tells** me to do so many things that are against my core values as a person.
22. Ed **makes** me think horrible things about myself; it takes away my self-esteem.

As the above corpus excerpts clearly demonstrate, the lexical collocates of *ED* are frequently verbs whose agency is attributed to anorexia or a personification of anorexia as the *ED voice* or *ED voices*. Reference to anorexia as a 'voice' occurs in 19 per cent of the sampled message threads, confirming recent research that points towards the experience of a distinct voice or persona as a salient aspect of the condition (Williams et al. 2016). For the members of *anorexia.net*, the voice of anorexia is clearly presented as a powerful presence; where *ED* or the *ED voice* is the agent of a transitive process, the forum users present themselves as the direct object who is either spoken to (ex. 19–21) or made to 'think horrible things' (ex. 22) by their condition. Extract 20 describes the 'ED voices' as 'convincing' while the authors of extracts 18 and 19 use the reporting verbs 'screams' and 'yell' and capitalized reported speech to convey the intensity of the 'ED voice'. The replication of direct speech in these extracts also represents the 'ED voice' as communicating specific content about the forum members' diets, exercise and personal lives rather than an urge towards eating disordered behaviour more generally.

These excerpts go beyond euphemisms such as 'losing my mind' that are typically used to articulate a perceived loss of mental control (Allan & Burridge 2006) and explicitly attribute responsibility for chaotic thoughts to an external speaking agent; as the author of extract 17 states, 'We all have a ME and an ED'. This personification of anorexia as an independent entity provides a powerful means for the forum users to convey the experience of living with a condition that is felt to be beyond their control. Rather than them 'living with' or 'suffering from' anorexia, 'the ED' and the 'ED voice' are construed as directly acting upon the sufferer, hectoring them and commanding them to act in ways that are incompatible with their views of themselves (ex. 21; Tierney and Fox 2010; Williams and Reid 2010).

Having illustrated the agency that forum members readily ascribe to anorexia, we are in a better position to re-evaluate the 'odd' discursive separation they enact between themselves and their eating disorder through the expression *the ED* (Cassell 1976: 145). In the face of a condition that is described as deceptive, manipulative and beyond their control, it is unsurprising that the forum users typically avoid encoding grammatical ownership of anorexia; if anything, it is construed as something that possesses and controls them. Indeed, the agency that forum members attribute to anorexia in the foregoing extracts stands in stark contrast to descriptions of anorexia as 'self-engendered weight loss' (Beumont 2002: 162) and public perceptions of anorexia as a condition that is deliberately maintained by the sufferer (Stewart et al. 2006); for the majority of the forum members, the 'ED' that is responsible for their starvation is not an entity that they would identify as their 'self'. Seen in this light, the recurrent personification of anorexia as either 'the ED' or the 'ED voice' can be seen to play an important role in accounting for the sufferers' anorexia and hence managing the stigma associated with the condition. That is, by recurrently personifying anorexia as a grammatical actor that 'lies', 'convinces' and makes them 'feel' certain ways, the forum users displace agency for the onset and continuation of their anorexia onto an external entity. In so doing, they are also able to elide the fact that it is reproduced through their emotions and behaviours, including their verbal behaviours when discussing anorexia itself (Giordano 2005 and see Wenger 1998: 58). Congruently, by presenting themselves as (grammatically and semantically) passive, the forum users evince a limited capacity to resolve their situation or accurately perceive its gravity. In short, anorexia is presented as an entity that happens to them, rather than a condition over which they have any control or responsibility (Eivors et al. 2003; Hardin 2003; Galasiński 2008); as one forum member writes: 'being ill with an eating disorder is to my mind the OPPOSITE of being in control of your self'.

4.4 Anorexic behaviours, restriction and control

Having highlighted the emphasis on impaired personal agency that attends the forum users' representation of anorexia, the following analysis continues with these issues in examining members' accounts of a central anorexic practice, dietary control. The recurrent discussion of aspects of bodily regulation is indicated by the keywords *behaviours* and *restricting*, as well as by references to exercising (*exercise, exercising, exercised, exercised*), which occur in 5.46 per cent of the sampled messages. Of these, the most frequent and salient keyword is *behaviours* (*n* = 123, *log ratio* = 9.82).[1] In keeping with the use of

ED to refer to anorexia, *behaviours* constitutes a superordinate, euphemistic term that signifies a range of different activities. However, unlike *ED*, *behaviours* constitutes an example of vague language that is required by the strictures of the forum; *anorexia.net*'s forum rules proscribe specific descriptions of purging, laxative use and intensive exercise regimes that are typical of individuals with anorexia. The use of a hypernym therefore serves as a response to this while also functioning to amalgamate various unspecified activities and represent them as equally constitutive of the same condition. In parallel with *the ED*, then, the use of *behaviours* is suggestive of an attempt to establish a sense of common experience among forum users who likely engage in a variety of different disordered practices. Extended concordances of *behaviours* from the corpus allow a more detailed illustration of its use in the forum:

23. to go cold turkey on **behaviours** wouldnt work for me because i still feel i need them. but through therapy i'm slowly learning to replace them with new better coping skills. if they were taken from me on day one i would have had nothing to replace them with. in IP i've had this done to me and the minute i left **behaviours** were worse than ever.

24. I talked about that on another post, there is the underlying issues theory and the habit theory, yet you can stop, I stopped **behaviours** for several years.

25. There is no way that outside of IP I would have dealt with those feelings without resorting to **behaviours**.

26. I think for the **behaviours** to truly disappear, the thoughts have to change. Usually the **behaviours** are symptoms of an emotional state. Butttt i also think that as the **behaviours** get better, thoughts will start to become more positive.

27. It is true that thoughts precede feelings and **behaviours**, and this is the premise behind CBT.

28. What we want to know is how you are feeling, what you are using your **behaviours** to say, avoid, etc.

As with *ED*, the excerpts above illustrate a naturalizing discourse in which 'behaviours' are presented as a homogenous category and are grammatically dissociated from their enactors. For instance, in extract 23, the zero-article nominalized form 'behaviours' in 'the minute i left behaviours were worse than ever' backgrounds any sense of agency and does not clearly attribute the deleterious anorexic practices to the author (van Leeuwen 2008). Compared with feasible alternatives such as 'I engaged in anorexic behaviours more acutely than ever' or 'I behaved in a more disordered way than ever' (invented examples), extract 23 uses an existential process to state that 'behaviours' were simply 'worse' of their own accord. In addition, the verbal metaphor of going 'cold turkey' (ex. 23) and claim that 'behaviours' may be part of a 'habit' (ex. 24) frame 'behaviours' using the language of drug use and addiction, a metaphor that medicalizes *behaviours* by construing them in relation to physical and psychological dependency. The implication that 'behaviours' are a form of irresistible, self-destructive dependence clearly coheres with the obfuscation of agency behind 'behaviours' in extract 23. In each case, the way *behaviours* are presented in the messages masks the volition of the sufferer who engages in them.

Extracts 25 to 27 also illustrate a perceived relationship between anorexic *behaviours* and two of its lexical collocates, *thoughts* and *feelings*, in which mental distress precedes carrying out *behaviours*. This association is a consistent feature of the semantic profile (Orpin 2005) of *behaviours* in the forum messages (see Table 4.3). Accordant with the forum users' description of the *ED voice* as undermining their self-esteem and convincing them to act in undesired ways, the forum users ascribe precedence to their mental states and present these as precipitating particular behaviours.

Table 4.3 Top Twenty Collocates of *Behaviours*, Ranked by MI[3]

Rank	Collocate	Frequency	MI[3]
1	*the*	51	16.71
2	*to*	55	16.3
3	*and*	46	16.07
4	*thoughts*	14	15.94
5	*your*	25	15.45
6	*using*	7	14.76
7	*my*	25	14.65
8	*of*	21	13.77
9	*change*	7	13.36
10	*I*	29	13.29
11	*ED*	12	13.16
12	*rules*	5	13.1
13	*feelings*	7	12.94
14	*stop*	6	12.8
15	*on*	12	12.67
16	*without*	6	12.46
17	*for*	13	12.27
18	*so*	12	12.07
19	*through*	6	12.06
20	*these*	5	11.89

Forum messages associating 'behaviours' with 'thoughts' and 'feelings' support previous findings that anorexic practices function as mechanisms for managing stress and negative affect (Woolrich et al. 2006; Skårderud 2007a). For the forum members, presenting 'behaviours' as a means to 'deal with' otherwise intolerable feelings also offers an implicit justification for their use as a last resort rather than a wholly irrational practice. The author of extract 23, for example, constructs an extreme case formulation (Pomerantz 1986) of resorting to 'worse than ever' behaviours 'the minute' she finished in-patient treatment that left her with no other coping skills. Similarly, in extract 25, the author thematizes a categorical adverbial clause – 'there is no way' – to exclude the possibility of managing certain feelings without resorting to behaviours. Where food restriction, exercise and compulsive weighing can seem specious to people who do not have anorexia, these extreme case formulations imbue the forum users' behaviours with an 'internal logic' that legitimizes their actions as a reasonable means of controlling psychological distress (Harris 2000).

Alongside the discussion of *behaviours* using the language of addiction, construing *behaviours* as a consequence of difficult emotions underscores the psychological discourse explicit in the above references to 'CBT' and an 'underlying issues theory', in which conscious and unconscious thoughts are believed to give rise to external actions. As extract 28 demonstrates, members use this psychological model to engage in a proto-professional therapy with other users (de Swaan 1990), attempting to identify psychological motivations behind their behaviour and framing anorexia within a model of individual psychodynamics.

Following *thoughts*, the strongest lexical collocate of *behaviours* is *using* (table 4.3). Whereas behaviour is ordinarily considered a relatively unconscious process, collocations between *behaviours* and *using* represent *behaviours* as deliberate actions. Examples of these collocations are provided below, along with clauses in which *behaviours* are the object of other material processes.

29. No one would pretend that recovery is easy - in fact life will get much harder without **using** ed **behaviours** to cope.
30. Taking a step back into **using behaviours** just keeps the cycle going and you dependent on them [to manage 'feelings'].
31. Maybe you can use the fact that you are under strict doctor's orders NOT to engage in **behaviours** to alleviate some of the guilt and talk down your urges.

32.   i had tons of bad,scared thoughts but focused on eating and forced
      myself to trust her. as thougths raced through my head and as i wanted
      to practice **behaviours** i hung on tight to her words and the words of my
      new t.

The processes 'using', 'engage' and 'practice' in extracts 29 to 32 represent anorexic
behaviours as actions that individuals intentionally engage in. Indeed, 'using' or
engaging in 'behaviours' is presented in extracts 28 to 31 as a purposeful way of
performing other activities; 'behaviours' are used 'to cope', 'to say something',
to deal with 'feelings' and 'to alleviate some of the guilt'. The purposeful 'use'
of behaviours to achieve a desired end provides a relatively rare example in
which forum members ascribe goal-oriented material processes to themselves
and each other. This representation of agency stands in marked contrast to the
discussion of *the ED* and *ED voice* above, in which users are often in the role of a
grammatical patient affected by the actions of their eating disorder. Concordant
with this agency are several corresponding claims that activities such as food
restriction result in feelings of emotional self-control, for example:

33.   I feel as if **restricting** is making me more powerful. Like when i **restrict**, i
      am in **control** and when i eat, i lose all **control** [...].
34.   my **eating** can get so out of **control**, so on the days that I can totally **restrict**
      it, and like go the whole day without **eating** anything, I feel so IN **control**.

Extracts 23 to 34 provide varying depictions of *restricting* and *behaviours* as both
sources of control and accountable actions arising from intolerable thoughts
and feelings (Giordano 2005). The conflation of restriction and self-control
exemplified in excerpts 33 and 34 exists in tension with other users who claim
that 'behaviours' such as food restriction arise in reaction to their uncontrollable
'thoughts', 'feelings' and 'ED voice' and serve only to entrench sufferers in their
condition. For example, responding to extracts 33 and 34, one user states 'EDs take
all the control so we dont have it even tho we have the illusion of control'. While
acknowledging her addressees' perceptions of self-control, this forum member
counters the foregoing posts by recasting dietary restriction as a divestment of
control to anorexia itself; 'behaviours' are reconfigured as 'a form of control that is
itself out of control' (Malson 1998: 145) and ultimately initiated by anorexia itself.

This position is reiterated in instances of collocations between *behaviours*
and its statistically significant collocates *change* and *stop* (see Table 4.3), which
offer examples in which forum members discuss ways to escape the cycle of
uncontrollable thoughts and subsequent disordered behaviour (included here

are also instances of comparable collocations of *behaviours* with *changing* noted during manual reading of the corpus):

35.   The only way I have really ever been able to **change** my **behaviours** was by telling someone who could actually **stop** me.

36.   I would have to be forced to **change** my **behaviours** externally. I don't see myself **changing behaviours** through any sort of will power of my own, without something big happening, just like you said.

37.   I knew I couldn't deal with the thoughts until I had the support of a T to work through them, so I didn't **change** the **behaviours**.

38.   I should add though, that as I was **changing** my **behaviours** I was receiving therapy and learning healthy ways to cope with my feelings.

39.   It's possible to control and **stop** the **behaviours**, but it may never be possible to fully control our thoughts or feelings.

40.   Yes but how are many of us able to step in and **stop** the **behaviours** when we realize the damage they've caused......and then the illness slides back years later when we think we're recovered?

In keeping with the participants' alleged powerlessness over their thoughts and actions, collocations of *behaviours* with *change* or *stop* co-occur with reference to users' incapacity to alter their behaviour by themselves. Accordingly, throughout these excerpts, the forum members express a dependence on external help, professional interventions and therapists as means of altering 'behaviours' (ex. 35–38). Tellingly, the forum users do not clearly state that therapy prevents their psychological distress, but rather that it offers alternative coping mechanisms with which to manage their difficult emotions (Eivors et al. 2003). This results in a sceptical position among some forum users regarding the potential for complete recovery from anorexia; as the author of extract 39 states, although anorexic behaviours may stop, the 'thoughts or feelings' that encourage dietary restriction may not. Similarly, the author of excerpt 40 raises the possibility that anorexia 'slides back' of its volition even after someone has been able to 'stop the behaviours'.

    For those forum members who have not yet received psychotherapy sessions, the perceived prospect of discontinuing anorexic behaviours and the expected concomitant loss of control is viewed with acute trepidation. Directly following the content of excerpt 36, the same forum user states:

41.   I would not, at this point, make the choice to relinquish control to someone else in an 'IP' setting, or any other way. I would really, really not be ok if I did that. I would rather not live than give up control, at the state I'm in right now.

The notion that treatment necessarily entails surrendering control to healthcare professionals is also apparent in messages from sufferers who are currently undergoing therapy or have done so in the past (see ex. 23). These users identify discontinuing 'behaviours' and the identity shift involved in recovery as primary obstacles to improving health:

42.   I went to treatment for six weeks. It was by far the hardest thing I've ever done. [...] I had to completely surrender control.

43.   today i had one of those days... i miss my ed soooo much [...]right now i don't know who i am, i don't even know what i like. i don't have an identity. at least before i began the recovery process i was [username] the anorexic, i had something, i had a way to cope. now all i have is this huge confussion.

Extract 43 demonstrates the additional difficulties for those forum users who define themselves through their anorexia or attendant body shape. In marked contrast to the use of *the ED* discussed above, in which anorexia is represented as a separate entity, the author of extract 43 identifies directly with her condition, realizing this through an intensive copular construction, 'I was [...] the anorexic'. In this case, recovery not only requires discontinuing her anorexic coping mechanisms but also necessitates erasing the basis of one's self-identity, resulting in a 'huge confussion' (i.e. 'confusion'). This additional fear of identity loss illustrates a double bind involved in treatment and recovery from anorexia. That is, the identity crisis precipitated by giving up their anorexic identity creates further anxiety towards recovery; for those who identify directly with their anorexia, 'the possibility of "recovery" collapses into the threat of self-annihilation' (Malson et al. 2004: 483; Tierney and Fox 2010). Further, the increased food consumption prescribed during in-patient care for anorexia requires patients to do the opposite of their habituated mechanism for dealing with stress by eating more at a time when they feel compelled to restrict their diets. Indeed, the posts above reiterate the finding that fear of accepting professional dietary control and stopping anorexic practices is a key factor in dropout from anorexic treatment services (Eivors et al. 2003).

Analysis of the use of *behaviours* and its collocates reveals several contrasting perspectives on the performance of anorexic practices. The articulation of 'behaviours' as a nominalization permits potentially unfavourable activities to be presented without reference to a performing agent (ex. 23 and 26) and, like *the ED*, as disconnected from the individual who enacts them. Attempts to obscure responsibility for 'behaviours' or present them within extreme case scenarios signify efforts by some users to discursively legitimize their conduct. Other users, however, explicitly encode their agency in using, practising or engaging in 'behaviours' in order to 'cope' and 'alleviate … guilt'. In conjunction with its collocates *thoughts* and *feelings*, *behaviours* are therefore presented as a psychological resource for controlling emotions and external stressors. When contextualized against the earlier discussion of the *ED voice*, however, the motivation to 'use' or 'engage' in 'behaviours' can be seen to stem from 'ED' thoughts that are experienced as uncontrollable; as one forum member writes: 'the voice makes me second guess myself and I feel badly about myself or triggered and think engaging in behaviours will help'. The eventual powerlessness over their own disordered behaviour is reiterated in the users' discussion of attempts to *change* or *stop* their disordered actions, which are consistently associated with receipt of external assistance. Despite this, forum members remain ambivalent about dispensing with their behaviours during professional treatment and perceive this as a direct threat to their 'control' and, in some cases, personal identity.

4.5 *Eating, eating more* and *not eating*

Fear of eating and weight gain is a primary source of personal distress and interpersonal conflict for people with anorexia. It is therefore unsurprising that words relating to food consumption pervade the corpus, and particularly the keywords *food* (n = 256, *log ratio* = 2.64), *eat* (n = 352, *log ratio* = 2.52) and *eating* (n = 367, *log ratio* = 4.21), which appears 258 times outside of the bigrams *eating disorder(s)*. The strongest lexical collocate of *eat* is *more* (n = 27, MI^3 = 14.13), which occurs fourteen times as the bigram *eat more* and in the three-word cluster *to eat more* six times. Examining how sufferers discuss the process of increasing the amount of food they eat offers insight into their experiences of resisting their anorexic 'behaviours':

44. the part of me that so desperately wants to feel safe keeps saying that I need to just **eat more** of what I am already doing.
45. i need **to eat more** i know i do but i find it hard to go against the ed but i dont want to be in hospital.
46. unfortunately, when you need to gain weight, you have **to eat more** than normal, which results in a lot more guilt.
47. I am scared **to eat more** and ***********% of my meal plan, not only because of having to eat the food and gain the weight; but also because of the major fear of feeling my hidden, buried feelings.

48. everyone says trust your body so i think sometimes i am full ill stop
     now, they tell me over eating is bad yet i try not over eat and they tell me
     eat more that i have to eat what they tell me but yet trust myself im am
     sooooooooooo confused ahhhhh!

49. I am really scared right now. I am confused about what to do. I really do
     want **to eat more.**

50. I feel ashamed of it [anorexia] and think people will judge me/ question
     how it will impact on my children, try to make me **eat more** without
     really understanding that it wont help.

In contrast to 'using behaviours', eating and particularly eating 'more' could be
expected to signify a step towards recovery from anorexia. Nevertheless, the
forum members associate attempts to 'eat more' with negative emotions such
as feeling guilty (ex. 46) and being 'scared' and 'confused' (ex. 47–9). Eating
more is construed as both a source of distress in itself (ex. 46) and associated
with 'feeling my hidden, buried feelings' (ex. 47), reiterating a direct association
between physical satiation and overwhelming emotions (Skårderud 2007a).
Forum users' attitudes towards eating more are also conveyed by the phrasal
structures in which *eat more* occurs. For instance, the excerpts above include
two examples of 'need to eat more' (ex. 44–5) and 'have to eat more' (ex. 46) as
well as 'tell me [to] eat more' (ex. 48) and 'make me eat more' (ex. 50). These
are recurrent phrasal patterns around *eat*, with *need to [just] eat* and *have to
[learn to] eat* being used eight and thirteen times, respectively, throughout the
corpus. Both of these modal structures construe eating as an act of obligation
and necessity. The obligation to 'eat more' appears both as a means to meet a
specific goal, for example 'when you need to gain weight' (ex. 46), and as an
unspecified end in itself (ex. 44–5). Despite the necessity associated with eating
in these examples, extract 50 includes a claim that being made to eat more 'wont
help' her anorexia, which implies that simply increasing food intake is not, for
this user at least, a route to recovery.

Ambivalence towards increasing eating is further conveyed through
representations of internal conflicts around eating. In extract 44, the author
refers to a 'part of' her that tells her to keep eating, invoking a division of
the self into conflicting parts that echoes the internal battle with the ED voice
presented above. Similarly, in extract 45, the author's chain of disjunctive
clauses situates eating in a conflict between what she knows, going 'against
the ed' and the overarching threat of hospitalization. A similar pattern of
contrasting coordinate clauses characterizes extract 48, in which indirect

speech representation is used to show inconsistencies in professional advice to simultaneously trust her body, not overeat and to eat what she is told. In both cases, clause coordination using 'but' or 'yet' demonstrates conflicts with 'the ED' and between competing desires and professional instructions. The layering of these disjunctive clauses construes trying to 'eat more' as a conflicting process that reflect the ambivalence of anorexic individuals towards recovery. This pattern is also reproduced throughout the forum, with *but* being a significant and strong collocate of *eat* ($n = 30$, $MI^3 = 13.03$), typically occurring after *to eat* as forum members situate eating against a countervailing motivation to restrict.

The strong collocations of both *eating* and *eat* with *feel* ($MI^3 = 11.86$ and 11.13, respectively) provide further evidence that food consumption is semantically associated with emotional states in the corpus. Examinations of the concordances in which these collocations feature provide a clear insight into the forum users' attitudes towards food consumption:

51. *to be able to accept the attention of being made love to
    *to be able to **eat** and not **feel** ashamed and criminal afterwards
    *to be able to go out and not feel ashamed of myself

52. I really cant **eat** anything at this party, its a fondue party, and I really dont **feel** at all comftorable **eating** that, and i dont think it would match with my MP.

53. I do this all the time - especially when I'm homesick or **feel** ashamed of **eating**. It's just a spiral into feeling worse.

54. I really try not to **feel** guilty when I **eat** what I've alloted for that's my idea of GOOD and what I've craved....

55. I've stayed the same [weight] since I saw [my therapist] last, which actually made me **feel** okay about **eating** 'normally' tonight and having wine with my dinner, as she actually recommends for me.

The discussions of feelings in these posts associate the process of eating with powerful negative emotions of shame, guilt and discomfort. These collocations establish a strongly negative semantic prosody (Louw 1993) for *eat* and *eating* within the forum messages, creating a semantic overlap between food consumption and difficult psychological states. Repeated references to feelings of criminality, guilt and shame (ex. 51, 53 and 54) also associate eating with morality and represent food consumption as an act of moral transgression that must be balanced against the physical inclination to eat.

Extract 55 diverges from the prevailing negative semantic prosody of *eating*, with the author claiming to 'feel okay' about consuming food. However, this description is grammatically subordinate to stating that she has maintained her weight and the adverbial 'actually' with which it is prefaced denotes that this is in clear contrast to expectations (Carter and McCarthy 2006). Feeling 'okay' about eating is therefore presented as both unexpected and brought about – 'made' – by neither gaining nor losing weight. Consequently, despite representing a more positive experience of eating, this post reiterates the relationship between weight, food consumption and emotional responses that is characteristic of the other excerpts in this section. As with the foregoing analysis of *behaviours*, then, these posts exemplify a psychodynamic relationship between weight, eating and affect in which food is strongly invested with emotional significance and bound up in a system of deliberately regulating distressing emotions (Malson 2008). This representation of *eating* contrasts sharply with the second range of attitudes, prevalent in some users' explanations of choosing to 'not eat':

56. I am terrible at relaxing and whenever I try, the ED comes in full force, telling me that I am lazy, gross, unproductive and therefore should **not eat** or feel okay about myself.

57. How do I make myself **eat** when the anorexic voices in my head are screaming at me that I don't deserve to **eat**?

58. this [exam disappointment] kinda caused me to **not eat** and restrict because I told myself I didn't deserve food if I didn't get good grades...

59. I was relying on ed now because I was mad that I got a ninety-five on a test. I wanted to get higher then that. And at my school that grade is only a B....which makes me very upset. [...]And when I consider that a failing grade then I wanted to punish myself..by **not eating** and resorting back to the eating disorder.

Rather than construing restriction as a strategy for managing emotions, these extracts represent restriction as a means of self-castigation for individuals who believe they are somehow unworthy of eating. These messages therefore reverse the beliefs above, in which food is viewed as a source of guilt, and instead portray eating as a reward that the authors feel they do not deserve (Skårderud 2007a). There are several drivers of food restriction represented in these excerpts: in extracts 56 to 58, responsibility for 'not eating' is located outside the individual with 'the ED' or 'anorexic voices' telling the authors they do not deserve to eat, and with the exam results that 'caused' the author of extract 58 to 'not eat'. However, later in the same thread of messages the author of extract 58 claims that she 'wanted to punish herself' (ex. 59), representing food restriction as a volitional, reflexive process driven by her perception of exam failure. Over the course of this thread, then, this forum member comes to implicate herself in her dietary restriction, seeing it as a deliberate punishment. While only accounting for a small minority of the uses of *eating*, these two posts provide a more uncompromising representation of anorexia as a form of self-punishment for perceived personality flaws. This is a severe view of the condition and one that offers little hope of recovery for the individual. Accordingly, the author of extracts 58 and 59 elaborates her feelings later in the same thread, saying 'No..i guess I never want to get better. I deserve to be miserable and unhappy'.

Analysis of keywords related to eating consistently reiterates the relationship between restricting the body and restricting difficult emotions found in the concordances for *behaviours* and *restricting*. This association is linguistically realized through the consistent co-occurrences of *eating* with references to negative emotions, particularly guilt and shame (ex. 46, 54 and 53) and *eating* is also described as a precursor to other 'hidden, buried feelings' (ex. 47). The prospect of 'eating more' is regarded ambivalently; the repeated clusters *need to eat* and *have to eat* construe eating as an obligation or necessity, while the messages involving *eat more* reveal a picture of conflicting impulses from parts of the self, 'the ED' and the prospect of coercive treatments. However, other collocations indicate a greater degree of variation. The bigram *not eat*, in particular, serves as a reference point for a contrasting account of disordered eating, with some members presenting not eating as a self-inflicted punishment. While the relationship between dietary restriction and emotional regulation is a well-established facet of anorexia, these messages indicate the danger of making generalizations regarding anorexic individuals' relationships with food and the degree of volition they claim over restricting their diets. Instead, the corpus data testifies to the complex and frequently contradictory experience of anorexia (Rich 2006), with sufferers' accounts varying both in relation to each other and over the course of an individual's posts in a single message thread (Rimmon-Kenan 2002).

4.5.1 Meal plans: A guide to recovery?

A further significant facet of the forum members' discussion of eating was the concept of meal plans, which are referred to in over a third of the discussion threads. Meal plans are professionally or personally designed diets intended to allow patients with anorexia to safely gain weight while responding to their attendant anxieties towards eating. In keeping with the community's pervasive use of initialisms to refer to healthcare professionals and practices, *meal plan* ($n = 50$) is often abbreviated to *mp* or plural *mps* (thirty occurrences), along with less frequent use of *food plan* (three occurrences) and the compound *mealplan* (four occurrences). Examples of these are presented below.

60. just know it can and will get better if you take the steps to follow a good **meal plan**.
61. So I can't go IP but I CAN start making more of a step forward. I mapped out a good **meal plan** that is healthy so I can follow it and I have set aside some time for each day to do something that I enjoy despite all the chaos with my classes.
62. I feel really proud of myself for yesterday and last night. I really did not want to follow-through on my **meal plan** […]. But I then remembered all the things I want for myself and my life […]
63. I am following my **mealplan** very well and have made great strides in letting go of rigid rules and ED behaviours.
64. I may still be able to pay for a few visits to get a good **meal plan**. I am actually willing to try a real **meal plan** which is real progress.
65. Well done for sticking to your **meal plan** and for being honest and open with your t.
66. If there is a specific reason you don't want to go [to hospital], keep reminding yourself that if you don't stick to your **mp**, you will eventually have to go.
67. I started worrying about what i had eaten (even though saturday was also over my 'normal/safe' **meal plan** i didn't let it affect sunday and ended up eating over my 'normal' **meal plan** anyway) […]. Big mistake there and i shouldn't be surprised. The past few days have been pretty terrible **MP** wise and i have definitely noticed a difference.

As the extracts indicate, a number of the forum users construe meal plans as integral to the amelioration of their anorexia. This meaning is conveyed through the repeated presentation of meal plans using a conceptual metaphor of movement (Lakoff and Johnson 1980). More specifically, recurrent references to users' 'steps' (ex. 60 and 61) and 'strides' forward (ex. 63), having 'mapped out' a meal plan (ex. 61) and making 'progress' (ex. 64) each instantiate the conceptual metaphor RECOVERY IS A JOURNEY. This metaphorical mapping is also realized by the keywords *taking* ($n = 84$, *log ratio* = 1.53) and *step* ($n = 74$, *log ratio* = 3.60) – as in 'taking a step' – and *ways* ($n = 66$, *log ratio* = 2.74), which are common across the users' discussions of treatment and recovery. While this conceptual metaphor is by no means exclusive to the *anorexia.net* community (Atanasova 2018), the metaphor is extended here by construing meal plans as a guide or facilitator of the journey towards recovery. This can be seen through collocations of *meal plan/mp* and *follow/following* (*n* =10 and see ex. 60–3), with meal plan adherence conceptualized as moving forward in accordance with a set route. Along with being 'followed', extracts 65 and 66 present meal plans as the object of the process 'stick to' (a phrasal verb that itself collocates with references to dietary choices and both literal and metaphorical journeys in the general spoken English of the BNC2014). Accordingly, meal plans are represented as the basis for praise when adhered to (ex. 62 and 65) and negative consequences when contravened (ex. 66 and 67). As a result, alongside this largely positive depiction there is also an alternative representation of meal plans as a source of potential anxiety:

68. i thought i had it under control again. and my dinner was items on my **MP** so i didnt feel too guilty.
69. Do try to stick to your **meal plan** during the day - regular eating means that you are less likely to guilt-eat and then get those voices nagging you about it.
70. I am telling my therapist and my nutritionist that I am struggling and not being compliant with my **MP**.
71. When I felt self-conscious about eating around others but wanted to maintain fidelity to my **MP**, I would pack a meal bar or two that fit my meal requirements and have veggies (salad) with others.
72. If I ate more than the allotted calories I would be breaking the rules.
73. I know you are right, but I feel like if I ate something, I would start to break down. I like sticking to my **mp** exactly.

As noted in the analysis of *eat* and *eating* above, co-occurring references to 'guilt' (ex. 68–9), 'complian[ce]' (ex. 70) and 'fidelity' (ex. 71) frame eating as an act of moral significance, obligation and potential transgression. Eating in excess of a meal plan is equated with 'breaking the rules' (ex. 72) and as leading to conflict with internal 'voices' and personal collapse (ex. 69 and 73). Non-prescribed eating is also associated with negative consequences, regardless of whether this eating is defined technically in terms of 'calories' or vaguely as simply eating 'something' (ex. 72 and 73). By framing meal plans in this way, the *anorexia.net* participants present meal plans as both nutritional guidelines and a moral index that frames unplanned food consumption as a culpable violation. Consequently, although they are discursively realized as a guide towards recovery, the dietary rules of a meal plan also constitute another avenue for investing eating with moral and emotional significance. In this regard, professionally sanctioned meal plans reiterate the practices of the condition they seek to alleviate by codifying dietary control and providing an index of permissible and transgressive eating (Malson 2008). Investigation of the use of the community members' discourses of *meal plan* therefore illustrates a further double bind for an individual with anorexia, in which a fundamental component of an individual's physical recovery from anorexia – regulated food consumption – perpetuates the debilitating emotional investment in eating that characterizes the condition.

4.6 ED as a discursive resource

The foregoing sections have illustrated the ways in which forum members represent anorexia, their disordered eating practices, relationships with food and conceptions of professional dietary plans. While some findings from these sections – such as sufferers' association of eating with emotional regulation – are acknowledged aspects of anorexia, the ways in which the forum users consistently personify anorexia as a speaking entity, anchored around the bigrams *the ED* and the *ED voice*, is less well elucidated in existing research. This representation is, however, pervasive across the forum and used by sufferers to convey the experience of having their thoughts and actions compromised by anorexia. The predominance of this representation indicates that these accounts of suffering from anorexia emphasize experiences of psychological difficulty rather than, for example, the unfeasible expectations of female bodies that characterize sociocultural interpretations of anorexia. This partiality is itself revealing; Hardin argues that presenting anorexia as primarily an issue of psychopathology 'reinforces the idea that anorexia nervosa is a legitimate disorder deserving treatment' (2003: 213) and aligns with the prevailing medical and psychological contention that a person with anorexia is 'cognitively impaired' (Boughtwood and Halse 2010: 85). As noted above, aligning with a psychological understanding of anorexia also has implications for how the participants represent their responsibility for anorexia and their own actions. As Hardin further claims, 'having anorexia nervosa surface as the result of psychological problems […] implies a lack of awareness/conscious choice and, paradoxically, unaccountability' (2003: 213). The forum's prevailing construal of anorexia, therefore, is also one which legitimizes users' experience as one of illness and mitigates their responsibility for a stigmatized condition by presenting the individual as a passive victim of the disease.

In order to fully apprehend the implications of the discourse of *the ED*, this section considers instances in which this dominant discourse is challenged by alternative accounts of anorexia. Perhaps unusually for corpus linguistic research, our analysis here is motivated by the claim from conversation analysis that interactional norms are sharply revealed by the ways in which discourse participants seek to account for their transgression (Schegloff 1968; Hutchby and Wooffitt 1998). In keeping with this theoretical motivation, our analysis here seeks to illustrate the ways in which the *the ED* discourse is strategically deployed during forum interactions rather than within isolated, decontextualized messages. This involves focusing on *the ED* and *ED voice* not simply as frequent collocations but rather as discursive resources with which *anorexia.net* users can achieve communicative goals (Willig 2000: 548); our interest is in identifying the 'interactional work' *the ED* is 'being used to do' (Hutchby and Wooffitt 1998: 99). Methodologically, this necessitates a departure from an analysis driven by keywords, collocates and concordance lines. Indeed, in challenging the community's prevailing *ED* discourse, messages such as that reproduced in extract 74 below use different lexical choices to present anorexia than those discussed previously in this chapter. As a result, they are less easy to identify using processes such as automated collocation analysis that highlight statistically typical word combinations. Although infrequent in the corpus as a whole, then, these moments of tension between forum members demonstrate both efforts to define anorexia as a fundamentally biomedical problem and the contextual utility of *the ED* for managing interactional difficulties.

The most overt challenge to the concept of anorexia as a medical or psychological pathology takes place in a message thread titled 'Anorexia – illness or choice?'. The thread consists of twenty-eight messages posted over three days, of which four messages are written by the user who began the thread. As the thread title anticipates, the content of the first message interrogates the notion that anorexia is an involuntary illness:

74. I don't think it is fair to say that anorexia is an illness, because didn't I CHOOSE to do this to myself? It is not a physical sickness. There is nothing wrong with my body that is making me starve, or take laxatives, or puke, or exercise. You can't take an eating disorder blood test. It is not physical. So, that leaves it to personal responsibility, right? Or wrong? I would like to hear your opinions.

This forum user's argument that anorexia is not an illness is here premised on excluding anorexia from the category of 'physical sickness'. She claims that her engagement in anorexic practices does not arise from any bodily necessity and that anorexia is not amenable to medical assessments such as a 'blood test'. The absence of a physical problem, she argues, entails 'personal responsibility' for anorexia and the conclusion that anorexia is a self-inflicted choice rather than an 'illness'.

Responses in this thread largely attempt to refute the first post, re-categorizing anorexia as a medical condition and therefore also not a matter of individual choice. Six separate responses compare anorexia to cancer or autoimmune diseases, using this comparison to imply that anorexia is just as involuntary. Similarly, the first reply opens with, 'No one chooses to have an ED. It chooses you'. This universalized claim bluntly denies individual agency in the onset of anorexia. Like many of the excerpts reproduced above, this response attributes agency to a singular 'ED' in choosing 'you' to be affected. Similarly, throughout the course of the message thread, the acts of convincing, taking over, taking control, sliding back and coming upon the sufferer are attributed to anorexia, presenting the onset and maintenance of anorexia as determined independently by the disease itself. In other messages, forum users draw explicitly on biomedical discourse in order to categorize anorexia as a physical illness:

75. People who are chemically balanced and don't have ED's know these are not normal behaviours and don't do them.
76. We don't choose our genes (many people with ED's are pre-dispositioned because of heredity) and brain chemistry.

Rather than implying that anorexia is only analogous to cancer, these excerpts go further in claiming a fundamentally organic basis for eating disorders. In extract 75, practising anorexic behaviours is presented as determined by whether or not the individual is 'chemically balanced', construing mental illness as a hormonal or neurochemical instability. A few messages later (ex. 76), the same author denies that anorexia is a choice by repeating her explanation of anorexia in terms of 'brain chemistry' and genetic disposition. Both factors further situate anorexia beyond individual choice, presenting it in terms of unalterable chemicals or determined by hereditary factors predating the individual's birth (Easter 2012). From a rhetorical perspective, these aetiological explanations are also highly effective in this forum context; challenging the claim that anorexia is the result of genetic disposition or neurological imbalance would require a forum member to show that their disorder exists despite a lack of genetic or neurological markers. Given that anorexia-specific genetic and neurological tests are scarcely available to lay individuals, forum members have little evidence with which to undermine such biomedical explanations and this account remains unchallenged throughout the rest of the thread. The potency of the forum users' prevailing representation of anorexia therefore rests both in its utility to insulate sufferers against attributions of personal responsibility and to subsume subjective explanations of anorexia within an overriding narrative of biological determinism.

This rhetorically powerful biomedical discourse also cues a specific role for the individual sufferer who wishes to recover; having defined anorexia as a biomedical malfunction, the author of extracts 75 and 76 then describes recovery in terms of contact with healthcare professionals and receipt of clinical treatments:

77.   You get better by doing what anyone else with an illness does. You get help. If you have an ED you see a T, pdoc, and N. [...] You get medication for the chemical imbalances, and you get a MP to help you get your eating stabilized. If you had an autoimmune disease or cancer you'd do the same thing.

This post constitutes a turning point for the discussion in this thread and it is worth considering its construction in some detail. As well as describing recovery, this post is noticeable for the way in which its author establishes a sense of expertise on treating anorexia. She presents stages of recovery in a chronological, stepwise fashion that moves from the vague 'get help' to detailing specific aspects of recovery – 'stabilized' eating and chemical balance – and their clinical precursors. She also demonstrates knowledge of various professional roles involved in eating disorder treatment – expressed using the forum's abbreviated sociolect 'T, pdoc, and N' – and implies an awareness of physiology through reference to 'the chemical imbalances'. Finally, the validity of medical treatment for anorexia is underscored by the claim that the addressee would themselves follow the same course of action for cancer or an autoimmune condition. In parallel with the presentation of anorexia as an individualized biological pathology, the author depicts recovery as a categorical, single course of action involving the adjustment to the individual's organic state through professional interventions. This post presents a paradigmatic example of medicalization (Conrad 1992), in which a problem is defined in biomedical terms and the sufferer is obliged to take up a 'sick role' (Parsons 1951) by seeking professional intervention. Accordingly, later in this post, the author claims that patients with anorexia are accountable for '[n]ot the illness, but the way you handle it'; even though anorexia is construed as biologically predetermined and beyond individual choice, this user claims that sufferers are nevertheless responsible for acting as patients by seeking and adhering to professional help. In broadly aligning behind a biomedical understanding of anorexia, the forum's dominant *ED* discourse is therefore significant in categorizing sufferers as patients and establishing a normative responsibility to seek professional help.

Online anorexia support is sharply divided between pro-recovery support and pro-anorexia networks that promote – or at least tolerate – disordered practices. As part of the former category, the explicit rules of *anorexia.net* oblige users to support one another towards medical recovery and proscribe messages that present anorexia as a positive or admirable condition. This means that messages that disclose members' reluctance towards recovery (a common experience among sufferers) or which explain the benefits they get from their anorexia risk contravening the forum's pro-recovery foundation. At the same time, overtly criticizing another member who says that they are struggling to come round to the prospect of recovery could well be seen as unsupportive. The result is a particular set of interactional expectations in which both anti-recovery messages and the responses that criticize them infringe upon the forum rules. Although there are relatively few instances in the corpus, it is notable that forum members repeatedly draw on the concept of 'the ED' as a controlling, speaking subject in order to negotiate interpersonal disagreements while still adhering to these interactional constraints. This occurs, for example, during responses to a forum member who describes his ambivalence towards gaining weight:

78.   I am now out of Hospital and am in a much better position both physically and mentally, although i am still finding it difficult to deal with the prospect of increasing my weight to a healthy level.[…] I still have the feeling as though i'm eating too much and getting too big, but i am getting help from my T for this.

In challenging this post, the next message in this thread draws on the discourse of 'ED' as a personified speaker:

79.   I'm glad to hear that you're out of hospital and are able to do what you need to do to keep out of hospital.

It's really hard to eat and gain weight. I think the large majority of us feel that we're eating too much and getting to big, but that's your ED talking.

Before challenging the addressee's feelings about being overweight, the author of this post prefaces her message with numerous features that function to mitigate explicit disagreement. For instance, the author expresses positive regard for the addressee's situation, acknowledges the difficulty of gaining weight and includes the addressee within 'the large majority of us' who experience doubt about weight gain. Rather than directly contradicting the addressee's fears, his concerns about weight gain are then attributed to his 'ED', thereby undermining their legitimacy on the basis that they are another instance of anorexia 'talking'. A similar strategy is employed in a separate thread, which is opened by a forum member describing a conversation with her psychotherapist, who has stated that she does not believe they should have a further appointment and that the forum member does not need to continue to gain weight, even if she is below the 'target weight' set at the outset of her therapy. While many responses criticize the therapist's purported suggestions, another forum member offers a more challenging position:

80.   You've got some really good support from the [others] but I just want to insert a gentle [nudge] here.

I'm not saying what your T said was necessarily right... but it does sound as though you have misinterpreted and distorted her message. As you say - you know she cares... and she wouldn't want to hurt you. But the way you've reported the conversation suggests she's both nasty, incompetent and downright dangerous!

I would imagine that's not the case... but that your ED mind has twisted her message in way that says your T doesn't believe you are 'sick enough'. This seems to be the message you are reading into many situations at the moment... and I just wondered to what extent this has happened here. […] I am suggesting that you look at any distortions and ED inspired misinterpretations that are going on here.

As with excerpt 79, extract 80 displays features of a heavily attenuated disagreement. The author acknowledges the contributions of the other users and provides a metapragmatic description of her response as a 'gentle' nudge. She also offers a partial agreement with the addressee's post ('I'm not saying what your T said was necessarily right') before claiming that it may also constitute a 'distorted' version of the therapist's recommendations. In accounting for this position, the author employs a representation of a distinct 'ED mind' that has caused the addressee to misinterpret the psychotherapist's message. While articulated somewhat differently to instances of 'the ED', this representation of anorexia as a separate part of the addressee is employed for the same interactional purpose of indirectly disagreeing with another forum member by categorizing her post as the product of 'ED inspired misinterpretations'. In a similar exchange in a different thread, another forum member who talks positively about the 'willpower' required for weight loss is told that their message 'is totally ed using your voice to express itself' (see Hunt and Harvey 2015). In each case, messages that express disagreement with professional recommendations or which discuss weight loss favourably are attributed to their authors' 'ED voice' or 'ED mind'.

When situated in these sequences of disagreement between members of the forum, therefore, we can see that the community's prevailing personification of anorexia serves a further two related functions; first, it enables forum members to redirect criticism from another member onto their anorexia and thereby preserve a position that is supportive of the individual sufferer. That is, by displacing overt criticism from the individual onto anorexia, group participants are able to delegitimize problematic messages without directly challenging another forum user or the supportive ethos of the wider group; the focus of criticism becomes their 'ED' rather than the community member themselves. Secondly, attributing authorship of an anti-recovery post to another user's 'ED' simultaneously neutralizes their culpability for writing a message that contravenes the forum's rules. Both a user's doubts about recovery and the message in which they have expressed them are attributed to 'the ED', allowing the forum member to avoid personal censure from the forum moderators or other group members.

As argued elsewhere (Hunt and Harvey 2015), it is hard not to see parallels between the use of 'ED' in the messages above and texts outside the corpus in which diagnostic labels are employed as a resource with which medical professionals enact control over patients. For example, in Malson et al.'s (2004) interviews with people whose eating disorders had led to hospitalization, anorexic in-patients claim that doctors see their resistance to treatment as part of their 'illness talking':

> Julie: Everything I say he [a doctor] just like, he laughs at you kind of thing. Like you say one thing and he just laughs and he goes: Oh it's not her talking, it's the illness.

> Jessica: And they don't listen to you at all. And whenever you try and like rationalize anything with them they just, you get told to sort of shut up because it's the illness talking [...]

(Malson et al. 2004: 482)

The similarities between the *anorexia.net* corpus and Malson et al.'s (2004) research are striking here. Both cases illustrate the way scepticism towards professional treatment or recovery from anorexia are categorized as signs of the psychological distortion that characterizes anorexia itself. In Malson et al.'s study, attributing agency to a patient's eating disorder affords clinicians a means to subvert their arguments during points of interpersonal conflict and thereby subject patients to professional interventions. In the *anorexia.net* forum, the discursive resource of the 'ED talking' emerges as part of an interactional repertoire (Wenger 1998) for meeting the local interactional goals of managing conflicting points of view, discrediting messages that problematize recovery, and mitigating direct criticism of others. In doing so, this representation of anorexia is also consistently used to foster compliance with professional interventions, even at the expense of expressing doubts about professional practice or articulating personal difficulties with recovery.

4.7 Chapter summary

The analysis of the *anorexia.net* corpus has illustrated that the forum members consistently recount experiences of disordered eating in which anorexia is personified in the role of an autonomous entity. This quantitatively dominant notion of *the ED* is largely concordant with medical discourses of diseases as discrete entities and the focus on cognitive impairment in psychological research on anorexia. When used by the forum members, these concepts linguistically distance the individual from their condition, emphasize its impact upon their thinking and actions and, in doing so, mitigate their agency and responsibility for a stigmatized illness. A similar mitigation of responsibility is apparent in the users' discussions of their experiences of 'behaviours', in which forum members frequently present their participation in anorexia-related practices either as part of an irresistible addiction or as happening of its own accord. Presenting anorexia as a single entity also serves to anchor the online community, homogenizing users' respective pathologies into a common condition. In addition, the analysis in this section has demonstrated that the forum members explicitly defend the view that anorexia is a medical condition that should be treated through submission to professional therapy. Forum members also medicalize expressions of resistance to professional treatments by pathologizing others' posts as examples of anorexia 'talking'. Consequently, as well as a means for forum members to populate their own narratives of suffering from anorexia, the notion of the 'ED voice' facilitates delicate interactional processes such as tactful disagreement that are specific to *anorexia.net*'s local rules and vital to its existence as a mutual self-help community. At the same time, these instances of disagreement in the forum illustrate a collective intolerance of alternative conceptions of anorexia, including those that present anorexia as a choice and imply a more empowered role for the sufferer in their own recovery (Giordano 2005; Sandaunet 2008b). While the community is intended for 'pro-recovery' support, the dominant representation of anorexia articulated within the forum therefore also functions to preclude alternative understandings and limit the expression of concerns that are meaningful for particular individuals.

The arguments presented above contend that the frequency of particular lexical items and collocations in the corpus can be attributed in part to their polyvalence in the context of the *anorexia.net* community. That is, the frequency of *the ED* far outweighs that of *my ED* because, among other functions, the former construction enables users to establish a sense of shared experience in this online context. In addition, the final section of analysis highlights the salience of *anorexia.net*'s community rules, which provide criteria for acceptable contributions to the message boards. A pro-recovery group that discourages explicit confrontation between members provides fertile conditions for its members to develop alternative approaches to disagreement, such as categorizing problematic posts as their author's 'ED talking'. Along with the qualitative analysis required to identify these functions, explanations of the discourse patterns within the *anorexia.net* corpus are enriched by considering their relation to anorexia-related texts outside the corpus itself. The parallels between the forum users' posts and psychotherapy practices that encourage 'externalizing' anorexia serve as a reminder that the content of the *anorexia. net* corpus is situated in relation to other discourse contexts which arise from members' embedment in online and offline milieus. Systematically charting these intertextual parallels could be achieved through the compilation of a multimodal corpus capturing the forum members' discourse, their encounters with clinicians and peers, and representations of eating disorders in other on- and offline media. The ecological perspective provided by such a corpus would provide further insights into the intersecting contexts and discourses that constitute and reflect anorexic individuals' experiences. An alternative – and more feasible – point of comparison for the *anorexia.net* corpus is the online interactions of speakers with contrasting mental health difficulties, which are examined in the following chapters.

Being 'sick of it'

Depression, medication and self-injurious behaviour

5.1 Introduction

This chapter presents the analysis of the *depression.net* corpus. The analysis proceeds in a comparable way to the previous chapter, beginning with a thematic grouping of the corpus's keywords before analysing how a number of these keywords are used in the forum's messages. This contextualized analysis centres on frequent collocations as a means of considering discourses around depression and to illuminate the meanings of keywords. In an inevitably limited space, it is only feasible to address a sample of the keywords and the broader topics to which they relate. The subsequent analysis focuses on the discursive representation of depression, antidepressant medication, and suicide and self-harm, which are salient topics of discussion for the support group participants and, as established in Chapter 2, also prevalent in existing research on depression. In parallel with Chapter 4, the concept of medicalization (see also Chapter 1, Section 1.2) provides a useful theoretical lens through which to interpret the ways in which users of the forum discuss depression. Indeed, the ensuing analysis reveals that the forum users linguistically represent depression in a manner that frequently coheres with an objectifying medical model of depression and use this concept to construct a separation between themselves, their condition and its medical management.

5.2 Establishing themes for analysis

A thematically and lexically grouped list of the corpus's keywords is presented in Table 5.1. The keywords reflect an impressionistic summary of the forum messages, encompassing depression, suicide, medication, lexis related to emotions and mental experiences, and contact with health services. As well as

Table 5.1 Key Thematic and Lexical Categories and Associated Keywords of the *depression.net* Corpus, Ranked by Log Ratio (Frequencies in Brackets)

Thematic/lexical category	Associated keywords
Depression, mental disorder and depressed behaviours	*depression* (429), *thoughts* (136), *depressed* (124), *problems* (122), *sleep* (145), *bed* (145), *work* (491)
Feelings and emotional responses	*feeling* (334), *feel* (763), *worse* (123), *felt* (104), *hard* (194), *better* (292), *understand* (118)
Healthcare services	*GP* (239), *therapy* (141), *appointment* (109), *doctor* (116)
Hedging	*may* (155), *seem* (103), *seems* (108)
Medication	*meds* (175), *medication* (145), *taking* (163)
Narratives	*2* (120), *life* (275), *since* (129), *although* (94), *sometimes* (180), *moment* (137), *weeks* (151), *work* (491), *days* (169), *told* (184), *until* (108), *times* (120), *today* (156)
Online advice-giving exchanges	*hugs* (118), *hi* (123), *hope* (259), *post* (111), *thanks* (126), *care* (118), *anyone* (133), *try* (293), *moment* (137), *will* (609), *understand* (118), *talk* (147), *best* (127)
Self-harm and suicide	*self* (114), *life* (275)
Self-management and recovery	*support* (134), *help* (422), *try* (293), *hard* (194), *better* (292), *talk* (147)
Other grammatical	*OK* (101), *its* (439), *myself* (377), *am* (670), *yourself* (155), *my* (2,206), *me* (1,691), *also* (237), *being* (305), *someone* (209)

discussing professional treatments for depression, the thematic group we have labelled 'self-management and recovery' encapsulates lexical items with which the forum users commonly describe their efforts to improve their well-being and to accrue different means of social and emotional support.

In addition to the thematic categories that broadly orient to the content of the forum members' discussions of their experiences of depression, there are several related groups of keywords that index the register and communicative genres that characterize interactions on the forum. Much like the keywords in the *anorexia.net* data, a group of high-frequency grammatical words indicates the highly (inter) personal nature of the forum interactions (*my, me, myself, yourself*) as well as the discussion of events in the present tense (*am* and *its*, a large proportion of which are non-standard versions of the contraction *it's*). The keywords *may, seem* and *seems* also point towards a preponderance of low epistemic modality in the forum when compared to interactions in the Spoken BNC2014, with these hedging strategies characterizing forum members' assessments of their own and others' behaviour.

More substantially, the thematic group labelled 'Online advice-giving exchanges' in Table 5.1 contains words that constitute phrasal expressions used in the exchange of advice between forum members. These phrasal structures include an initial salutation, 'hi everyone', as well as a grammatical cluster used to pose a question to the forum as a whole, 'does anyone else …?', a common feature of advice-seeking posts. This group also includes keywords that typify response messages that include expressions of empathy – 'I understand how you feel about' – as well as advice in the form of an imperative beginning with 'try'. The inclusion of *moment* in this category reflects the tendency for contributors to offer a general formulation of other users' narratives – 'You are having a tough time at the moment' – in such a way as to present the addressee's difficulties as temporary and, perhaps, therefore more surmountable (though the phrase 'at the moment' also features repeatedly in contributors' accounts of their own problems). These advice-giving messages frequently close with expressions of positive regard, such as 'I wish you all the best', or offers of further help, such as 'I'm here for you if you ever want to talk'.

Closely related to this group of keywords is a second category that indexes the frequent posting of personal narratives to the forum. Keywords in this category are used in the temporal ordering of events and descriptions of their duration and frequency (*2, weeks, days, life, sometimes*) as well as the verb *told*, with which users mark the reporting of indirect speech in the social interactions they narrate. These keywords also indicate that users seek help in relation to events that have recently taken place or are ongoing at the time of posting (*today, moment*) as well as events happening repeatedly (*times*). Finally, the keyword *although* features in concessive structures repeatedly included in users' narratives, such as 'This last week side effects have been less terrible, although I still sometimes find myself crying for no reason' and 'during this time I have managed to keep working, although not always as well as I would like'. Appearing after a main clause, these dependent concessive clauses are used to introduce an often-negative caveat that either qualifies the author's account of a more positive event or marks their experience as diverging from an expected norm. Accounting for their experiences in this fashion enables support group members to convey a sense of rationality and to signal their awareness of social norms, even while highlighting their own departure from them. Although the *depression.net* corpus contains descriptions of severe and long-term mental distress, therefore, its authors reliably narrate these experiences in such a way as to present themselves as reasonable and conscious of social expectations that they feel unable to fulfil.

As with the previous chapter, there are a number of overlaps between the categories and their constituent keywords; keywords related to antidepressant medication also imply forum users' contact with healthcare services, for example. However, we have grouped them separately here, as although antidepressant medication is sometimes discussed in relation to the healthcare professionals who prescribe them, antidepressant 'meds' are more commonly the focus of message threads that do not refer to professional healthcare. In addition, the keyword *depressed* occupies an ambiguous position between a non-medical description of an emotional state and something more closely synonymous with the diagnostic label 'depression'. The ambiguity between lay and medical meanings of *depression* and *depressed* in the keyword groups is paradigmatic of the following analysis which, beginning with *depression*, identifies the negotiation of depression's medical status as a recurrent feature of the forum interaction.

5.3 Verbalizing a relationship to depression

This corpus contains an expectedly high frequency of words relating to depression itself, with the most common being *depression* (n = 433, *log ratio* = 8.18) and *depressed* (n = 126, *log ratio* = 5.85). In what follows, we analyse the specific lexicogrammatical patterns and associated meanings in which these terms occur, focusing particularly on the grammatical relations between the forum users and their condition.

5.3.1 Having and suffering from *depression*

The respective frequencies of *depression* and *depressed* demonstrate the forum users' preference for referring to their condition with a noun rather than as a description of their feelings such as 'I feel depressed'. This preference aligns with the more pervasive tendency for Western cultures to construe illnesses as nouns rather than adjectives, not least in medical discourse (Warner 1976). When using this nominal form, the forum users present *depression* in a number of recurrent multiword constructions that encode grammatical relations between depression and themselves, as summarized in Table 5.2.

With the exception of *diagnosed with depression* (see Section 5.3.2), the forum users' attributions of depression coalesce into two main types. First, they refer to depression using attributive clauses such as *have had depression*; secondly,

Table 5.2 Recurrent Multiword Constructions
Involving *Depression*

Phrase	Frequency
suffering from depression	12
diagnosed with depression	10
have had depression/ I've had depression	8
suffered from depression	6
suffered with depression	4
suffer from depression	4
suffered depression	3
I had depression	3
suffered on and off with depression	2
suffering with depression	2

they refer to depression as an element of the behavioural process *suffer*. Both of these types of constructions are relatively unmarked ways of describing illness or psychological discomfort; Halliday (2002) observes that it is quite common to refer to 'having' some form of pain, and *depression* collocates strongly to the right of *suffer* (MI^3 = 12.08), *suffering* (MI^3 = 12.71) and *suffered* (MI^3 = 13.63) in the Spoken BNC2014.[1] Nevertheless, it is worth considering the specific grammatical relations each phrase encodes and the insights this grammatical analysis can offer into the experience of illness (Harvey 2012). In particular, those clauses involving *HAVE+depression* express a relational process in which depression is a possession attributed to the sufferer. In contrast, those involving *SUFFER+from/ with depression* present the forum user as a participant in a behavioural process – 'to suffer' – that is 'intermediate between material and mental processes' (Halliday 1994: 128). In *SUFFER+from depression* constructions, depression plays a causal element in the clause. That is, depression represents the reason that the speaker's suffering takes place. In the less frequent *SUFFER+with depression* clauses, depression occupies an accompaniment role, implying some form of joint participation in the suffering by the writer/speaker and the disease (Halliday 1994: 140–1).

Common to both the relational and behavioural processes is an implied separation between the individual and their condition. In *HAVE+depression* and *SUFFER+from+depression*, depression is externalized and either possessed by or inflicted on the speaker rather than being a change in their own internal processes (Warner 1976; Fleischman 1999). Dowrick (2004: 192) also argues that *HAVE+depression* and *SUFFER+from/with depression* constructions objectify depression as a definite medical entity and, when they occur without modifiers such as 'postnatal' or 'severe', homogenize the numerous medical and personal forms of depression. Of these two phrasal patterns, the forum users more frequently choose to refer to their condition as a process of 'suffering from' rather than 'having' depression. That is, the forum participants more frequently express their relationship with depression in terms of suffering rather than possessing depression, and simultaneously attribute this suffering to an externalized cause. Galasiński (2008) argues that verbally separating depression and the self is a recurrent feature of depression narratives, and one that enables individuals to mitigate the stigma of illness by avoiding explicitly identifying themselves with their condition. Since the forum participants demonstrate a stronger preference for those constructions that convey greater distance between themselves and depression, Galasiński's reading would also seem a plausible explanation for these linguistic choices on *depression.net*.

When examined in the forum messages, there are also contextual difference in the use of *SUFFER+with* and *SUFFER+from* phrases (as with the previous chapter, examples that exemplify wider trends across numerous concordances are presented throughout this chapter):

1. Hi there my name is [username] and i am from the uk. I have been **suffering with depression** for a number of years now and started to treat my condition around 6 months ago.

2. I'm new to all this so sorry if I should have put it elsewhere.
    I have **suffered with depression** on and off for about 8 years now, and the latest episode (starting about 2 years ago) has been my most severe so far […]. My question really is for those who have **suffered with depression** and then become preganant.

3. One of my college professors was epileptic and he also **suffered with depression**....that is until his doctors got the epilepsy under control. Apparently the worry about having a seizure, especially in public, was a big part of his depression.

4. Hi im new to this site
    ive **suffered on and off with depression** for 20 years ..... have just been diagnosed with it again after 2and half years being fine.

The extracts above suggest that messages which present depression as something to be suffered *with* are authored by users who are posting their first message to the forum. These new forum members also include statements regarding the duration of their condition, in two of these instances seeing their depression as something that occurs 'on and off', details that help to warrant their nascent membership of a depression community (Stommel and Koole 2010). In the third example, 'suffered with depression' is ascribed to a third party but is also presented as finite and successfully treated. 'Suffering with depression', then, appears to express a situation in which the condition can be relieved, albeit temporarily. These instances contrast with examples of *SUFFER+from*:

5. I've been **suffering from depression** for around three years and during this time I have managed to keep working, although not always as well as I would like. […]but recently the meds have started to lose their effect and I can feel myself getting dragged down again.

6. Does it not make sense, then, that a fundamental change in one's behavior, ESPECIALLY someone **suffering from depression**, is going to take longer than 3 hours?

7. have you told your boss or anyone at work that you are **suffering from depression** ..... i have as i was scared that if i broke down at work (which i have a couple of times) that they may think i was stupid ....

8. When I first **suffered from depression**, a girl I loved got pregnant by someone else, and eventually married him.

9. I also found that people started to disert me when they found out I **suffered from depression**, but that was over 20 years ago, and times have changed I think more people are aware of the illness and what it entails.

10. I've been **suffering from depression** since I was about 10, I think. I'm now 28. I cannot pinpoint a moment when I started feeling 'down' but I do remember wanting to cut myself when I was about 15 and trying various other things to harm myself.

Participants' posts including *SUFFER+from depression* address issues arising from their condition, most noticeably regarding its effects upon their employment and interpersonal relationships, as well as seeking and providing emotional support for other forum members. In contrast to those suffering *with* depression, instances of *SUFFER+from* depression are written by more established members of the *depression.net* community. This suggests that long-term forum users begin to adopt linguistic choices which further distance themselves from depression, seeing it as an external cause rather than a co-participant in their unhappiness. Although these users do still refer to the duration of their suffering (ex. 9–10), depression is also never presented as curable or as going into remission, indicating that these long-standing users are also less likely to discuss experiencing relief from their symptoms, a factor that in turn explains their long-term use of the forum itself.

Depression's strongest and most frequent collocate is *the* ($n = 153$, $MI^3 = 17.94$), with 32.7 per cent of these collocations ($n = 50$) arising in the noun phrase *the depression.* As noted in the previous chapter, this collocation is somewhat surprising given that mental health conditions are less obviously amenable to grammatical concretization; to repeat the quotation used in Chapter 4, 'it would be odd to hear someone speak of "*the* depression" when speaking about his own depression' (Cassell 1976: 145). Nevertheless, there are abundant examples of precisely this collocation in the corpus, which in turn provide a rich illustration of users' experiences of depression:

11. After that it went completely to hell. **The depression** got a lot worse, my tutors were all supremely disinterested and the doctors up at uni all kept telling me I was just a 'little bit stressed', not depressed. Uh huh.
12. It's **the depression** which is hiding the point [in living], not that there isn't one..
13. I have felt like that too, like an outsider looking in, and everyone seems to be happy, in a couple, going on holidays etc - just makes you feel worse, but I think **the depression** magnifies things also, because when you are 'well' it doesn't seem to upset so much, lol being around happy people, in my case, doesn't work […].
14. Now, 11 years on..**the depression** is really taking its toll and ive got to do something about it.
15. The rest of the time I've struggled along with St John's Wort or nothing. (I was worried that if I admitted to **the depression**, after I had children, the social workers might take my children.)

These concordances further convey the personal difficulty depression entails for the members of the forum, again situating depression as a factor that problematizes educational and professional activities and maternal roles, which shades the way they perceive themselves and other people, and which obscures their reasons for wanting to live. What is particularly noticeable – or, in Cassell's terms, 'odd' – here is the way in which *the depression* is personified as actively performing processes such as 'hiding' the value of living, 'magnif[ying] things' and 'taking its toll' (ex. 12–14). Processes in which *depression* or *the depression* is an agent also encode forum members' perceptions of acquiring and recovering from their condition:

16. I think, but did not realise it at the time, that was **the depression** starting.
17. I also feels there's not necessarily any reason for **depression hitting**: it may be that there was one event that tipped the balance and your mind could no longer cope, but there is probably a lot of underlying stuff that you may not even be aware of.

18. Strangely I never had post-natal depression with either of my children, and **depression didn't rear its head** again until I was in my early thirties.
19. prozac did wonders for next 2 years, then **depression came** back.
20. though it was after life events changed at the age of 12, I started to experience real senses of oppression, injustice, hatred and **depression came** after that.
21. Many doctors now recommend remaining on a maintenance dose for a full year after the symptoms of **the depression** lift.
22. I got depressed seriously after my first child was born nine years ago and it is only the past few years **the depression** has lifted but the anxiety is still here, now and again Damn panic attacks!!

Ordinarily we may euphemistically speak of 'catching', 'falling' or 'getting' an illness in which we are, however involuntarily, agents (Johnson and Murray 1985). On *depression.net*, however, sufferers repeatedly remove themselves from descriptions of the onset of their depression by using intransitive ('starting' and 'hitting' in ex. 16 and 17), reflexive processes (ex. 18) or spatial metaphors (ex. 19 and 20) to describe the start of their distress. Representing depression in this manner also constructs the forum participants as passive, with neither control over nor responsibility for the onset of their condition. This lack of agency during depression's onset is clearly demonstrated in extract 20; whereas the author constructs himself as grammatically agentive in experiencing feelings of oppression and hatred, depression comes by itself, seemingly beyond the forum user's control, even if implicitly resulting from his feelings. A related pattern holds for the forum participants' descriptions of recovery in extracts 21 and 22; rather than being an active process of struggling against depression, the figurative intransitive process 'lifted' presents the alleviation of depression as independent of actions taken by the authors.

Further instances in which *depression* or *the depression* are presented in an active role offer an insight into the ways in which the forum users present depression as affecting their subjective experience, not least by impairing sufferers' assessment of themselves and their capacity to make informed decisions affecting other health conditions:

23. Has anything happened? Or is it 'just' **depression** biting hold? We are here for you.
24. I find I cannot make a sensible decision because I can't work out whether the need to make that important choice is being driven by **the depression** or by common sense.

25. Its so hard to recognise when your thinking is being skewed by **depression**, I know. I'm a great believer in writing things down, be it lists, posting on forums or journalling.

26. I've learned that when I'm depressed I make a lot of black and white judgements because that's the way **depression** makes my mind work.

27. I went a whole year of mapping my mood swings to my cycle and sometimes it fit and sometimes it didnt so I dont know what to think. I think maybe **the depression** makes the PMS worse, but the mood swings are also extra.

As these corpus extracts attest, even while they describe the ways in which it affects their lives, forum members do so in ways that mitigate or minimize their own involvement in depression's actions. For example, in extract 23 and extracts 14 and 17 above, the figurative material processes of 'biting hold', 'taking its toll' and 'hitting' are each expressed without a direct or indirect object role that could be filled by an explicit reference to the forum member (as, for example, 'taking its toll on me'). Likewise, in extracts 24 to 27, depression's actions directly affect 'choice', 'thinking', 'my mind' and 'the PMS', but never explicitly the forum participants themselves. Extract 26, for example, could have been articulated as 'that's the way depression makes me think', thereby encoding a transitive relation between the speaker and their depression. Instead, the clause constructions frequently hold depression at a slight remove from the forum members, articulating its influence over their actions or, in extract 26, a discursively separate 'mind'. This separation is particularly clear in extract 27 above, in which 'the depression' is said to 'make the PMS worse'. Not only is depression objectified using a definite article rather than a possessive pronoun, but it affects 'the PMS' which is also grammatically disowned by the speaker. In extract 25, this distancing effect is also realized through the contributor's choice of pronouns; although their post is written in response to a specific forum member, they opt for a non-specific second person 'your' when referring to the effects of depression on thinking before switching to a specific first-person pronoun to describe the actions they take to ameliorate such effects. In keeping with these posts, there are few instances in which the support group members present *depression* as directly affecting them:

28. Can't say may **depression gives me those sort of symptons** although I do often feel very detached from what is going on around me and regularly get the exhausted feeling.

29. Sometimes, reading over what I've written, I can see what **depression is doing to me**. Everything becomes black or white. I obsess and over

analyse. I get a little paranoid that there are 'rules' out there for social interaction and I just don't know them.

Extracts 28 and 29 provide the only instances in the corpus in which forum participants explicitly encode themselves as an object of a process attributed to *depression*. Of these, extract 28 contextualizes this interaction with a negated modal verb, and thus refers to something which depression in fact does *not* do to the author. Extract 29 is therefore the only example in which a forum member explicitly positions his/herself as the recipient of a process attributed to *depression*, with this action again reporting the effect of depression upon the speaker's perception and cognition.

While depression is discursively construed as a volitional entity, its agency is only seldom presented as directly extending to the depressed individual themselves. Much like the forum participants' accounts of *suffering from depression*, then, their descriptions of depression's actions typically distance it from their own identity; depression may 'take its toll' or 'bite hold' but the group members seldom present themselves as the direct recipients of these actions. Even as sufferers disclose the damaging effects of depression on their thoughts and behaviours, therefore, they make transitivity choices that distance themselves from the stigma of illness and imply their passivity rather than rendering it explicitly. This is a finding that has been noted previously (Galasiński 2008: 53–5). Galasiński claims that this distancing depression from the self is a prominent feature in the narratives of men and allows them to preserve a sense of masculine identity untrammelled by depression. However, this same discursive practice features across messages by both male and female users of *depression.net*. It is also hard not to see similarities between the examples above and the discussion of *the ED* in the previous chapter. While members of *depression.net* seldom refer to 'depression talking' ($n = 4$) and do not share a comparable discourse of a 'depression voice', they do repeatedly engage in the same personification of their mental health condition. Although it may not be specific to men's narratives of depression, therefore, like Galasiński (2008), we also interpret this discursive distancing as functioning to mitigate the stigma of illness by enabling forum members to depict their identity as at least partially independent of depression, despite the deleterious effects it has on their lives.

In contrast to messages involving *the depression*, which objectify the condition and verbally distinguish it from the speaker, *depression* also collocates strongly with *my* ($n = 61$, $MI^3 = 15.31$), of which 32 cases (52.46 per cent) form the bigram *my depression*. The relative frequencies of *my depression* and *the depression* here are comparable with those for *my ED* and *the ED* in the *anorexia.net* forum (see Chapter 4, Section 4.3), with nominalization using the definite article occurring more frequently in each corpus than with the first-person possessive. *Depression* also has several other frequent L1 collocates, including *of* (*n* = 32) and *with* (*n* = 51). These recur in a number of repeated clusters involving *diagnosed with* and *SUFFER+with*, discussed above, and the noun phrases *symptoms of depression* (*n* = 6), *signs of depression* (*n* = 2), *episode(s) of depression* (*n* = 3) and *bout(s) of depression* (*n* = 2). Concordances for *my depression* demonstrate that it is often situated in a particular discursive context which is not shared by *the depression*:

30. Thats exactly the reason why my parents don't know of **my depression**, I saw it with my brothers wife who was in a horrible condition, psych wards etc for a few years, they just don't understand.

31. Only three people know the extent of **my depression**, one of which is my boyfriend, who just this evening said 'I am fed up with your moods' which doesn't really help.

32. I tried that with my ex. I sat her down on our third meeting and told her all about **my depression**, the treatment, the psychiatrist - all of it. I was convinced that she would run a mile, but she didn't.

33. However, I do now feel resolved to do something. Having taken such positive steps to deal with **my depression** and stop drinking [...] then it would be silly not to deal with all the other issues at the same time.

34. My therapist is honestly heaven sent [...]. She helped me realise what it is that I need/want to do to be able to put the initial cause of **my depression** behind me.

Whereas *the depression* is employed when forum members are discussing the indirect effects depression has upon them personally, forum users adopt *my depression* when discussing its impact on their relationships with family members or partners. Depression is construed as having an adverse effect on these relationships due to uncomprehending or unsympathetic responses from others (ex. 30-31) or anxiety about divulging the secret of mental illness – 'I was convinced that she would run a mile' (ex. 32). Forum users who report witnessing the stigma of depression also claim that the expectation of non-comprehension from others leads them to remain secretive about their condition (ex. 30). Seen in this light, the choice of a possessive determiner explicitly associates the sufferer with their condition and underscores the personal nature of the problems it produces.

Messages involving reference to *my depression* also provide a riposte to concerns that online support groups lead their members to neglect supportive relationships in their daily lives (Wright and Bell 2003; Baker and Fortune 2008). Following an account of a failed relationship, one forum participant asks if he should refrain from romantic engagements altogether. The responses, including the message from which extract 32 is taken, acknowledge the fear engendered by revealing depression to a loved one and use personal narratives to claim that this anxiety can be misplaced:

35.   When i met my partner, before we officially became a couple i sat him down and told him about **my depression**, and how life with me wouldn't be easy. […] I was pretty scared about that conversation before hand, but i thought if he backs off afterwards at least i've saved myself the heartbreak […]. That was 19 months ago, and we're about as perfect as a couple gets.

In these cases, the choice of *my depression* conveys a greater proximity between the speaker and condition but does so in a more positive context. Using a possessive determiner also validates the author's subsequent advice to pursue relationships cautiously by signifying its basis her own experience of illness. *My depression* is also used in a positive discursive context in extracts 33 and 34, in which forum members explicitly verbalize their ownership of depression while referring to steps they are taking towards recovery. Similarly, one forum member uses *my depression* three times in a post describing the onset, duration and management of their condition, before using *my depression* in a subsequent post five days later in which they state:

36.   I guess I'm lucky as most of the time nowadays I cope pretty well although I still have down days. […] Anyone who has read my post about how **my depression** began will recognise that I imagine.

These examples suggest that *my depression* may have a more positive semantic prosody if the collocation is examined in the wider context of the messages in which it appears. That is, as with examples of *my ED* in Section 4.3 of Chapter 4, these examples of *my depression* that explicitly verbalize the sufferer's possession of the condition correlate with users reporting a movement towards recovery or with those who experience depression in a way that they find manageable.

5.3.2 Being *depressed*

Having examined the discourse surrounding the noun *depression*, we now turn our attention to its adjectival equivalent, *depressed*. The keyword *depressed* occurs

126 times in the *depression.net* corpus across 34 per cent of the message threads. *Depressed* functions most frequently as a complement in intensive attributive clauses, predicating depression as an attribute of the speaker ('I have been depressed from about the age of 15'), rather than a feeling ($n = 15$) or possessed object, *depression*. By incorporating depression into the speaker's identity rather than construing it as a distinct phenomenon, phrases such as 'I am depressed' posit a closer relationship between speaker and condition than 'I have depression' or 'I suffer from depression'; instead of depression being an external possession, it is a way of describing the self (Fleischman 1999). During focus groups with depressed patients, Epstein et al. (2010: 958–60) found that sufferers deliberately avoid expressing this closer relationship, with one participant explicitly comparing 'having depression' and 'being depressed' to 'having cancer' and 'being cancerous'. The latter of each pair was believed to construe the condition as an enduring trait and was explicitly identified as more stigmatizing than the possessive clause (cf. Harvey 2012: 363–4). The stigma that Epstein et al.'s participants associate with 'being depressed' could also explain the frequency of *depressed* in the corpus, which has 316 fewer occurrences than *depression*.

Other than *i*, the two strongest collocates of *depressed* in the *depression.net* corpus are the copula forms *was* ($n = 33$, $MI^3 = 21.41$) and *been* ($n = 19$, $MI^3 = 19.15$), examples of which are below.

37. The first time I **was depressed was** when I **was** 13, I was terribly shy
    and self conscious and was tall and fairly advanced for my age. [...]
    I eventually got through that phaze after a few years, without it ever
    really being diagnosed as depression, at the time it was said that I had an
    inferiority complex.
38. I've **been depressed** since I was in my late teens/early 20's. Back then, I
    just assumed everyone felt the same way and dealt with the same feelings,
    etc. It wasn't until I was in my 40's that I began to discover what was going
    on and not until lately have I gotten counseling with a psychiatrist and
    proper diagnosis and medication which has helped a lot. I just have to
    accept the fact that my brain chemicals don't work like most people's and
    that I react differently to stimuli differently because of that.
39. I think I have **been depressed** from about the age of 15 when I used to lie
    on my mums bed and cry for hours. I would plead with her to take me to
    the doctor as I knew something wasn't right.
40. I realise now with the benefit of much reading and soul searching that I
    have **been depressed** most of my adult life but not been able to properly
    articulate what I was feeling.

In the messages above and other instances of *depressed*, *was* and *been* collocate to the left of *depressed* as part of copula constructions of the form *have+been+depressed* or *was+*[adverbial intensifier]*+depressed*. These account for 88 per cent of left-sided collocations of *been* with *depressed* and 90 per cent of left-sided collocations of *was* with *depressed*. Expressions of previous uncertainty over the nature of depressed experiences are consistent in the concordances containing *been depressed*, not least in extract 38, whose author states that it took two decades 'to discover what was going on'. Similarly, extract 39 refers to knowing only that 'something wasn't right' and the author of extract 40 describes the 'soul searching' that helped him to realize he is depressed. These three posts thus all convey that depression may not immediately present itself as an explanation for personal unhappiness and may also be misinterpreted by others as a reflection of their personality (Karp 1996; Wittink et al. 2008).

These extracts also demonstrate that *been depressed* and *was depressed* typically occur in messages where sufferers are discussing the duration of their depression. Seventy per cent of the total occurrences of *was depressed* and *been depressed* appear in one message thread, titled 'How long… …have you suffered from depression?' This is also the third longest thread sampled from the forum and contains seventy-three posts. As the title anticipates, posts in this thread overwhelmingly consist of short narratives of each author's condition. Accordingly, *depressed* collocates significantly with words such as *when*, *since*, *years* and *life* that signal recurrent and chronic periods of unhappiness. For members who describe experiencing depression since their childhood, these narratives often include reference to unstable family lives, physical and/or sexual abuse or unspecified 'stuff that happened' during childhood, as well as incomprehension from their parents. Those who identify the onset of depression during adolescence describe feelings of sadness, anxiety, shyness and social isolation but do not often offer any causal explanations for their feelings (ex. 37–9). Forum members who describe the onset of depression in adulthood frequently refer to postnatal depression, parental death, abusive relationships and the demands of work. The majority of these narratives recount engagement with health professionals followed by antidepressant and/or talking therapies which have not helped the users to recover. Three further examples are offered in extracts 41 to 43:

41. Looking back myself I really have **been depressed** since I was about 15. I also had slight anorexia at the time […] It was left untreated till I was about 22 my previous job didn't help and made it worse, thats when I realised I actually had depression and anxiety.

42. Although I was dx'ed with depression when I was 18, I think I **was depressed** for some time before that. I was actively suicidal throughout my teens, and my first attempt was when I was 16.

43. I was diagnosed with depression in my teens.......I had trouble sleeping too. [...] I've **been depressed** since but although I'm taking Anti-depressants now, I have no current diagnosis.

Within these narratives, forum participants draw on medical and psychological discourses to contextualize their experiences with reference to depressive symptoms of sleeplessness (ex. 43) and suicidal behaviour (ex. 42) or psychological concepts such as 'an inferiority complex' (ex. 37). These narratives thus frequently take on the form of proto-diagnoses, in which participants adopt a position of rational self-observation over their past lives and integrate medical concepts within their 'unique biographical frame of reference' (Pilgrim and Bentall 1999: 268). Finding a similar tendency among depressed interviewees, Galasiński (2008) argues that the process of retrospective self-diagnosis positions depressed individuals as capable of detached and rational reflection on their condition. This in turn permits sufferers both to demonstrate their ability to reason about their experiences and to reframe previous difficulties as symptoms of depression rather than personal imperfections. Schreiber (1996) also claims that situating depression within a wider personal history that includes periods of relief and instances of positive behaviour is an important aspect of recovery. A recovering individual, she argues, is more likely to accept depression and internalize it as part of their personality, eventually being 'able to see [themselves] as a whole person, complete with inconsistencies, strengths and shortcomings' (Schreiber 1996: 486). The act of personal narration prompted by this thread may therefore itself be therapeutic for users, with copula constructions such as *have been depressed* that attribute depression to the sufferer offering a verbal index of this integration in the context of participants' self-reflection.

The high frequency of *was depressed* in this particular thread is somewhat surprising given that the thread title under which participants are posting verbalizes depression as an external entity. Forum participants who use *was depressed* in this thread are therefore opting to express their relationship to depression in a way which differs from that established by the thread's title as well as the community's verbal norms more generally. Extracts 39 and 43 to 45 above hint towards an explanation for this; in each extract, the authors distinguish between being or feeling 'depressed' and subsequently 'having depression', a grammatical shift that follows their interactions with clinicians.

Table 5.3 Unique Lexical Collocates of *Depressed* and *Depression*, Based on Their Top Fifty Strongest Collocations (MI^3)

Node	Unique lexical collocates
Depressed	*feel, feeling, just, people, really, say, think, time*
Depression	*anxiety, cause, diagnosed, illness, natal, post, suffer, suffered, suffering, symptoms, treat*
Shared lexical collocates	
since, years	

This distinction is reflected in the respective semantic profiles of *depressed* and *depression*, established by the unique lexical collocates each word carries (Orpin 2005). These are summarized in Table 5.3.

Their distinctive sets of lexical collocates confirm that, despite an ostensible similarity, *depressed* and *depression* have markedly different semantic profiles in the forum discourse. *Depressed* is represented as an affective state associated with feeling, thinking and measures of time as well as a label for classifying *people*. In contrast, *depression*'s unique collocates situate it firmly within a medical register through collocation with specific diagnostic labels such as *anxiety* and *post-natal* and reference to *symptoms*, diagnosis (*diagnosed*) and treatment (*treat*). The movement from *depressed* to *depression* presented in the examples above thus involves resituating feelings of despair within a medical discourse via a process of professional diagnosis (Karasz 2005; Harvey 2012). Likewise, the narrative presented in extract 38 recounts the author receiving 'counseling with a psychiatrist and proper diagnosis and medication', before he defines his depression as 'my brain chemistry doesn't work like most people's'. In this case, contact with healthcare professionals clearly correlates with the uptake of a biomedical model of depression.

As noted above, such grammatical shifts are neither arbitrary nor inconsequential when viewed in relation to the sufferers' sense of self. The process of medical diagnosis in the extracts above correlates with a change in users' identities from 'being depressed' to 'having' or 'suffering from depression', a change that also alters depression from a personal attribute to an externalized possession or antagonist. The prevailing tendency to refer to depression nominally as *the depression* permits it to partake in a wider range of verbal relationships than *depressed*, which is limited to copula constructions and behavioural processes such as 'I don't feel depressed anymore'. Most notably, *depression* is frequently represented as a grammatical agent and the analysis in Section 5.3.1 above reveals that messages which construct depression as an external object frequently also depict it as autonomous and having a powerful, deleterious effect upon sufferers' lives. In this respect, even while it may bring substantial relief for individuals struggling to understand and legitimize their distress (Karp 1996), professional diagnosis concretizes subjective distress into a clinical entity and corresponds with a position of diminished personal agency for the participants in our data (Schreiber and Hartrick 2002). To put this another way, the process of diagnosis appears to render sufferers both as medical patients and as grammatically patient as they come to view themselves as affected (however indirectly) by a depression that acts of its own volition. However, we are cautious of suggesting a causative rather than correlational relationship between diagnosis, a medicalized view of depression and a diminished belief in one's ability to recover (Knudsen et al. 2002). As Karp (1996) observes, adopting a medical understanding of depression and regarding it as beyond individual control are potentially independent characteristics of chronic depression, in which the condition endures despite the sufferer's efforts to recover. It may also be that sufferers pursue diagnosis because they already experience their feelings as beyond their control. Nevertheless, in moving from 'being depressed' to 'having depression', sufferers evince an increased sense of powerlessness over their condition.

5.3.3 Lay diagnosis in (inter)action

Although the foregoing discussion foregrounds the close association between the label of 'depression' and diagnosis by a health professional, the process of lay diagnosis between forum peers is also apparent in the corpus. User-led diagnosis is most visible in threads in which new forum members describe their experiences for the first time. These initial posts seldom invoke the category of depression explicitly, leaving open the possibility for responses to negotiate whether or not the individual is categorized as having depression (although the fact that a new user has posted on a website with 'depression' in its title indicates that this is a label to which they are themselves already orienting). Examining the responses of more established members can therefore illustrate how new users are greeted into the online community as well as how existing members negotiate the category of 'depression' in their own replies (Stommel and Koole 2010).

In one such instance, a new member discusses feeling 'down' and 'burned out', lacking in motivation or interest in activities, having 'trouble sleeping' and 'all kinds of irrational thoughts', but claims her GP diagnosed her as 'just tired'. Although the post concludes with the question 'Does anyone have any suggestions as to what to do?', a response from one of the forum moderators begins by diagnosing the individual:

44.   It sounds like you are experiencing a number of the classic symptoms of depression. You've lost interest in things you used to enjoy, have felt really down for several months, and continue to feel tired even after sleeping. I agree, a second opinion is in order...the sooner the better.

The brevity of this post belies the sophisticated ways in which it constructs the addressee's experience as one of depression. Although this proto-diagnosis is initially hedged ('It sounds like'), the pre-modifier 'classic' signals knowledge of established diagnostic criteria and, in doing so, implicitly validates the categorization of the addressee's experiences as 'symptoms of depression'. The subsequent description offers a gist formulation (Antaki et al. 2005) of the addressee's narrative in the form of a tripartite list, using intensifiers ('really down') and adverbials ('for several months', 'even after sleeping') to emphasize the prolonged and anomalous nature of her experience. This description also presents the addressee's experiences in the form of the diagnostic criteria in the *DSM*. By imitating official psychiatric discourse (Antaki 1994), this diagnostic formulation further warrants the moderator's recommendation – 'a second opinion is in order … the sooner the better' – which presents the need for further medical attention as a matter of urgency. As suggested by 'I agree' in the moderator's response, the advice to seek a second opinion is persistent in this thread, with six out of the seven responses from other forum participants advocating a change in doctor and one recommending seeking support within the addressee's workplace. By situating the original message in terms of symptoms of depression and constructing their own medical expertise, responding participants are able to formulate the experience described by the newcomer as one of medical pathology – that is, as 'depression' – even when this contradicts the report of a trained medical professional. As a result, the non-diagnosis of depression is constituted as a deficit of the original doctor's clinical acumen rather than as an indicator that the original poster does not have the condition. As Barker (2008) notes, such interactions illustrate a paradox of lay-driven medicalization in which lay forum members employ medical discourse to define a new member's experience as one of pathology, even while denying the view of a medical professional.

   The phrase 'classic symptoms of depression' is used by the same moderator in relation to another new member of *depression.net*. This new participant describes weeping, 'feeling very alone' and thinking 'about how rubbish i am' and expresses a reluctance to seek medical help. Again, although the new forum member does not explicitly request a diagnosis or advice, she receives the following response from the community moderator:

45. You have most of the classic symptoms of depression. Please get help, dear. Depression is a very real illness, no different than another other illness other than the fact there are no outward signs such as a broken bone or a horrid cough with fever. Depression can be successfully treated. But you need to be in the care of a physician to get the diagnosis and the proper treatment.

This post offers a formulation of the new user's message by directly attributing the 'classic symptoms' of depression to the new forum member (an interpretation that is, incidentally, not supported by the original post, which does not mention anhedonia, weight changes or trouble sleeping). The moderator then orients to the addressee's reluctance to seek medical help by legitimizing depression as 'no different than another other illness'. By conveying an apparent knowledge of depression's symptoms, nosology and amenability to treatment, the moderator is able to construct a position of expertise on depression and warrant her diagnostic formulation (Drew and Sorjonen 1997). Further, her designation of depression as an illness which has 'no outward signs' makes a diagnosis of depression virtually unavoidable; external normality is reconfigured as evidence of internal pathology as the absence of visible signs of depression is itself classified as a sign of depression. Having construed the new user's narrative as a description of depression, the moderator then reiterates the notion that depression is a medical condition with specific symptoms, and that the successful treatment of the illness – rather than the individual – is the preserve of medical professionals. The response therefore serves to socialize the new member into the interactional norms of the forum, in which they will receive unsolicited advice from others, and into the forum's normative model of depression, a model that transforms, through formulation, personal difficulties into symptoms of an underlying psychopathology (Antaki et al. 2005; Vayreda and Antaki 2009).

In both the above illustrations, the moderator's lay diagnoses of depression are used to encourage the addressee towards seeking further professional treatment. As Vayreda and Antaki (2009: 936) argue, new members of online support groups who accept such recommendations also commit themselves to the particular model of the disease with which it is packaged. Although the addressee of extract 83 does not contribute further to the thread, in the case of extract 84, this commitment is exemplified by a subsequent response from the original poster. In this, she describes a trip to her GP in which the forum members' diagnoses were ratified by a health professional, resulting in a prescription of the antidepressant Citalopram. In more theoretical terms, the messages above present medicalization in interaction, in which new members seeking help come to view their emotional experiences in medical terms (Conrad 2005; Barker 2008) and regard themselves as someone in need of professional medical help (Bartlett and Coulson 2011).

As well as being deployed when responding to new members' posts, a medical model of depression is also to reassure long-term members who report experiencing renewed difficulties. Prior to the example below, an established member of *depression.net* has posted a message consisting solely of 'i am not good in a real mess'. In response, another user writes:

46.   You're not a mess, you may feel like it, things may be getting to you and you might be feeling like you can't cope BUT this is what depression (for me anyway) feels like. Its a disease, a chemical imbalance in your brain. Be kind to yourself, you're ill!

Here, defining depression as a malfunction of brain chemistry provides a means of countering the addressee's self-criticism and prefaces the advice to '[b]e kind to yourself'. By categorizing difficult experiences as symptoms of a biomedical anomaly, the biomedical model of depression facilitates mutual peer support and encouragement on the forum, offering a way of caring for others through alleviating their self-reproach and legitimizing their experiences (Giles and Newbold 2011). As we argued in Chapter 4, the potential for this medical model of depression for supporting the forum's core activities of peer support provides a clear motivation for the uptake and deployment of this discourse on *depression. net* (Horton-Salway 2004).

Having illustrated the forum's prevailing representations of depression, the following section analyses how sufferers represent its treatment through antidepressant medication.

5.4 Antidepressants and 'the right medication'

Although *depression.net* has a separate 'Medication' message board, the main 'Depression' section from which the corpus was compiled is replete with references to antidepressant and mood stabilizing pharmaceuticals. Questions about dosages, latency periods and side effects as well as discussions of the desire to overdose were apparent even during the process of corpus compilation. In this regard, the relatively small number of keywords related to medication in Table 5.1 is somewhat misleading; forum members frequently refer to specific brand names for sedatives (*diazepam*), antipsychotics (*risperidone, seroquel*) and various branded SSRI antidepressants (*citalopram, venlafaxine, sertraline*) along with referring to *antidepressants* and *pills* more generally. However, the range of brand names used to refer to antidepressants means that each has a comparatively low frequency and dispersion in the corpus and so does not meet our keyness criteria. When taken in sum, however, references to medication, dosages or effects occur an average of around once every 200 words in the corpus, indicating that they are a recurrent feature of the forum interactions. Of these keywords, by far the most frequent are *meds* (*n* = 175, *log ratio* = 11.80) and *medication* (*n* = 145, *log ratio* = 8.18). Notably, the forum users prefer these superordinate nouns over the specific *antidepressants/anti-depressants/anti depressants* (seventy-five occurrences in total), and their abbreviated forms *AD* or *ADs* (*n* =13). The use of *medication* permits speakers to refer to various differing antidepressant, bipolar and antipsychotic products using a single term that emphasizes their medicinal purpose. It also offers an alternative to the superordinate term *drugs* (*n* = 38), which is used in the forum to refer to both prescription and recreational narcotics and hence carries the risk of misinterpretation.

Despite both *meds* and *medication* appearing a total of 320 times throughout the corpus, there are only nine instances in which either collocates with *depression* itself, examples of which are reproduced below.

47. You are tackling the **depression** with **medication** and hopefully, you will feel physically better and begin to put on weight etc, which is step 1.
48. Are you currently taking any **medication** for the **depression**?
49. R u on any **meds** for ur **depression**?
50. 3 months ago i was feeling depressed but didn't want to take **medication** because i feel **medication** long term changes the person. Obviously hormone related **depression** can benefit from **medication.**

As these examples show, references to medication feature in longer stretches of advice (ex. 47), questions to new forum members (ex. 48-49) and narratives of users' experiences of chronic unhappiness (ex. 50). Both extracts 47 and 48 utilize the *the depression* bigram which is identified above to establish a discourse of depression as a separate entity. In each case it is for *the depression*, rather than the individual patient, that antidepressants are taken. Extract 50 also divorces depression and medication from individual sufferers, stating that hormone-related depression itself benefits from antidepressants rather than the individual sufferer. This reduction of the therapeutic process to one between medicine and illness rather than medicine and patient is a long-standing characteristic of medical discourse (Poirier and Brauner 1988; van der Geest and Whyte 1989). Extract 49 uses 'ur', a common rebus meaning 'your' that makes explicit that medication is for depression which is associated with her addressee. Nevertheless, the implied target of antidepressants remains depression itself, rather than the individual or their subjective feelings of unhappiness. Indeed, there are only two instances in which medication is described as positively affecting the emotions or cognition of a forum member.

This medical discourse is further established in extract 50 by the statement that medication benefits 'hormone related depression'; that is, when depression arises from an imbalance of organic hormones. This forum user also presents antidepressants as a threat to their sense of self – 'medication long term changes the person' – with this danger offering a justification for avoiding medication (McMullen and Herman 2009). This reasoning also encodes a separation of depression and antidepressant effects from the sufferer; rather than seeing personal alteration as, in fact, the intended aim of antidepressants, a change to 'the person' is construed as an adverse effect of 'long term' medication use, which should ideally only affect depression in isolation. The result is a mixed discourse of antidepressants that combines characteristically medical representations of the therapeutic process with lay concerns about a self who will be changed in the process of recovery (Stephens et al. 2004; Maxwell 2005).

These examples contrast with instances in which antidepressants are ascribed as being directly 'for' sufferers, instantiated in collocations between *meds*, *medication* and personal pronouns:

51. you have made the first steps and got help from your GP so well done - lets hope these are the right **meds for you** in the end.
52. what works for one person doesn't work for the next and it may take a few attempts before you find the right **medication for you** X
53. If you get the right **medication**, and help, **for you** then things will improve
54. […] because I have been on quite a few diff meds over the years I have been referred to a psychiatrist to sort out best **meds for me**.
55. I agree with [username]. -- I think you need to find another doctor that is willing to listen and work toward finding the right **meds for you**.

The repeated collocations *right meds* and *right medication* are apparent in the extracts above. Along with 'right dose and medication' and 'best meds for me', these collocations appear nine times in the corpus. While the antidepressants discussed in extracts 47 to 50 above were intended for 'the depression', medication which is intended for an individual is pre-modified as the 'right medication' or 'best meds'. Repeated references to the *right medication*, defined broadly in extracts 52 and 53 as that which 'works' and improves 'things', demonstrates that the forum users are aware there are different antidepressants available, including those that could, by implication, be 'wrong' for the individual. The above concordances construe finding the *right medication* as a valuable goal for the forum members, even if this can mean a process of trial and error with ineffectual drugs lasting 'years' (ex. 54) and where the benefits are only vaguely defined. The repeated discussion of the *right medication* also suggests a faith in antidepressant therapies that explains a lack of improvement as a mismatch between the individual and a specific pharmaceutical product or dosage. Accordingly, the *right medication* is something to be hoped for (ex. 51), is a precondition for improvement (ex. 53) and is worth breaking continuity of care to pursue (ex. 55).

Although the notion of right and wrong medication may simply reflect many forum users' negative experiences of different antidepressants, the search for an elusive, uniquely suited antidepressant may also lead patients to approach therapy as a matter of consumerism, demanding medical commodities from clinicians in pursuit of recovery (van der Geest and Whyte 1989; Barker 2008). Indeed, just as the previous section illustrated that a new forum user was encouraged to seek a second opinion after their doctor did not diagnose them with depression, here an ethos of patient consumerism is apparent in the recommendation to pursue a personally suited antidepressant. While promoting the notion of a 'right medication' may usefully encourage patients to be proactive in their healthcare choices and to persevere if their mental health is not improved by one antidepressant, it may also lead to conflict with doctors who prescribe treatments with which the patient disagrees or who withhold treatments that the patient believes they should have. For example, in extract 55, a forum user who has been refused antidepressants by her doctor is encouraged to change doctors in order to pursue the 'right meds'. While criticizing the addressee's general practitioner for not listening, this response nevertheless conveys the forum members' dependency on medical professionals who act as drug gatekeepers. This extract is also typical of responses in this thread, which endorse changing doctors in order to fulfil the member's medication preferences. The *depression.net* community's collective faith in finding the 'right medication' is such that none of the responses claim that the doctor may be correct and pharmacological therapy may in fact be unnecessary or unhelpful. Indeed, the advice to pursue the 'right' medication may also preclude sufferers from addressing situational, relational or psychodynamic issues that contribute to their psychological distress (Lewis 1995). The prevalence of discussion of antidepressants on the forum is also somewhat surprising in light of the narratives that users provide of their depressive experiences. That is, while the onset of depression is situated in relation to family dysfunction, histories of abuse, bereavement and work-related stress, it is medication rather than employment advice or familial and psychosexual therapies that comprise the bulk of sufferers' treatment discussions. Though the corpus data does not provide a clear explanation for this, the disconnection between the situational factors that the group members cite as causes of their depression and the biomedical interventions used to treat it may well reflect their experiences of healthcare. That is, the forum users' discussion of antidepressants rather than talking therapies correlates with the relative prescription rates and availabilities of these interventions in primary care (Chew-Graham et al. 2002; Conrad 2005). At the same time, it is also congruent with the community's dominant representation of depression, which construes the condition through features of medical discourse and advocates a biomedical treatment to alleviate it.

5.5 Discourses of self-injurious behaviour

The *depression.net* forum contains specific password-protected sections intended for the discussion of suicide and self-harm that were not used to compile the corpus. Nevertheless, like *meds* and *medication*, references to forms of self-injurious behaviour are common occurrences in the corpus. This is demonstrated by the keywords *self* ($n = 114$, *log ratio* = 3.73) and *life* ($n = 275$, *log ratio* = 2.24), which form collocations such as *self-harm* and *END*+[possessive pronoun]+*life*. Beyond these keywords, the phrases *kill myself* and *hang myself* occur six times and once, respectively, while *cut* and *cutting* are used to refer to specific means of self-injury on a total of thirteen occasions. The corpus also contains thirty-eight instances of *suicidal* and twenty-six instances of *suicide*, with either term occurring at least once in 26 (17 per cent) of all the threads sampled. Despite the social taboos that might proscribe references to suicide and self-harm (Coggan et al., 1997), *suicidal* or *suicide* appear in the first message in twelve (46 per cent) of these threads, suggesting that forum users do not shy from discussing suicidal ideation.

This unusual candour means that the *depression.net* corpus represents a valuable source of first-hand, naturally occurring descriptions of self-injurious behaviour and the meanings individuals and groups attach to it through their own unsolicited accounts. This is particularly the case given that previous studies of suicidal ideation have been forced by ethical considerations to rely on simulated discussions with actors (Reeves et al. 2004; Feldman et al. 2007) or have used notes written by people who have attempted suicide (Galasiński 2017). These foregoing studies identify that discussion of self-injurious behaviour is often approached indirectly, which prompted a search for additional euphemistic references to suicide. This revealed two instances of the euphemism 'topped myself' and phrasal constructions such as 'go to sleep and never wake up'. Forum participants also employ spatial metaphors for suicide and death such as 'wanting out', 'I'm still here, although I'm getting close' and '... still here, despite trying not to be'. Finally, more ambiguous intimations of suicidality are evident through phrases such as 'sick of it' and seven instances of *end it [all]* in which endophoric antecedents for 'it' are not explicit. The absence of a definite reference renders such expressions ambivalent, particularly in lieu of any other verbal context. For example, one long thread of messages entitled 'me again ...' begins with a post comprised solely of '.. sick of it.', in which 'it' has numerous possible exophoric referents. Nevertheless, forum members constitute this message as an example of suicidal thinking by responding with imperatives to 'try and stay safe and focus on each hour separately'. This – admittedly single – example offers some indication that the support group participants orient to suicidality in the interpretation of ambiguous posts.

The diverse constructions through which the forum participants refer to self-injurious behaviour make them less amenable to corpus-driven analyses that are designed to identify recurrent single words and n-grams rather than one-off expressions such as 'I want desperately to jump on to the [train] track'. The following analysis is therefore based predominantly on qualitative investigation of concordance lines and whole messages and includes analysis of messages identified through manual reading and corpus-driven methods.

While it is possible to see self-harm and suicide existing along a cline of self-injury, *suicide* and *suicidal* occur only three times in the same conversational threads as references to self-harm. This general lack of mutual occurrence suggests they have largely exclusive discursive contexts in the forum. As such, we initially consider self-harm and suicide separately before comparing their use in the forum directly.

5.5.1 Discourses of self-harm

As noted above, explicit reference to self-harm is a relatively frequent occurrence in the data; a search for *self harm**, *harm** and the abbreviation *SH* returns fifty concordance lines related to self-injury from twenty-two (15 per cent) conversation threads, signifying that self-injury has a relatively common role in experiences of depression discussed in the forum.

The functional nature of self-harm stands out strongly as a recurrent motif of the forum users' descriptions of self-harm and their intentions to injure themselves:

56. I don't feel that any form of **self harm**, from anorexia, to **cutting**, through to alcoholism and stockpiling medication is cowardly. We are driven to find ways to cope and often those methods seem bizaare but they are not cowardly.

57. and the **self harm** as they call it, i call it self relief, i really dont want more scars i have to many already but i cant live like this much more, i have no one i can talk to and even if i did i would not know what to say.

58. The urge to sleep or **cut** or any other form of release that we have found useful over time will fight our efforts and whilst giving in can be easier, it may not help in the long term.

59. is so hard not to get the knife out and start **cutting** my arms my legs my chest anywhere, just to feel something thats not pain.

These extracts illustrate that self-harm is presented as functional when it is construed as a mechanistic form of 'release', a 'relief' from otherwise intolerable pain and isolation, or as a way 'to cope' by managing affect (Boynton and Auerbach 2004; Laye-Gindhu and Schonert-Reichl 2005; Klonsky 2007, 2009; Victor et al. 2018). Extract 57 demonstrates that recourse to self-harm is explained as arising from a lack of other, less damaging outlets such as verbal expression and provides a necessary channel for otherwise uncommunicated emotions. For this sufferer, the relief that injury permits also seemingly outweighs the dismay caused by physical records of self-harm: 'i really dont want more scars i have to[o] many already but i cant live like this much more' (ex. 57; Boynton and Auerbach 2004).

Framing self-injurious behaviour as beneficial despite drawbacks such as scarring serves to de-pathologize self-harm and present it as a legitimate, considered activity. Self-harm is presented by these contributors as part of a 'situated internal logic' (Harris 2000: 169); it is a way 'to cope' in an intolerable or lonely context, even though it can seem 'bizaare' to others. In a similar vein, extract 57 renames self-harm as 'self relief' and thereby elides any sense that it is damaging, while the author of extract 59 paradoxically equates self-harm with *removing* pain, even when it is carried out in a seemingly arbitrary manner: 'my arms my legs my chest anywhere'. While equating self-harm with an analgesic is uncommon both in the forum and more widely (Horne and Csipke 2009), doing so similarly legitimizes this extreme behaviour, however maladaptive it may appear to others. It also shows self-harm can fulfil distinct functions for different individuals (Horne and Csipke 2009), thus problematizing the possibility of finding a single therapeutic remedy for self-harming behaviour.

As the last of the above extracts also suggests, a further prevailing theme of these messages is the repetitive and compulsive nature of self-harm. Sufferers' compulsions to injure themselves are encoded in several ways across different messages, not least through references to self-harm as the object of an uncontrollable 'urge':

60. I've self harmed 6 times in the last 14 days usually cutting my stomach, its such a mess.
61. My mind seems to work so that if anything goes wrong, even slightly, I will immediately have the **urge** to take a handful of tablets. […]But, I can't seem to get control of my mind. I so much want to take them its such a strong pull for me. It like I would imagine an addiction to feel like.
62. It sounds insane in my own ears but it is how I feel. Just thinking about taking them fills me with warmth. A real **urge**. I need to get control of my mind.
63. so as usual I'm fighting the **urge** to take some extra tablets.
64. I am an artist so I do try to express it that way, and i do also write alot down. And yet I still **self harm**.
65. It's [twisting hair] better than SH right, but i just don't know how to **stop** myself doing it.
66. Self destructive self has taken over. Dunno how to **stop** it, I can see it but not stop it. Self harming again. Just hate me.
67. i cut b/c i have to hurt.

These posts make clear that, despite the functionality described in the previous extracts, self-harm also engenders internal conflict and regret as it becomes habituated. The author of extract 60, for instance, specifically details both the repetitive nature of his self-harm and its perseverance over an extended period of time, despite his explicit dismay at the results: 'its such a mess'. The experience of self-harm as a long-term or consistent behaviour is evinced elsewhere through adverbials ('as usual I'm fighting the urge') and simple present tense verbs that convey an unchanging state of affairs ('I still self harm'). Concomitant with this are claims that self-harm continues unabated despite their awareness of its irrationality ('It sounds insane in my own ears' in ex. 62) and efforts to pursue other, less deleterious forms of self-expression (ex. 64).

Rather than functioning to regulate their emotions, these posts suggest that continual self-harm has taken on an addictive quality for some forum users. Extract 61 conveys a sense that self-injurious impulses arise 'immediately', with this forum user thrice describing her compulsion to self-harm as an 'urge' and once explicitly comparing the feeling to an addiction (Boynton and Auerbach 2004). The language of diminished self-control is present elsewhere in expressions such as 'i just don't know how to stop myself', 'I can't seem to get control of my mind' and 'Dunno how to stop it' (ex. 62 and 65–6), implying that insurmountable impulse has replaced purposeful choice (Harvey and Brown 2012). While conveying the authors' sense of helplessness, construing self-harm in terms of an addiction or overwhelming desire also has clear implications for their degree of responsibility for self-injury, establishing a position of powerlessness over their own behaviour (Bennett et al. 2003). This representation of helplessness is vividly expressed in extract 66; paralleling anorexia sufferers' representation of 'the ED' in the previous chapter, this forum user attributes her actions to a distinctive 'self destructive self', circumscribing her own agency to verbal processes of perception but not material action to prevent self-harm: 'I can see it but not stop it'.

This disempowered subject position makes clear the cruel irony of self-injurious behaviour; while the foregoing posts (ex. 56–59) claim there is an immediate benefit from self-harm in terms of the 'release' or control of negative emotions, habitual or recurrent injury is construed in terms of impaired control over actions, thoughts and even oneself. Reflexive coping mechanisms such as self-harm also fail to offer sufferers any control over the causes of their unhappiness and may well arise from a perceived inability to change situational causes of distress (Rogers and Pilgrim 1997). Therefore, although self-harm presents an opportunity for active emotional control, sufferers nevertheless remain in a passive position 'driven to find ways to cope' (ex. 56) by external factors. Indeed, the use of an agentless passive structure in extract 56 to avoid naming a cause for emotional distress is telling, as discussion of the specific situational factors that lead to individual sufferers' initial self-injury is rare on the forum. Rather, the interactional focus gravitates towards the immediate desire to self-harm and the problem it comes to signify for the individual. In one respect, this constitutes a limit to the forum members' construction of self-harm as ultimately an issue of subjective control and responsibility (or a lack thereof), rather than behaviours situated with complex personal and social causes (Roen et al. 2008).

5.5.2 Suicidal ideation

Contrary to our expectations that references to suicide would co-occur with *commit* and *committed*, *thoughts* is the sole lexical collocate of *suicide* ($n = 5$, $MI^3 = 12.55$) and *suicidal* ($n = 18$, $MI^3 = 17.54$). These collocations denote a strong association between suicide and patterns of cognition, as demonstrated below:

68.   I'm really at the end of my tether now, **suicide thoughts** are dominating and I feel like it's only a matter of time. I'm terrified.
69.   **Suicidal thoughts** seem to be returning, and that is not very welcome.
70.   I stay at work for 10 hours, plagued constantly by fatigue and **suicidal thoughts**.
71.   Cannot deal with stress at all and any type of pressure just makes me have **suicidal thoughts**.
72.   Although depressed I have never had **suicidal thoughts** until I started my tablets. […] I have twice had serious **suicidal thoughts** and can thinking about the pleasure of dying on a regular basis
73.   If I get twisted in them thoughts [about his children] it always seems that **suicidal thoughts** are not far behind.

As with the discussion of self-harm above, these posts consistently emphasize the persistence of suicidal ideation. This is realized through adverbials such as 'constantly', 'always', and 'on a regular basis' (ex. 70, 72–3) and also by choice of simple present tense verb forms (Carter and McCarthy 2006), which present suicidal ideation as part of a general, unchanging state of affairs (ex. 70–1).

   In parallel with the discussion of anorexia in Chapter 4 (Section 4.3) and depression in Section 5.4.1 of this chapter, the forum users here also attribute a range of processes to their suicidal thoughts, which are presented using transitive and intransitive processes as 'dominating', 'returning' and 'plaguing' the authors. These processes convey a lack of agency on the part of the support group members to prevent their suicidal ideation, which acts upon them in a physical manner. In the same vein, extract 71 employs the absolute qualifier 'at all' and determiner 'any' to frame the author's suicidal feelings as an extreme case (Pomerantz 1986) in which the onset of suicidal ideation is an inescapable consequence of a complete inability to manage stress. Similarly, the author of extract 73 makes use of the absolute adverbial 'always' to indicate the unavoidable nature of suicidal ideation which arises from concerns over the welfare of his children. By including such 'defensive detailing' in their accounts (Drew 2006), the authors of these posts each construe suicidal ideation as inevitable, regardless of whether it arises from the apparent volition of suicidal thoughts themselves (ex. 68–70), prescribed medication (ex. 72), or seemingly insurmountable external factors and emotions (ex. 71, 73). The effect is to legitimize suicidal ideation by rendering it as the inexorable result of each sufferer's particular circumstances rather than a volitional process for which they are accountable (Bennett et al. 2003).

A similar rationalizing process is also evinced when the forum users discuss the influence of other people on their suicidal behaviour:

74. i often feel like just throwing myself under a bus but then the thoughts of others who will be hurt keep me here i dont know why i feel like this.
75. Only reason i haven't finished myself off is because i'm staying with my mum and what it would do to her.
76. Why am I here, why do I exist etc. Then come thoughts of suicide, followed by tears, followed by guilt as to how it would hurt my children so much if I were to carry these thoughts out.
77. Ending your life is not the answer to your depression. And think about the pain and horror it would inflict on your survivors.
78. I'm scared that if I mess up [marital relations] again I will be left with nothing. It seems that **dying** would be the best solution for **everyone**.

As these extracts attest, the discussion of suicidal ideation is also marked by the frequent use of if-conditional structures and the epistemic modals 'will' and 'would' that signify authors' consideration of the potential effects of a suicide. As suggested by extracts 74 to 76, the desire to avoid the effects of suicide on surviving family members and social relations is the most frequently cited reason for resisting suicidal impulses. This finding runs parallel to a number of existing studies, in which participants who have attempted suicide identify familial and interpersonal responsibility as inhibiting further suicidal behaviour (Chesley and Loring-McNulty 2003; Roen et al. 2008). A comparable preventative measure is advocated by the author of extract 77, who advises another forum member to think of 'the pain and horror it would inflict on your survivors' as a guard against suicidal desires. As a caveat to this, however, it is important to note that a sense of obligation to spare others pain is not presented as helping to resolve depression or suicidal ideation, but only as inhibiting suicidal actions. Additionally, the narrative from which extract 76 is taken complicates the value of this familial obligation, indicating that it can be a source of guilt for suicidal ideation and thereby increase sufferers' distress. In the case of extract 78, the same obligation to others is reversed and considered a reason for pursuing suicide. Although thinking about a responsibility towards others may therefore help to prevent suicide in some cases, the complex causes of each individual's suicidal ideation and the reasons through which they rationalize ending their lives mean that no single reason to avoid suicide will apply in every case (Reeves et al. 2004; Roen et al. 2008).

When considered together, the discussions of self-harm and suicide in the *depression.net* corpus reveal a number of discourses around self-injurious thoughts and behaviour with attendant subject positions that differ in terms of personal agency and responsibility. Suicidal ideation and self-harm are described as occurring both acutely and chronically, and as originating in factors seemingly beyond forum members' control. Once they begin, however, forum members are able to evaluate their self-injurious impulses and their outcomes, allowing the construction of a reasoning and considerate identity even within descriptions of profound personal crises. In contrast to the view that suicidal and self-harming individuals are incapable of rational thought, these messages highlight that sufferers' descriptions of profound subjective crisis are underpinned by efforts to construct identities as reasoning and considerate parents, children and friends (Drew 2006; Galasiński 2017). This rationalizing does not take place through monologue, however. Rather, members of the community provide accounts of self-injurious behaviour collectively. This collective opinion explains self-harm as a 'means to cope' in an intolerable situation and thereby justifies behaviours that would otherwise be regarded as pathologically irrational. In contrast, sufferers guide each other away from suicide by encouraging their peers to consider the undesirable consequences of ending their own lives. While online contexts that facilitate discussions of self-injurious behaviour have been criticized for encouraging suicide (see Baker and Fortune 2008), the *depression.net* corpus demonstrates the value of online support groups as a place to which people can turn when they feel like they have no one else, where their concerns will be acknowledged, and where others will provide reasons to avoid suicidal behaviour that respond to each sufferers' unique suicidal crisis (Robinson et al. 2016; Wiggins et al. 2016).

5.6 Chapter summary

What emerges from the forum interaction is ultimately not a single discourse of depression but several mixed and at times contradictory ones (Kangas 2001).

Depression is frequently verbally separated from the individual as *the depression* but is also represented as a possession, *my depression*, in the context of discussing strained relationships with friends and family members. The difficulty of personal relationships to which depressed forum members testify provides a clear warrant for their use of online media in which disclosure, empathetic understanding and community solidarity are explicitly encouraged and repeatedly demonstrated.

Taken in sum, these findings point towards the construal of depression as a condition that arises from a sufferer's 'life world' (Mishler 1984) but which comes to be viewed from a biomedical perspective and treated using a biomedical approach. That is, although members of *depression.net* identify situational and psychodynamic antecedents of their illness, their discussions of treatment options focus prevailingly on the individualized pharmacological intervention of antidepressants (Lewis 1995). The confidence expressed in the *right medication* on the forum is particularly surprising, given that individuals for whom the *right medication* facilitates recovery are presumably less likely to use a depression forum for ongoing support. Given that the vast majority of forum members do not claim to be recovered, the value of the *right medication* may therefore lie in its capacity to partially relieve depression, rather than cure it outright (Knudsen et al. 2002).

Constant across each of the aspects of depression presented above is the way in which sufferers' narratives and interactions are suffused with the negotiation of agency, accountability and stigma, both for depression itself and for specific behaviours such as self-harm and suicidal ideation (Lamerichs and te Molder 2003). In this regard, the messages from *depression.net* parallel those of *anorexia.net* and users of both fora draw, moreover, upon biomedical discourse as a resource with which to achieve this negotiation. We return to this issue substantively in Chapter 7, along with the discussion of diabulimia discourse, which we analyse in the next chapter.

Diabulimia

Discourses of chronic illness and mental distress

6.1 Introduction

This third and final analytical chapter explores the discourse surrounding the contested eating disorder known as diabulimia. Echoing the format of the previous chapters, our analysis of the diabulimia support group messages begins with an overview of characteristic words and themes in the corpus using the keywords technique. The analysis then takes a more qualitative turn, utilizing the perspectives of collocation and concordance to explore the wider discourses that surround and constitute the interconnected themes of diabulimia, insulin and diabetes. This chapter therefore addresses diabulimia's status as a dual pathology (involving both insulin restriction and pre-existing type 1 diabetes), which distinguishes it from the other mental disorders explored in this book.

6.2 Establishing themes for analysis

Using the same parameters and reference corpus as in the previous chapters (see Chapter 3), we began by generating keywords for *diabulimia.net*. This yielded a total of seventy-two keywords, which we then grouped into thematic and lexical categories (Table 6.1). As in the preceding chapters, this categorization was based on manual, qualitative analyses of the keywords within their wider contexts of use.

The first thing to note is the thematic overlap between the keywords in this corpus and the other corpora examined in this book. As might be expected, the keywords for all three corpora include those which are related to the management of personal relationships during advice-seeking and advice-giving interactions, including *thanks*, *hope* and *understand* (as in 'I understand'), and

Table 6.1 Key Thematic and Lexical Categories and Associated Keywords of the *diabulimia.net* Corpus, Ranked by Log Ratio (Frequencies in Brackets)

Thematic/lexical category	Associated keywords
Body and weight	*gain* (127), *weight* (559), *loss* (83), *exercise* (77), *body* (161) *lose* (161), *fat* (87), *lost* (89)
Diabetes	*DKA* (72), *complications* (83), *diabetes* (328), *sugars* (68), *diabetic* (117), *diagnosed* (72), *control* (217), *blood* (127), *low* (132), *sugar* (92), *type* (168), *high* (152), *life* (152), *years* (247)
Diabulimia and disordered behaviours	*diabulimia* (202), *disorder* (140), *problems* (74), *since* (109), *less* (85), *months* (84), *problem* (95)
Feelings and emotional responses	*needs* (68), *hard* (123), *feel* (199), *difficult* (62)
Food and eating	*carb* (86), *carbs* (122), *diet* (83), *eating* (316), *food* (136), *eat* (187)
Forum-related	*luck* (70), *hi* (104), *others* (66), *post* (73), *wish* (69), *hope* (122), *thanks* (69), *anyone* (89), *understand* (95), *keep* (154), *best* (95)
Healthcare and health professionals	*doctor* (98), *care* (122)
Insulin	*insulin* (791), *pump* (73), *taking* (173)
Pronouns	*im* (122), *myself* (140), *yourself* (91), *my* (1,402)
Recovery	*healthy* (95), *support* (85), *health* (104), *help* (330)
Other	*etc* (70), *am* (347), *its* (88), *may* (14), *young* (73), *also* (208), *without* (70), *will* (421), *found* (90)

markers of low epistemic modality used to mitigate advice. The consistent theme of 'Feelings and emotional' responses testifies to the discussion of challenging emotional experiences (*hard*) and external phenomena that influence the way contributors feel (*makes*, as in 'makes me feel'). More positively, there are also several repeated keywords related to recovery in each corpus, including *better*, *support* and *trying*. In the diabulimia and anorexia data there are also shared keywords related to body size, food and eating, with both corpora containing significantly frequent uses of *body*, *weight*, *food* and *eating*. However, the differences in keywords between the *anorexia.net* and *diabulimia.net* corpora are equally revealing; the forum moderators on *anorexia.net* prevent users from specifying how they have lost weight, resulting in the use of generic *behaviours* rather than the more explicit *exercise*, which is key in the diabulimia messages. Users of *diabulmia.net* also frequently talk about the specific nutritional content of food using the keywords *carb* and *carbs*. Finally, *fat* is a keyword related to the discussion of the body in the *diabulimia.net* data but not in the *anorexia.net* corpus. These keywords not only point towards the widespread concern with food and body weight in the diabulimia-related messages but also indicate that a concern with the appearance of fatness pervades these messages to a greater extent than those authored by individuals with anorexia.

Like our grouping of the anorexia and depression keywords in the previous chapters, the diabulimia keyword categories are interconnected and overlap with each other. In the interests of space, our focus in this chapter is necessarily selective and will explore the discourses surrounding the interconnected themes of diabulimia, diabetes and insulin. We elected to analyse these themes on the basis of both their statistical salience in the corpus (the lexical instantiations of these themes represent some of the most key, and so most statistically salient lexical items in the data), as well as their significance to the fundamental experience of diabulimia, as a condition that necessarily affects people with pre-existing diabetes. Nevertheless, Table 6.1 provides a clear overview of characteristic words and themes in the messages.

6.3 Lexicalizing diabulimia: Proximity, agency and medicalization

While all of the keywords presented in Table 6.1 are related, more and less directly, to the topic of diabulimia, the keyword *diabulimia* most explicitly instantiates this topic since as it is used to denote or lexicalize the condition across the support group messages. Although this is a relatively small category (in terms of number of keywords), its precise lexical relation to the concept of diabulimia itself renders its constituent keywords as useful analytical entry points for studying the discourses around this contested condition. *Diabulimia* occurred a total of 202 times across 147 individual messages and is also the highest-ranking keyword in the corpus with a log ratio score of 139.79. The salience of this term is to be expected, given that it matches the search term *diabu** that was used to sample threads for the corpus (see Chapter 3, Section 3.2.1) and because *diabulimia* does not appear at all in the reference corpus. However, this was not the only word used to lexicalize diabulimia in the data, for the contributors also used other terms, many of which also matched the search term but did not meet our keyness criteria. Prior to carrying out the keyword procedure, we noted from the frequency output the presence of spelling variations of diabulimia, including *diabulimia*, which occurs twenty-six times along with *diabulima* and *diabullemia*, which each occur twice, and *diabelimia, diabulaemia, diabullimia, dibulemia* and *dibulimia* (once each).[1] As discussed in Chapter 3, this orthographic inconsistency is characteristic of much CMC (Barton and Lee 2013) but also likely reflects the non-official status of the term 'diabulimia' and the condition it denotes. In the remainder of this section, we will explore the discourses surrounding the keyword *diabulimia*.

Before proceeding further, it is important to bear in mind that, despite the readiness with which the contributors appear to use the terms *diabulimia* and, to a lesser extent, *diabulimic* ($n = 23$) in their messages, these terms do not constitute medically legitimate terminology. Consequently, the ascription of experiences and behaviours to *diabulimia* or description of such experiences as *diabulimic* here is unlikely to have followed any medical diagnosis. Due to this, the labels *diabulimia* and *diabulimic* (including their spelling variants) will not necessarily encapsulate the same set of institutionally recognized experiences or behaviours on each occasion of their use across the forum messages. This feature of the data does not present an obstacle with regard to the present study, since its aims are neither to diagnose nor to determine the clinical validity of the experiences contributors construe as being part of *diabulimia*. Whatever the case may be, the initial inspection of word frequency and keyword output suggests that these terms provide a useful interactional resource for the forum contributors, affording them the means for making sense of and communicating about their own and others' experiences and understandings of this health phenomenon.

Our examination of *diabulimia* began with collocation. Like our analysis of anorexia and depression in the previous chapters, we were interested in both the grammatical and lexical collocates of *diabulimia*, and are particularly mindful of the potential for the former to reveal the ways in which the support group contributors encode not only the condition itself but also themselves in relation to it.

The collocational strength of the first-person pronoun, *i*, is particularly noticeable in Table 6.2. *I* was assigned the highest MI[3] value, occurring within the five words preceding or following *diabulimia* a total of sixty-three times across fifty-one support group messages. Along with the first-person possessive, *my*, the prominence of *i* as a collocate of *diabulimia* provides yet further evidence, following the emergence of first-person pronoun keywords earlier in this chapter, of the tendency for contributors to frame diabulimia from their own, first-hand perspectives and experiences, for example:

1.   Hi, yes, **I** had **diabulimia** when **I** was about 18 years old.

Another feature of Table 6.2 worth mentioning at this point is the presence of collocates which reflect messages seeking advice and descriptions regarding

Table 6.2 Top Twenty Collocates of *Diabulimia*, Ranked by MI³

Rank	Collocate	Frequency	MI³
1	*i*	63	14.94
2	*with*	33	14.49
3	*is*	38	14.31
4	*of*	39	14.22
5	*and*	46	14.06
6	*about*	24	13.98
7	*to*	46	13.87
8	*suffered*	9	13.87
9	*have*	31	13.85
10	*a*	39	13.78
11	*from*	20	13.72
12	*the*	40	13.51
13	*called*	8	12.72
14	*years*	14	12.69
15	*had*	16	12.47
16	*struggled*	5	12.37
17	*my*	23	12.33
18	*as*	18	12.25
19	*it*	24	12.16
20	*for*	21	12.13

diabulimia, which in many cases indicate a lack of awareness about what diabulimia actually is. This includes the collocates *of* ($n = 39$, $MI^3 = 14.22$) and *about* ($n = 24$, $MI^3 = 13.98$). In such messages, contributors either inquire about diabulimia or confess to not knowing much about it, even if they then proceed to offer advice and support:

2. I had never heard **of 'diabulimia'**, but I sure know that teenagers, especially girls, are very anxious about their weight.
3. I don't know much **about diabulimia**, but know that there are a lot of us here who are always willing to listen if you just need to vent.

When analysed more qualitatively, then, these collocates help to reveal some of the functions of the messages submitted to the *diabulimia.net* fora. Like *anorexia.net* and *depression.net*, messages are written from contributors' subjective perspectives, including both advice-seeking and advice-giving messages. The collocates *of* and *about* largely feature in messages within which both advice-seekers and -givers indicate that they do not seem to know much about diabulimia, attesting its offline status as a contested and largely unknown phenomenon. Having established this, we turn our attention towards collocates which reveal more about how diabulimia is itself construed and how the contributors position themselves in relation to it.

Examining messages in which the terms in Table 6.2 collocated with *diabulimia*, we observed how some were used by the contributors to either align themselves with diabulimia or distance themselves from it. One manifestation of the distancing constructions, observed earlier in relation to the discourse around anorexia and depression, is the use of the definite article, *the* (n = 40, MI^3 = 13.51). *The* features overwhelmingly as a left-sided collocate of *diabulimia* (n = 36), most frequently in the L1 position, resulting in the expression 'the diabulimia' (n = 10). So, just as contributors to the anorexia and depression fora frequently spoke of 'the ED' or 'the depression', so too do participants in our diabulimia corpus refer to 'the diabulimia', arguably construing the condition as a discrete and countable entity that is detached from the individual experiencing it. For example:

4.   Getting over **the diabulimia** was quite possibly one of the hardest things that I have ever had to do. I was in therapy for quite a while and learning to eat normally again was really hard. I'm really glad that I confronted it though and I wouldn't want to go back down that path again.

5.   I juust wanted to offer you support with **the diabulimia** if you want it. I struggled with Diabulimia for a long time but I've been in recovery for the past 2yrs.

Two other collocates in Table 6.2 which encode this separation between diabulimia and the self are the verb *have* (n = 31, MI^3 = 13.85) and its past-tense variant *had* (n = 16, MI^3 = 12.47), which function as main verbs (Lipták and Reintges 2006), rendering diabulimia as a discrete entity that is possessed by the person experiencing it, rather than being an inherent part of them (Semino 2008: 182) (see, for example, ex. 1). As Fleischman (2001: 491), elaborating on the work of Warner (1976), argues, 'the genitive construction ("I have") casts the pathology as an external object in one's possession' and relocates the pathology *outside* the patient.'

Another, less frequent way in which the forum contributors created distance between diabulimia and themselves (and others) was through a discourse of suffering. As Table 6.2 indicates, the past participle *suffered* (MI^3 = 13.87) co-occurred with *diabulimia* a total of nine times across nine individual messages, in each case as a left-sided collocate. If we consider all realizations of the lemma SUFFER across the corpus (including *suffer*, *sufferer*, *sufferers*, *suffering* and *suffered*) (n = 85), just over half (n = 43; 50.58 per cent) refer either to diabulimia directly or to some perceived consequence of it. This trend also helps to explain the high frequency and strength of *with* and *from* as collocates of *diabulimia*. As discussed in the previous chapter, the dative construction 'SUFFER+*from* diabulimia' implies a degree of separation between the condition and the sufferer, who is here construed as being negatively affected by it (Staiano 1986). In such constructions, diabulimia takes on a causal role in relation to individuals' suffering and is thus distinguishable from them (Fleischman 2001: 491). Likewise, although 'SUFFER+*with* diabulimia' construes the act or state of suffering as a joint experience that involves both diabulimia and the individual experiencing it, it nevertheless conceptualizes diabulimia as an independent agent who, in this case, shares the negative experience of the human sufferer. Examining messages in which the lemma SUFFER was used in reference to diabulimia, we observed the tendency for many of the contributors to construe their suffering as having taken place within more and less specific time periods in the past, as the extracts below demonstrate.

6. Hi guys..I've been type 1 diabetic for almost 5 years...I **suffered** from **diabulimia** (insulin skipping to lose weight) for probably 2.5 years..I stopped this awful habit in August of 2008 but my recovery was followed by the development of gastroparesis and malnutrition as a result.

7. Hi, I **suffered** from **diabulimia** for over 20 years and have been in solid recovery now for close to 4. You are definitely not the only one! Ask any questions you want, I am very open about my journey to recovery and recovery! PS... Welcome to [forum name]!!!

8. I **suffered** quite badly with **diabulimia** when I was younger. Started missing injections and would lose weight as my sugars rose. I then started skipping meals and, before long, was living on not much more than an apple a day. […] It was a really hard thing to conquer but I did manage. I was 15 when it all started and even now, 15 years on, I still find it easy to slip back into old habits if I'm not careful.

The time periods over which these individuals describe suffering diabulimia vary quite significantly. The contributor of extract 6 describes their suffering from diabulimia as lasting for '2.5 years'; a figure that is quite precise, expressed here using a decimal, despite the tempering modality of the preceding adverb, 'probably'. The contributor of extract 7 states that their suffering lasted for over twenty years up to four years before the time of writing. The contributor of extract 8, meanwhile, describes their suffering with diabulimia as occurring 'when I was younger'. Furthermore, while some of the contributors appear to situate their diabulimia-related suffering as impermanent and occurring firmly in the past, others would seem to be more acutely aware of the prospect of the condition returning. As these extracts demonstrate, common to all of the messages in which contributors describe *suffer*[*ing*] with diabulimia is the sense that, rather than being a fixed aspect of their lives, diabulimia is construed as something that can be pinpointed to a more or less specific period in their lives (usually in the past). Even in extract 8, where the time period in which diabulimia-related suffering occurs is vague ('when I was younger'), the experience was situated in a past time; emphasized further by the consistent use of past participles elsewhere in this post. This pattern can also be observed in messages in which *diabulimia* occurs alongside the aforementioned collocate *had*, as well as *years* ($n = 14$, $MI^3 = 12.69$), which tends to feature within the wider context of diabulimia recovery (a theme which we return to later in this chapter):

9.   I've spent 4 **years** getting better from **diabulimia**, I'm only just now
      starting to take regular injections, rather than just one or 2 a day.

It might be that discursively confining their diabulimia-related suffering to a particular period of time, usually in the past, enables these contributors to adopt an ontological perspective on diabulimia and so assume the subject position of a rational observer who is sufficiently detached from the condition so as to be able to examine, and so draw conclusions about, their past experiences of it (Pilgrim and Bentall 1999). This observation was also made in relation to depression in the previous chapter, where we drew parallels between this finding and the work by Galasiński (2008), who argued that the ability to situate illness within a specific past time period allows sufferers to create distance between it and themselves.

As well as allowing the contributors to create temporal distance between diabulimia and themselves, constructions of diabulimia-related experiences as *suffer*[*ing*] also allowed various contributors to adopt the role of experienced expert and to give diabulimia-related advice to other forum members (see, for example, ex. 7). Similarly, despite the distancing function of the 'the diabulimia' formulation, the contributors of extracts 4 and 5 also exhibit a degree of familiarity with diabulimia in their messages for the purposes of giving advice to other members of the support group. In this sense, as well as separating the self from diabulimia, the kinds of distancing constructions discussed above therefore have the potential to figure in users' constructions of themselves as so-called expert patients (Fox et al. 2005), who adopt an arguably more objective tone when referring to 'the diabulimia' when sharing their experiences and giving advice to others members of their respective support groups.

Another way in which the contributors distance themselves from diabulimia is through the past tense verb collocate *struggled* ($n = 5$, $MI^3 = 12.37$), which functions as a lexical instantiation of a violence metaphor. Because they generally lack obvious physical consequences, mental illnesses, including contested conditions like diabulimia, are likely to pose acute problems for sufferers in terms of understanding and communication (Semino 2008: 179). In such cases, metaphor can offer valuable linguistic resources for understanding and articulating subjective experiences and understandings of illness due to their utility for communicating about phenomena that can be linguistically elusive and so otherwise difficult to describe (Sontag 1978; Kövecses 2005). As the examples below indicate, the collocate *struggled* was used to anthropomorphize diabulimia as an adversary against which sufferers were engaged in conflict:

10. Sorry but I think that is a harsh and insensitive comment. Especially for those of us who have **struggled**/are struggling with **Diabulimia**. It is part of a complex and deadly eating disorder that isn't about just omitting insulin.
11. I **struggled** with **diabulimia** for about 3 years before overcoming it. It was a vicious cycle of an eating-disorder and it really took a lot for me to overcome it.

As well as creating distance between themselves and diabulimia by construing it as an external social actor or force with which they were engaged in a struggle (Stewart et al. 2011: 587), the use of *struggled* also allowed the contributors to create temporal distance between themselves and diabulimia. In this sense, the past tense *struggled* functions in a similar way to the past tense *suffered* and the noun *years* considered above insofar as the suffering is located within the past and the contributors are writing in a context in which they consider themselves to have recovered or at least be in recovery. The subject position of the individual who resists and even fights diabulimia might therefore be interpreted as emphasizing the non-volitional nature of these individuals' predicaments (Seale 2001: 309) and their invariable desires to be rid of their condition (Knowles and Moon 2006: 30). They emphasize the violent and predatory nature of diabulimia, while at the same time implying that those experiencing it are acting in defence of themselves, thereby absolving them of responsibility for the onset of the condition (Lupton 1994). Collocates like *struggled* and *suffered* therefore not only create distance between diabulimia and sufferers but also help mitigate sufferers' culpability, challenging broader cultural discourses which conceive of eating disorders as self-inflicted (Crisafulli et al. 2008).

The distancing constructions of diabulimia examined so far can be interpreted as reflecting a broader dualistic framework for understanding and communicating about health and disease, according to which illnesses are commonly represented as external and separable from the individual, while good health is represented as an internal and integral part of the self (Herzlich 1973; Cassell 1976). As Gwyn (2002: 18–19) puts it, 'when we talk of "catching a bug", or of there "being a virus around", our understanding of illness at large is of an "it" that strikes the individual from outside, making him or her ill.' Fleischman (1999: 8–9) argues that this is also the product of a Western cultural tendency to nominalize illnesses and so to linguistically denote them as nouns; she writes, '[n]ouns congeal what is essentially a process into a static state that becomes superimposed on the individual rather than the individual being construed as an integral part of the development of the disease' (see also: Fleischman 2001: 489–90). It seems logical, then, that the distancing constructions examined so far have gravitated around reference to diabulimia using a nominal form. Its comparatively infrequent adjective, *diabulimic*, occurred just twenty-three times across twenty-three texts and thus fell short of our criteria for keyness. However, when we examined messages containing this term, we found that it consistently featured in advice-seeking messages and within the wider context of (attempted) recovery:

12. I am a **diabulimic** and need help. Can anyone suggest a forum for me, book or treatment? Anything? I'm desperate to get better.
13. I just found this web site and need counseling from someone who can relate. I've been a **diabulimic** for 14 years now and glad to know there is finally a name for it and others like me out there.

Although *diabulimia* and *diabulimic* share the same lexical root, they can be distinguished in terms of their discrete lexicogrammatical characteristics, which afford distinctive ways of discursively situating the self in relation to the condition (Fleischman 1999). Broadly speaking, *diabulimia* and *diabulimic* encode two essential means of representing experience, those of 'having' and 'being', respectively (Fromm 1976). By constructing diabulimia as something that they are (*am*) or have *been*, as opposed to something that they *have*, the contributors of these messages arguably convey the sense in which diabulimia is a part of their own (and other sufferers') lives. Indeed, Staiano (1986) argues that to state that 'I am + [condition]', as opposed to 'I have + [condition]' posits an identification with the condition in question, incorporating the pathology as a part of one's individual, personal identity (and see Davies et al. 2011: 175).

Just as contributors who described themselves as being *diabulimic* did so consistently in the wider context of (attempted) recovery, so did those contributors who construed diabulimia as something they possess – that is, 'my diabulimia' (*n* = 6):

14. I guess there's quite some time since I wrote, however I'm better, like I'm not 'cured' from **my diabulimia** however I've gotten a lot of help during the past 9 months, I'm in several groups at the hospital at the eating disorder unit also my D.nurse have been very helpful.

15. Like, when ever I would have my really bad episodes and would end up in dka they assumed that it was just me being irresponsible. Now if I was to tell them that I let that happen, that I made it happen? I'm pretty sure they would loose trust in me. They would support me no matter what but they would try to control every aspect of **my diabulimia** recovery.

Fleischman (1999, 2001) argues the distinction between impersonal, distancing representations of illness and the more personalized constructions in extracts 14 and 15 arises out of the contrast between experiences of acute and chronic illnesses. Perhaps due to being deeply intertwined with individuals' lives (Williams 2000), chronic conditions such as diabetes are more readily constructed in personalizing terms compared to often transitory acute conditions. If we accept this distinction, it might be the case that some of the contributors perceived diabulimia to be a part or even a complication of their (and others') pre-existing diabetes and accordingly constructed diabulimia in similarly aligning terms.

Overall then, and in parallel with the users of *anorexia.net* in Chapter 4 and *depression.net* in Chapter 5, contributors to *diabulimia.net* tended to construct diabulimia as something more aligned to themselves – either as something that they are or as something that they possess – within the wider context of recovery. Ridgway (2001: 338) observed a similar tendency in narratives of recovery from psychiatric disorders, and noted in particular the propensity for individuals to recast themselves, as part of their recovery, from the relatively passive role of sufferer to the comparatively more active role of owner of the illness concerned (see also: Deegan 1994). We return to this in the following chapter. For now, we turn our attention to the ways in which diabulimia was construed as a medical condition – that is, through medicalizing discourses.

Before considering the discursive features that indicate medicalizing conceptions of diabulimia in the support group messages, it is first worth thinking about the potential for the term *diabulimia* itself to perform the function of defining non-medical problems in medical terms (Conrad 1992).

As mentioned in Chapter 2, the label *diabulimia* is a portmanteau of the words *diabetes* and *bulimia*, each medical in origin and denoting diseases with more medical legitimacy than diabulimia. Similarly, the influence of medical language can also be observed in the associated adjective, *diabulimic* – a word whose morphology (particularly the suffix +ic) mirrors the terminology associated with other, medically legitimate diseases, such as diabetes (i.e. *diabetic*), bulimia (*bulimic*) and anorexia (*anorexic*). On the one hand, this appropriation of existing medical labels and morphological choices in the formulation of the term *diabulimia* (and *diabulimic*) could reflect the centrality of modern medicine's conceptual and linguistic frameworks to the ways that people living in Western cultures both think and talk in relation to illness. On the other hand, we could read a little more deeply into the distinctly biomedical tone of the label *diabulimia* (and its morphological variants) and interpret its use as signalling an understanding of diabulimia itself as a medically legitimate disorder like bulimia or anorexia. Further evidence for this interpretation can be seen in the foregoing analysis in this chapter, which has shown that the ways in which diabulimia is referred to in this corpus mirrors the lexicalization of medically recognized mental disorders, namely anorexia and depression, observed in the previous chapters. Specifically, in the collocation-driven analysis reported above, like the contributors to the anorexia and depression support groups, we observed how members of the diabulimia support groups formulated their experiences and understandings of diabulimia in distancing and objectifying terms, with sufferers' agency mitigated.

To explore this issue in more detail, it is necessary to go beyond the lexical item *diabulimia* and its immediate collocates to explore the wider medicalizing discourses and potential counter discourses across the support groups. Specifically, by widening the analytical lens to encompass the concordance lines and wider messages (and threads of messages) in which *diabulimia* is used, we found evidence of arguably more explicit manifestations of medicalizing discourses. For example, many contributors adopted what we interpret to be a diagnostic discourse, diagnosing themselves and others as having diabulimia, describing its symptoms and judging the prototypicality and severity of those symptoms. This discourse was particularly prevalent in messages describing the 'symptom[s]' ($n = 14$) and 'warning sign[s]' ($n = 4$) of diabulimia:

16. **Warning signs** for diabulimia include a change in eating habits – typically someone who eats more but still loses weight – low energy and high blood-sugar levels

The attested symptoms could also be judged in terms of their severity and prototypicality. For example, the contributors of the extracts below describe features of what they perceived to be (and not to be) diabulimia and the characteristics of their own 'severe' diabulimia.

17. **Classic diabulimia** is not a complete renunciation of insulin, that would just be suicide. Diabulimia do enough insulin to barely get by.
18. I had **severe diabulimia** from 20-33 (I was diagnosed at 15). I basically ate all the sugar I could get my hands on and barely injected any insulin.

In each thread in which a contributor disclosed so-called symptoms of diabulimia (namely, reducing insulin intake below practitioner-prescribed levels for the purposes of reducing or controlling their body weight (ex. 17), sometimes in conjunction with 'binge eating' sugar-laden foods, such as ex. 18), that contributor could describe themselves as diabulimic. Messages that included descriptions of insulin restriction and binge-eating practices could also be diagnosed as diabulimia by other forum users in subsequent posts:

19. **you are practicing something called diabulimia** please please talk to someone!! do a google search on this.we have a couple of members here who have gone through this im hoping they see this and answer you.
20. **It sounds to me like diabulimia** - she is eating whatever she wants and not taking enough insulin for the food to actually be absorbed. What she needs is professional help. Sorry, but threatening her in any way won't help.
21. you know what you're doing is dangerous and i think it's great that you are seeking support here, **are you able to do the same thing in 'real life'? are you able to go to your GP/endo/nurse?**

By diagnosing themselves and others as having diabulimia and judging and grading the severity and prototypicality of the attested symptoms, many of the contributors to these support groups can be interpreted as both adopting the position of expert patient (Fox et al. 2005) and propagating a medicalized understanding of diabulimia, subjecting it to the kind of classification that is routinely made of other, medically legitimate mental disorders. In the vast majority of cases, these so-called diagnoses were accompanied by warnings about the negative health consequences associated with diabulimia and the need to resolve the condition at all costs. As extracts 20 and 21 indicate, despite diabulimia lacking official medical recognition, some of the contributors nonetheless implored – or, in keeping with the theme of the expert patient, 'referred' – others to seek advice from a health professional, thereby situating diabulimia-related concerns firmly within the remit of medicine.

At other points across the data, the contributors contested the suggestion that they or another support group member actually had diabulimia. These contestations were made not on the basis of diabulimia's lack of official disease status but rather because the particular experiences or circumstances disclosed were judged not to satisfy the diagnostic criteria for diabulimia, presumably as established within these and other such online communities. Examples of three such passages are provided in extracts 22 to 24.

22. As long as you're not actually using less insulin to raise your BG levels to lose weight...then no, you're **not considered diabulimic**.
23. To [name] and other low carbers, **No, your approach is not diabulimia**, as you are not skipping shots in order to pee out sugar and lose weight. I really can't comment on your overall health, but that is **not diabulimia**.
24. My endo equated what I do with diabulimia, yet my own choices have been accompanied by weight loss, improved health, more energy, disappearing complications, better control (though my Christmas A1C slid back up to 6.0), and a much better prognosis. My war-torn retinas looked great once again last week! **What I do isn't diabulimia** yet I suppose it is close if you only consider it with ignorant eyes. I still take my insulin and have never contemplated not, but my current levels are just below half of what they were four years ago – <50u vs 120u.

The contributors of extracts 22 and 23 each resolve that because other group members' insulin restriction was not motivated by the desire to lose weight, they cannot be considered diabulimic. The contributor of extract 24, meanwhile, refutes an endocrinologist's suggestion that they have diabulimia on the grounds that they still take some insulin (even if not necessarily in prescribed amounts). Such is the influence of the medicalizing perspective within these contexts, then, that even when online diabulimia diagnoses are refuted, such refutations are made not because diabulimia is not officially an illness, but rather because the reported 'symptoms' do not fit with the diagnostic criteria established within and by such online communities. The expression, 'I suppose it is close if you only consider it with ignorant eyes' in extract 24 is tellingly disparaging of the practitioner's perspective (as 'ignorant'), perhaps enforcing the sense in which it is the contributors to this and other such online communities, rather than medical professionals, who are truly the knowledgeable 'experts' when it comes to diabulimia (an observation also made by Fox et al. (2005) in relation to online diabetes support groups).

Returning to Table 6.2, we initially suspected that the high-ranking collocate *called* (n = 8, MI^3 = 12.72) might signal a counter discourse to the kinds of medicalizing constructions identified so far in this chapter; one that reflected diabulimia's non-official status. However, upon analysing posts containing this collocational pairing we found that while the faltering modality implied by the word 'called' did seem to indicate uncertainty over the legitimacy of the term *diabulimia*, such messages did not call into question diabulimia's legitimacy as a disease. Indeed, even when pre-modified by *called*, *diabulimia* was nevertheless used to reify this condition as an eating disorder. Of the seven occurrences of *called diabulimia*, one was in reference to the establishment of a diabulimia thread. The remaining six are reproduced in extracts 25 to 30.

25. I misuse my insulin for years, had poor control and never tested. It can get you into a cycle **called diabulimia**, without realizing it.
26. I have been looking at various posts on so **called 'Diabulimia'** and feel for all Type 1 diabetics struggling with weight.
27. As others have stated, what you are doing is actually known as a dangerous eating disorder **called Diabulimia**. It's an easy trap to get stuck in but it IS a trap and is very difficult to get out of. Please take care.
28. Thousands of the approximately 1 million people with Type 1 (or juvenile-onset) diabetes are willing to take the risk. Mostly teenagers and young women, they suffer from a unique eating disorder **called diabulimia**.
29. Some people do, it's certainly not the norm and it is a dangerous thing to do. It's **called diabulimia** although I don't think it has an official clinical name.
30. you are heading towards a path that has severe trouble at the end.recently it is coming more and more to light you are practicing something **called diabulimia**.

As well as not explicitly questioning the medical legitimacy of diabulimia (despite using *called*), these extracts variously evidence some of the other medicalizing features witnessed in other posts, including describing it as a 'dangerous eating disorder' (27) and 'unique eating disorder' and offering prevalence figures for it (both ex. 28). So, the collocate *called* does not indicate hesitation or contestation of the perception of diabulimia as a medical disorder, or for that matter the legitimacy of others' suffering, but rather reflects the uncertainty surrounding its terminology.

Most of the foregoing analysis in this chapter has focused on the discourse surrounding the keyword *diabulimia* and, to a lesser extent, the adjective *diabulimic*. However, the final part of the analysis in this section will focus on the other keyword used to lexicalize diabulimia: *disorder* (see Table 6.1). As well as describing diabulimia as a *disorder* ($n = 12$, ex. 31–2), the support group contributors also described it as an *eating disorder* ($n = 123$, ex. 27–8 and 32) and, on one occasion, as a *mental disorder* (ex. 33):

31. I had Diabulimia and was seriously unwell with it. It is a horrendous **disorder** to have and the mortality rate is exceptionally high due to DKA and the complications associated with it.

32. I think what we might be missing here is that this is an **eating disorder**... not terribly different from anorexia or bulimia... it's not a healthy diet, it's a **disorder**.

33. It [diabulimia] is a complicated **mental disorder** that is absolutely terrifying not only for those suffering from it but for their friends and family as well.

In extract 32, diabulimia is not only described as an 'eating disorder' and a 'disorder', but is also likened to other medically recognized diseases (anorexia and bulimia) – 'not terribly different from anorexia or bulimia'. To further investigate this comparison between diabulimia and more recognized eating disorders, we examined messages mentioning *anorexia* and *bulimia* in this corpus. Some of these messages exhibited the terminological collectivization (Jones 2013) of diabulimia with these other disorders. Extracts 34 to 36 below demonstrate broadly the three ways in which this collectivization occurred.

34. With so many teenagers suffering from **bulimia** and **anorexia**, I suppose this is the same thing but in another form. I think teenager girls with diabetes need a lot more attention to make sure they don't fall into these pitfalls.

35. Myself I have suffered from **anorexia** and **bulimia**, for some reason never done the omitting insulin thing, just all the rest!

36. there are psychogenic causes, but I thought I had read something about altered brain chemistry, as well, in **anorexia** and **bulimia**?

Diabulimia is likened here to anorexia and bulimia, described in extract 34 as 'the same thing but in another form'. However, this connection is more implicit in extract 35, the author of which is seemingly at a loss to explain why they had not had diabulimia, having experienced anorexia and bulimia in the past, writing: 'I have suffered from anorexia and bulimia, for some reason never done the omitting insulin thing, just all the rest!' (where the expression 'all the rest' also serves to collectively group diabulimia with these other disorders). Finally, the contributor of extract 36 situates diabulimia firmly within a biomedical discourse by attributing its causes to biological and neurological complications – that is, to (vaguely worded) 'psychogenic causes' and 'altered brain chemistry', the latter presented, once more, as the cause of anorexia and bulimia.

The analysis presented so far in this chapter has revealed the tendency for members of the support groups in the *diabulimia.net* corpus to construe their subjective experiences and understandings of diabulimia using what we have interpreted as medicalizing discourses. We will return to this finding in the concluding section of this chapter. For now, we turn our attention to the theme of insulin.

6.4 Insulin: Restriction, abuse and (mis)use

The discussion of insulin was indexed most directly in this corpus by the keywords *insulin* (791), *pump* (73) and *taking* (173). Although this constitutes a small number of keywords compared to some of the other categories in Table 6.1, its top keyword, *insulin*, is one of the strongest keywords in the entire corpus (ranked fourth, *log ratio* = 11.66). This, coupled with the fact that restriction of insulin is diabulimia's most essential characteristic, means that this theme warrants closer focus. In this section, we analyse the discourses surrounding the word *insulin*, although *taking* also makes an appearance as a strong collocate of this keyword. Table 6.3 shows the top twenty collocates of *insulin* (L5>R5), ranked by MI^3.

The first collocates we want to explore in this section are those which denote weight and weight loss – namely, *weight* and *lose*. In the majority of posts containing these collocates, insulin was construed as causing weight gain, for example:

37. I was diagnosed with type 1 diabetes in 2004,,I educated myself very quickly on it through books and internet, thats when i discovered that **insulin** = **weight** gain...

38. That is why we T2 are usually fat, first we get insulin resistant then the pancreas pumps out EXTRA insulin to overcome the resistance now we have a lot of insulin in our blood and we gain **weight**. the extra **insulin**

also prevents us from berning the fat. I saw a study about 20 years ago where they tracked some 500 people. They found that people in the study that became diabetic would suddenly gain about 20 Lb with no change in food or exercise BEFORE being diagnosed as diabetic.

The representation of insulin as the cause of unwanted weight gain in these and other forum posts implies an uneasy relationship between the self and diabetes. Establishing insulin as the cause of weight gain also helps to rationalize the practice of insulin restriction for weight loss, while at the same time offering these and other members the opportunity to mitigate any culpability that might be attached to them for their attested gains in body weight (Markula et al. 2008). Indeed, presenting such weight gain as a corollary of insulin therapy allows the forum members to maintain the identity of the disciplined diabetic who has their chronic disease under control (Peel et al. 2005), since weight gain is framed as resulting from adherence to prescribed diabetes regimen and not, say, the consumption of sugary and calorie-laden food.

This positive self-presentation is re-enforced by references to scientific and medical forms of knowledge that could index an identity of expert patient. For

Table 6.3 Top Twenty Collocates of *Insulin*, Ranked by MI^3

Rank	Collocate	Frequency	MI^3
1	*to*	276	19.66
2	*taking*	93	19.43
3	*and*	196	18.37
4	*the*	189	18.27
5	*weight*	101	18.09
6	*i*	184	17.61
7	*of*	134	17.60
8	*on*	97	17.31
9	*my*	110	17.14
10	*take*	59	17.00
11	*your*	87	16.89
12	*not*	87	16.79
13	*that*	102	16.45
14	*is*	98	16.44
15	*a*	111	16.33
16	*for*	82	16.06
17	*skipping*	23	15.65
18	*less*	30	15.56
19	*lose*	37	15.54
20	*with*	66	15.52

example, the author of extract 37 describes educating themselves about diabetes following their diagnosis. Similarly, extract 38 supports the claim that insulin therapy induces weight gain with reference to a scientific study demonstrating this link. This post is also notable for its use of technical jargon to describe the internal biological processes involved in insulin-related weight gain, including invoking the concept of 'insulin resistance' (Reaven 1988). In drawing on such biomedical discourses, these and other forum members appropriate what van Leeuwen (2008) terms the 'authority of expertise' to legitimize through scientific validation the claim that insulin intake induces weight gain.

Descriptions of insulin-induced weight gain could also be quite detailed and specific. This pattern emerged in posts mentioning *insulin*, if not necessarily in conjunction with *weight*:

39. I'm so ashamed to admit this but yes, I have done this many many times before I went onto the pump. I was and still am very critical about my weight. A few pounds gained gets me upset but when I gained nearly 30 lbs when I went on **insulin** I went nuts. I would never do such a thing these days.

40. I've gained 30lbs in the past two months being on **insulin** and it's incredibly difficult to break the cycle.

41. Is it really more difficult to lose weight when you're on **insulin** than for non-d people? I've heard this before, but I have no experience. I was skinny as a rail by the time they put me on **insulin** 5 years ago, and I gained about 5 pounds in the first few months. Well, over the past year, since i got off of the EVIL mixed **insulin** and got my b/s under control I've gained another 5...and at 5 ft tall these 10 pounds ain't looking so hot! So I just want to know FOR REAL, if this is going to be some major uphill battle, or if it's really no different that before D.

The authors of these and other posts offer quantified presentations of themselves and their bodies, in each case describing in detail the number of pounds (lbs) gained as a result of taking insulin. Recalling the statistical ways in which bodies tend to be conceived of and talked about within society more broadly (Lupton 2016), this kind of precise quantification can also be compared to the level of numerical precision observed elsewhere in studies of sufferers' accounts of eating disorders (Day and Keys 2008). Yet, Potter et al. (1991: 333) argue that such numerical niceties can also perform a rhetorical function. In this context, we would argue that the kinds of precise quantification of weight gained because of insulin are not *just* a verbal flourish designed to underscore the extent of the weight gain but also have a kind of evidential quality. Forum posts postulating the causal link between insulin and weight gain thus, we would argue, exhibit features that help to legitimize their claims, including presenting the self as knowledgeable, invoking scientific and medical expertise and giving precise quantification of the amount of weight that individuals attest to gaining as a result of taking insulin. The reason why this discourse equating insulin with weight gain might require legitimation in this context is that, although it is a majority discourse, it was also contested. For instance:

42. I don't believe **insulin** in itself causes **weight** gain at all. when I was first put on insulin I had been eating everything in sight for months and months, and losing weight like crazy...I must confess that I would have enjoyed that freedom if I hadn't been so sick! But eating like that was a hard habit to break.

43. Hospitals sometimes give insulin to non-diabetic patients to induce appetite and weight gain. It works. I don't believe **insulin** needs to cause **weight** gain, but a cycle of too much insulin followed by increased caloric intake will lead to weight gain.

44. The part **insulin** plays in **weight** gain is where insulin has not been carefully matched to carb intake or basal requirements.

These extracts provide representative examples of the ways in which the discourse of insulin causing weight gain could be challenged, with contributors framing weight gain as being more likely to result from poor management of diabetes, including not matching insulin dose to calorie intake. The author of extract 43, for example, suggests that insulin-related weight gain is likely the result of 'a cycle of too much insulin followed by increased caloric intake', while the author of extract 44 proposes that insulin intake causes weight gain when 'insulin has not been carefully matched to carb intake or basal requirements'. Perhaps indicating their minority status in this context, such claims tended to be carefully hedged. For example, both the authors of extracts 42 and 43 state that they don't 'believe' insulin causes weight gain – a lexical choice which shrouds this proposition in relatively weak epistemic modality. It is worth bearing in mind that posts challenging the connection between insulin and weight gain were in the minority, and for every one of the posts like those above, we found four cases that asserted that insulin *does* cause weight gain. So, the majority discourse in this context equates insulin therapy with weight gain, but this too is a site of discursive contest, and not all contributors were in agreement.

The next set of collocates we want to consider are those which denote either the practice of taking or not taking insulin, including the lexical verbs *taking*, *take* and *skipping*. Relatedly, the negating adverb *not* tends to be used to modify *taking* in clauses like 'not taking insulin' or 'not taking enough insulin'. In fact, the majority of the collocates in Table 6.3 tend to feature in formulations which lexicalize the act of insulin restriction. For example, the collocates *take* and *taking* occur in tri-grams like 'not taking insulin' ($n = 33$), 'stopped taking insulin' ($n = 9$), 'stop taking insulin' ($n = 5$), 'not take insulin' ($n = 5$) and 'take less insulin' ($n = 4$). Similarly, and as this final example attests, the collocate *less* tends to function as a degree adverb to convey that someone is taking or has taken less insulin than prescribed. If we go beyond the collocates displayed in Table 6.3 and include weaker collocates of *insulin*, we find a plethora of other collocates which function as verbs or nominalizations denoting insulin restriction, including (minimum frequency 2): *skip* ($n = 18$), *stop* ($n = 17$), *reduce* ($n = 15$), *stopped* ($n = 13$), *reducing* ($n = 11$), *cut* ($n = 9$), *omitting* ($n = 8$), *manipulating* ($n = 6$), *skipped* ($n = 6$), *cutting* ($n = 4$), *decrease* ($n = 4$), *lower* ($n = 4$), *abusing* ($n = 3$), *adjust* ($n = 3$), *drop* ($n = 3$), *manipulation* ($n = 3$), *omission* ($n = 3$), *quit* ($n = 3$), *restrict* ($n = 3$), *stopping* ($n = 3$), *underdosing* ($n = 3$), *withhold* ($n = 3$), along with *abuse*, *avoid*, *limit*, *limited*, *lowering*, *minimizing*, *reduction*, *restricting*, *restriction*, *short* and *withholding* (each $n = 2$). Perhaps unsurprisingly, in the majority of cases these collocates occurred as part of the contributors' lexicalizations of their own or others' insulin restriction. In analysing these posts (such as ex. 45 below), we observed a curious tendency for support group members to describe (ostensibly their own) insulin restriction in conceptually vague and distancing terms. For example, contributors rarely gave details about how frequently they skipped insulin or about how much insulin they omitted (in fact, such information features in just 2 per cent of posts describing insulin-restricting practices).

45.   8 years ago, before hearing the term 'diabulimia' I decided to **reduce** my **insulin** intake as well in order to lose some weight. I maintained my basal injections, but hardly ever gave a bolus (regardless of correction bolus or food bolus). I did this for probably 4-5 months and ended up losing 40 pounds. It got to a point though where I started getting so thirsty that I would consistently eat more as well, and my portion sizes became outrageous. At 125 pounds, I could sit down and eat an entire large pizza and not think twice. Kind of crazy looking back.

This feature of the data becomes even more marked when we compare it to the types of quantification we saw earlier in descriptions of the amounts of weight gained from taking insulin. Similarly, the author of this post also gives precise figures pertaining to their body weight ('at 125 pounds'), the amount of weight they lost ('ended up losing 40 pounds'), and when and for how long their insulin restriction took place ('8 years ago', 'probably 4-5 months').

The general vagueness with which the contributors described their insulin restriction, at least relative to other aspects of their bodies and health, could constitute a strategy for downgrading or backgrounding the severity of their disordered practices. Such an interpretation is supported, moreover, by the tendency for the contributors to linguistically distance themselves from their insulin restriction. For example, by evaluating their insulin restriction as 'kind of crazy looking back', the contributor of extract 45 is able to situate themselves within the less stigmatizing role of rational and disapproving observer in relation to their previous insulin-restricting practices (Galasiński 2008). Another notable feature of this extract is the way in which this support group member distances themselves from the label 'diabulimia' itself, stating that their insulin restriction predates their 'hearing the term "diabulimia"', perhaps to anticipate the charge that they are engaging in something faddish or 'jumping on the bandwagon', such is often the public perception of diabulimia (Sharma 2013).

The vague and distancing constructions of insulin-restricting practices observed here as well as in the discourses surrounding *diabulimia* considered earlier might thus constitute a means for support group members to avoid critical responses from other forum users (Armstrong et al. 2011). Indeed, we can find evidence of such responses in this corpus; disclosures of insulin restriction were most likely to be met with warnings from other forum users who alluded to the risks associated with diabulimia:

46.   As others have said **omitting insulin** to loose weight is highly dangerous and is really not worth the risk.

In addition to being perceived as risky, insulin restriction was also construed as a form of deviance. According to Clinard and Meier (2011: 6), deviance can be considered 'a collection of conditions, persons, or acts that society disvalues [...], finds offensive [...], or condemns'. Deviance discourses manifested most explicitly in contributors' references to insulin-restricting practices using the lemmas ABUSE and MISUSE:

47.   I **misuse** my **insulin** for years, had poor control and never tested. It can get you into a cycle called diabulimia, without realizing it. Not saying that is what you are do or have, but that is what I did. For me, it last from my teens

into my thirties. Now am 35, and for the first time have been healthy for the last 4 years, with my diabetes in control, since my diagnosis age age 8.

48. My daughter was diagnosed with diabetes at 12 (not a great age with hormones kicking in :( ) and developed 'disordered eating' pretty soon after. She is nearly 18 and has been **abusing insulin** ever since. How she has managed to survive until now is beyond belief and is currently taking basal insulin to try and retain some stability. However, she is still abusing and has now confided she is taking it 3 days a week Mon,Tue, Wed, and then stopping. She is binge eating thur, fri, sat, sun and running deliberately with high ketones to get rid of the weight she has put on in those 4 days. She can lose anything up to a stone in a week. :(She has been staying with her father who is in complete denial there is a problem, but we have spent the weekend in tears where I have managed to get her to admit exactly the extent of what she is doing so will obviously be acting immediately. I am currently researching as much as I can to find the support she needs.

The author of extract 47 groups their insulin misuse with their 'poor' diabetes control, going on to equate recovery from diabulimia with being 'healthy' and having their diabetes 'in control'. Similarly, the author of extract 48 indicates that she is surprised that her daughter is still alive, such is the extent of her insulin 'abus[e]'. This contributor also constructs their daughter's actions as secretive and even shameful by lexicalizing her disclosure about her insulin restriction using lexical choices like 'confided' and 'admit'.

In contrast to constructions of diabulimia as a form of deviance, in a minority of the forum posts insulin restriction was actually represented as a normal means of effective and autonomous diabetes management, seemingly on the proviso that it occurs in conjunction with the appropriate reduction of calorie intake (i.e. not restricting insulin dosage to compensate for excessive calorie intake, or 'bingeing' (Littlefield et al. 1992)):

49. As long as he is **taking** enough **insulin** to cover what he eats then there is really nothing wrong with 'abusing' your insulin to 'eat things you shouldn't'. Personally, I don't have any forbidden food or drink list (I drink regular soda) and I keep my control perfect all the time. Your concern should be that he does take enough insulin when he eats higher carb/sugar foods. It will not harm him at all if he takes the right amount of insulin to cover it. I think your husband probably knows what he's doing, there is nothing wrong with what he is doing.

Forum posts construing calculated insulin restriction as a potentially normal and even medically legitimate means of managing one's diabetes were, however, in the minority, for, as we have seen, the contributors were more likely to represent diabulimia as a deviant and risky practice, even while there is some overlap between diabulimic and medically sanctioned insulin use in this context. Discussing different weight loss practices, Malson (2008) argues that it is through the labelling of certain practices as 'normal' that others come to be regarded as pathological. In the support groups represented in this corpus, 'normative' diabetes management tends to be construed as incongruous with insulin restriction except, for a minority of the contributors, if it occurs in conjunction with careful management of calorie intake.

6.5 Diabetes: Chronic illness, eating disorders and control

We now turn our attention to the discourse surrounding diabetes in this corpus. The salience of the theme of diabetes across the support group messages was initially indicated by the plethora of keywords surrounding this topic in Table 6.1. These are *DKA, complications, diabetes, sugars, diabetic, diagnosed, control, blood, low, sugar, type, high, life* and *years*.

That this category had the highest number of keywords (fourteen) might be expected, given that this corpus consists of posts from diabetes fora. This notwithstanding, the quantity of diabetes-related keywords also attests the centrality of this theme to many of the messages in the corpus. Owing to limitations of space, we cannot carry out a fine-grain examination of all of these diabetes-related keywords. Therefore, our analysis will focus on the most frequent of these words, *diabetes* (n = 328, *log ratio* = 8.61). By dint of its high frequency, statistical salience and direct lexical relation to the theme of diabetes, this keyword should afford a promising avenue through which to explore how the discourses surrounding this topic contribute to the broader discursive construal of diabulimia in the support groups. As in the previous section, our analysis of the keyword began with collocation. Table 6.4 lists the top twenty collocates of *diabetes*.

As in our earlier analysis of *diabulimia*, the use of MI³ to rank the collocates of *diabetes* has produced a mixture of lexical and grammatical collocates. *Type* features overwhelmingly in the formulations 'type 1 diabetes' (n = 16) and 'type 2 diabetes' (n = 5), *behavioral* consistently features as part of the phrase

Table 6.4 Top Twenty Collocates of *Diabetes*,
Ranked by MI³

Rank	Word	Frequency	MI³
1	*and*	107	17.02
2	*my*	77	16.86
3	*with*	60	16.37
4	*of*	65	15.73
5	*the*	78	15.71
6	*type*	28	15.54
7	*to*	73	15.17
8	*a*	56	14.64
9	*i*	62	14.17
10	*control*	22	14.13
11	*in*	39	14.07
12	*have*	36	13.80
13	*is*	39	13.73
14	*eating*	22	13.59
15	*behavioral*	6	13.27
16	*for*	32	13.26
17	*uk*	9	13.17
18	*clinical*	5	13.16
19	*disorder*	12	13.01
20	*managing*	5	12.70

'behavioral diabetes institute' ($n = 6$), an American non-profit organization focusing on social and psychological support for diabetes, while *uk* occurs in reference to the charity Diabetes UK. Several of the grammatical collocates indicate how contributors to the support groups linguistically situate diabetes in relation to themselves and others, including as something that people *have*, possess (i.e. *my*) and live *with*. Rather than engaging in a full analysis of how the support group members construe themselves and others in relation to diabetes (as we did earlier for diabulimia), we will use this space to explore the discourses around diabetes specifically as these relate to diabulimia. Therefore, the analysis in this section will first examine the link between diabetes and eating disorders by examining messages in which the keyword *diabetes* occurred alongside *eating* ($n = 22$, $MI³ = 13.59$) and/or *disorder* ($n = 12$, $MI³ = 13.01$). Since the frequencies of these collocational pairings are relatively low, to expand the scope of our analysis and account for a wider range of discourses, we also examined messages containing *diabetes* and *eating* or *disorder*, even if these co-occurrences did not necessarily occur within the collocation span stipulated earlier (in other words, in messages in which these words both occurred but more than five words apart).

In the majority of messages mentioning *diabetes* alongside *eating* and/ or *disorder*, contributors construed diabetes as a condition that heightens susceptibility to eating disorders, including, and in some cases specifically, diabulimia.

50.   Based on what you have written, it sounds to me that your fiancée's sister has a form of **eating disorder** which compounds (or is compounded by) her Type 1 **diabetes**. She found a way to lose weight while eating unhealthy highly refined carb food by fiddling with her insulin intake. It's a double whammy for her, as she has no control over her **diabetes** and has an **eating disorder**.

51.   I told my endo back in the 80's that having type 1 **diabetes** makes you ripe for an **eating disorder** (bingeing & purging was my specialty). She looked at me and said, 'You just don't let it control you.' Funny, that's just what they tell women in **eating disorder** programs.

52.   This doesn't shock me at all. The beginning of my **eating disorder** started probably around a year before my **diabetes** diagnosis, i then suffered from anorexia, but mainly bulimia from age 17-21. I think **diabetes** played a part in me developing a fully blown **eating disorder**. i felt very restricted in what i could eat, felt guilty for **eating** something 'bad'.

In these representative extracts, diabetes is variously construed as something that both 'compounds' and is 'compounded by' eating disorders, as well as something that makes people 'ripe for' and 'play[s] a part in' eating disorders. In extract 52, this heightened susceptibility is attributed, explicitly and quite precisely, to the demands of diabetes self-management, when the contributor describes feeling 'very restricted in what i could eat' and as feeling 'guilty for eating something "bad"'. The notion that disordered eating can be caused, or at least exacerbated (ex. 51), by the dietary restraint necessitated by diabetes self-management is considered as a possible cause of diabulimia by Goebel-Fabbri, who writes,

> [i]t may be that the current goals of intensive diabetes management increase the risk for developing an eating disorder. Some researchers argue that the attention to food portions (especially carbohydrates), blood sugars, weight, and exercise that comprises the standard recommended medical treatment for type 1 diabetes parallels the rigid thinking about food and body image that is characteristic of women who have eating disorders but do not have diabetes.

(Goebel-Fabbri 2008: 530)

Another theme in the discourse surrounding diabetes indicated by the collocates shown in Table 6.4 is diabetes control. Specifically, this theme is suggested by the frequent collocate *control* ($n = 22$, $MI^3 = 14.13$), which was also a keyword in this corpus. The concept of control is widely understood to be salient both with regard to the self-management of chronic illnesses, particularly diabetes (Broom and Whittaker 2004; Peel et al. 2005; Naemiratch and Manderson 2006), and in relation to subjective experiences of eating and purging disorders (Neumark-Sztainer et al. 2006; Burns and Gavey 2008; Evans et al. 2008). In the support group interactions represented in the *diabulimia.net* corpus, the concept of control was drawn upon in relation to diabetes and within the broader construal of diabulimia in various ways, which we will explore now.

In most cases, diabulimia was construed as something that constituted a lack of control over diabetes on the part of its sufferers. In these messages in particular, the keyword *control* took on a distinctly biomedical connotation, used mainly in reference to diabetes management in terms of controlling diabetes and the body, including blood glucose, diet, calorie intake, all in accordance with a practitioner-determined self-management regime. As such, diabulimia and other 'disordered' practices were frequently equated with poor control or a lack of control on the part of those affected:

53. I wish I had willpower to achieve the same, but with my eatng habits out of **control**, my **diabetes** out of **control** my last result was 14.6% I feel like a failure!! Im now attending counselling to battle my food demons, so hopefully I'll be on the road to recovery and get both the **diabetes** and eating disorder under **control**!!!

54. Sometimes, I look at the big picture and it's just so huge, scary and overwhelming and like I said before, I still don't have perfect **diabetes control**. But, instead, I try and take it on a day by day, sometimes an hour by hour approach. If I mess up, I accept I've done so and move on and try again.

Consistent with this logic, not having diabulimia – that is, not engaging in deliberate insulin restriction – was construed as an indicator that a person was in control of their diabetes or had 'good' or 'great' control over it. For example, in extract 55, diabulimia is judged to be 'out of the question' among the members of one of the support groups on the basis that its regular contributors have 'great control':

55. Many of the regulars here have great **control** so diabulimia is out of the question.

These types of messages can be interpreted as exhibiting a neoliberal discourse of chronic disease management. Neoliberalism is a contemporary political movement which advocates economic liberalization, free trade and open markets (Harvey 2005). As a theory of political and economic practice, it proposes that 'human wellbeing can best be advanced by liberating individual entrepreneurial freedoms and skills within an institutional framework characterised by strong private property rights, free markets, and free trade' (Kwan and Graves 2013: 5–6). Neoliberalism has played an increasingly central role in the ways that Western societies are governed, which has led to social services (including healthcare), state-owned enterprises and indeed some aspects of government itself, all working with, and in some cases being supplanted by, private industries operating in a context of economic deregulation and tax cuts (Steger and Roy 2010). The neoliberal political project is supported by, and supportive of, the reconfiguration of expert knowledge and power, whereby it is taken away from the 'bureau-professionals of the welfare state' and reassigned to managers, auditors, consumers and the market (Mulderrig 2018: 41). As a consequence, social relations are reshaped, whereby individuals are positioned as responsible and risk-prepared citizen–consumers, meanwhile the state acts as an enabling force which promotes a 'neoliberal political rationality' (Glasgow 2012: 1) by 'enticing or nudging citizens to "take responsibility" for their lives and their communities' (Peeters 2013: 584). Neoliberalism is underpinned by personal responsibility, with Foucault arguing that neoliberal governments maintain social order and prosperity by relying on citizens to manage their bodies and their health voluntarily rather than having to be coerced or threatened with punitive measures (Foucault 1973, 1979). From this perspective, the management of chronic illnesses (like health more generally) becomes the responsibility of the individual (Burchell 1993), more so than medical authorities or the state, to the extent that it is the individual who is held personally culpable when things go wrong and ill health occurs (Galvin 2002).

This sense of responsibility for failing to maintain health is evident across messages in *diabulimia.net*. For example, the contributor of extract 53 laments their lack of control over their eating and diabetes, citing their lack of 'willpower' which causes them to 'feel like a failure'. Tellingly, the level of control that this contributor exhibits over their diabetes is self-judged to be inadequate in accordance with the biomedical measurement of glycaemic control (Bray and Colebrook 1998), expressed here as a percentage figure of 14.6 per cent. In this very same message, the contributor also demonstrates their desire to (re)harness control, attesting to having attended counselling sessions in order to 'get both the diabetes and eating disorder under control'. Similarly, though seemingly not as self-condemnatory, the author of extract 54 appropriates the same neoliberal discourse of diabetes self-management when equating not having 'perfect' control with their 'mess[ing] up'; a responsibilizing construction which locates the duty of effective diabetes management and 'control' firmly with the individual experiencing the condition, in this case, the contributor themselves, who also assumes responsibility – or in this case, blame – when things go wrong (Gomersall et al. 2011).

Yet, as alluded to above, neoliberal frameworks apply not just to the management of illness but have the power to influence all aspects of our lives. Indeed, if we expand our analysis to consider messages which mention the keyword *control* (not just in conjunction with *diabetes*), we find evidence of diabulimia and other eating disorders being equated not just with a lack of control over diabetes but also over one's life more generally (see also Chapter 4, Section 4.4). For example, in the extracts below, diabulimia is linked with feeling 'so out of control' (ex. 56), while recovery from an eating disorder is equated to 'taking back control of your life, your eating disorder [diabulimia] and your diabetes' (ex. 57).

56. I've been saying I wish I could be committed for years because I feel so out of **control** :(I've got [name] on Facebook, I hope that this group helps to get this problem better recognised in the medical profession.
57. I'm glad you're taking back **control** of your life, your eating disorder and your diabetes.
58. You start by thinking that you are in **control** and can stop whenever you want to but before you realise what has happened you have been stripped of all **control** and the eating disorder seems to take **control** of your life and won't stop at anything.

The message reproduced in the final extract above contains three separate references to the keyword *control*, all of which testify to distinct but seemingly sequential stages of experiencing an eating disorder, which in this case is diabulimia. The contributor attests to 'start[ing] by thinking that you are in control', but then to having been 'stripped of all control' by the eating disorder, which ultimately 'take[s] control of your life and won't stop at anything'. Much like the representation of anorexia in Chapter 4 as something that 'take[s] all the control', the ultimate lack of control experienced by this diabulimia sufferer is rendered all the more striking by the anthropomorphization of diabulimia as an agentive and oppressive force which 'strip[s]' the sufferer of control, 'takes' control, and 'won't stop at anything'. This equating of diabulimia with a lack of control provides further evidence of the acute sense of powerlessness experienced by people with diabulimia, identified in our analysis of *diabulimia* earlier in this chapter, and which is comparable to the experience of powerlessness in some people with anorexia (see Chapter 4).

In analysing messages containing the keyword *control*, we also observed an alternative discourse to that explored in the previous section. Rather than construe diabulimia as signifying a lack of control, for a minority of the contributors, diabulimia actually offered a means for harnessing control over various aspects of their lives. For example, in the extracts below, diabulimia is construed as a means for people to control their weight.

59. Your daughter has worked out how to harness the power of insulin, or rather the lack of it, to help her **control** her weight. I'm certain she's bright enough to realise the lasting damage she will do to her body without insulin.
60. My hba1c went from 8 to 11 but I felt fine so I kept abusing the power I had to **control** my weight. I dread the thoughts of putting on weight.
61. Possibly for the first time in my life I feel I can **control** my weight, losing steadily and then reach a point where I can maintain the weight.

Tellingly, in two of the above messages, diabulimia, or at least the weight loss potential that it affords, is lexicalized as *power*, described in extract 59 as the 'power of insulin, or rather the lack of it' and in extract 60 as the 'power I had to control my weight'. As well as affording individuals a measure of control over their weight, the seemingly empowering properties of diabulimia could also take on a broader significance in the forum messages, construed as a means for individuals to take control over their lives more generally, typically where pre-existing diabetes and the demands of self-management were perceived to have taken this away.

62. We are burdened with an incurable condition and anything which gives us some degree of **control** over it can be abused without the right sort of long term care.
63. What some people dont seam to understand is that it feels like you dont have **control** of your life (I know this sounds strange to anyone reading it) you are constantly at the beck and call of your insulin and sometime you do forget (during stressfull times) I promice you it will get better but its not going to happen overnight.

Speaking in quite general terms, the author of extract 62 characterizes the experience of diabetes as being 'burdened' with an 'incurable condition' and goes on to suggest that diabulimia (or more specifically the weight loss induced by reducing insulin intake) gives people 'some degree of control' over diabetes. However, it is worth noting that despite this seemingly empowering discourse, this forum member nonetheless construes diabulimia in deviant terms (as 'abus[e]') and also suggests that diabulimia might result from inadequate long-term care. Furthermore, the author of extract 63, again in general terms, describes not having control of 'your life' due to the constant demands of diabetes self-management, that is, the 'beck and call of your insulin'. This discourse, of diabetes as burdensome and even controlling, or at least as depriving individuals of control over their own lives, echoes the findings of previous discourse-based research into subjective accounts of diabetes and chronic illnesses more broadly (Charmaz 1991; Gibson and Kenrick 1998; Peel et al. 2005). Rather than signifying a lack of control for these forum members, it is in this context of compromised autonomy that diabulimia can enter as a means of enacting power over diabetes.

In three of the support group messages containing the keyword *control*, extracts from which are reproduced below, the attested lack of control was attributed not to the demands of diabetes self-management, but rather to the role of family members who were perceived as exerting control over either the contributors themselves or other support group members who were the target of the advice-giving message.

64. Thanks, yeah, I'm actually going home this weekend to visit my family, and I'm still debating if I want to break it to them. Lately there was a lot of issues going on with my schooling and living situation. And my parents kept praising me for being so responsible and mature about dealing with everything, and I don't want to shatter this image they have of me now. Like, when ever I would have my really bad episodes and would end up in dka they assumed that it was just me being irresponsible. Now if I was to tell them that I let that happen, that I made it happen? I'm pretty sure they would loose trust in me. They would support me no matter what but they would try to **control** every aspect of my diabulimia recovery. Part of my issues in the first place is being able to actually **control** something in my own life.

65. In addition, it may help to talk about your relationship with your mother and it may even be related in someway to how you are feeling now.

Perhaps you are feeling controlled by her and this is one way to exert your independence and **control** something in your life.... Not saying that is what it is but you may be surprised at what you find out about yourself and in the end, you may find positive ways to live your own life under your rules with being happy and satisfied at the same time.

66. I think you are dealing with larger issue relating to freedom and **control**. I think you really want to be someone who can stand on their own two feet and take responsibility for yourself - and not managing your diabetes is to some extent demonstrating you're trying to make a break with your childhood condition.

The author of the message contained in extract 64 describes 'a lot of issues' relating to their school and living situation, and expresses the fear that disclosing difficulties in their personal life would 'shatter the image' of them being 'responsible and mature and dealing with everything' and result in their family 'try[ing] to control every aspect of [their] diabulimia recovery'. This contributor then concludes their message by proffering a lack of control over things in their life as a motive for, or at least a factor in the development of, diabulimia in the first place, when they write, '[p]art of my issues in the first place is being able to actually control something in my own life.' Issues with familial control are also evident in extracts 65 and 66, both of which were taken from separate responses to the same initial message in a thread about one sufferer's relationship with their mother. The author of extract 65 suggests to the author of the original post that they might be 'feeling controlled by her [i.e. their mother]' and that 'this [diabulimia] is one way to exert your independence and control something in your life'. Likewise, the author of extract 66, responding to the same message, interprets the attested diabulimia as relating to 'larger issue[s] relating to freedom and control', and as constituting a means for that contributor to demonstrate how they can 'stand on their own two feet and take responsibility for [themselves]' by 'trying to make a break with [their] childhood condition' (by adhering, once more, to the neoliberal ideal of effective chronic disease self-management). Common to all three of these messages is the representation of control as something that is possessed by someone other than the person experiencing diabulimia. Accordingly, diabulimia is construed, once more, as a means for individuals to take control of their own lives, in that such practices, although on some occasions openly acknowledged to be disordered or in some other way deviant, can be framed as means for individuals to take responsibility for their diabetes and to display autonomy (Peel et al. 2005).

In the final type of forum post we want to discuss in this chapter, the support group contributors actually construed insulin restriction not as a way of effectively managing their diabetes but as something that actually grants individuals a means of relinquishing the feelings of powerlessness, obedience, restraint and self-denial that they experience in relation to having to manage their diabetes. This discourse was evident in a small proportion of the messages (approximately 7 per cent of posts mentioning *diabetes*) and is exemplified by the representative example below.

67.   Anyway, since I am taking a bunch of premed classes now, I not only get to hear about all of the terrible things that happen with chronic high sugars, but I also learn a lot about cell bio and can use this info to further manipulate my insulin. All of this started out as just wanting to drop a few pounds, but now that I have tasted life without **diabetes**, I just don't want to go back. When I was diagnosed, I just accepted that this was the way it was going to be. I didn't ever consider just not doing it. It feels so good to not obsess over every carb that I put in my body, to not worry about testing, to not have to calculate corrections or meal boluses.

This support group member equates insulin restriction with relinquishing diabetes itself when they write, 'now that I have tasted life without diabetes, I just don't want to go back.' At the same time, this contributor also stresses to others that their actions are not careless or neglectful, presenting their insulin restriction as deliberate and even calculated, lexicalizing it as insulin 'manipulati[on]', and legitimizing it by foregrounding their knowledge of biomedical concepts like 'cell bio', acquired through 'premed classes'. Even in cases where insulin restriction is framed as relinquishing the burden of their diabetes, then, this does not preclude the subject position of 'expert' diabetic patient which, we suggest, can help to legitimize what might otherwise be perceived as reckless diabetes (mis) management.

6.6 Chapter summary

Based on a corpus of diabulimia-related interactions in online diabetes support groups, the analysis in this chapter has explored the discourses surrounding the keyword themes of diabulimia, insulin and diabetes. Our analysis of the diabulimia keywords, in particular *diabulimia* itself, found that the condition tended to be lexicalized in grammatically objectifying and distancing terms (except in contexts of recovery), experiences were presented using diagnostic discourse as 'symptoms', and diabulimia itself was described in explicit terms as a *disorder*, an *eating disorder* and a *mental disorder*, which included collectivizing diabulimia with medically legitimate eating disorders. Such was the dominance of this medicalizing perspective that in cases where diabulimia 'diagnoses' were refuted, these refutations were made on the basis that the disclosed 'symptoms' did not fit with the support group's diagnostic criteria, rather than having anything to do with diabulimia's medically contested offline status. These trends, which can be likened to the linguistic patterns we have observed in relation to the lexicalization of anorexia and depression in the previous chapters, are particularly intriguing in the context of conversations about diabulimia, given the condition's lack of medical recognition. We will return to this adoption of conceptual and linguistic medical frameworks and consider their implications for understandings of diabulimia, anorexia and depression in the next chapter.

The analysis of the keyword *insulin* in the second part of the chapter uncovered a range of discourses around this concept. Unsurprisingly, insulin was frequently construed as inducing weight gain, with insulin restriction in turn presented as helping people to reduce or control their body weight. However, this majority position was also challenged, mostly by posts arguing that taking insulin does not necessarily entail weight gain and that other lifestyle factors, including diet, exercise and diabetes management, are more likely to affect body weight. This section also showed how disclosures of insulin-restricting practices were commonly met with negative evaluative responses from other group members warning of the risks associated with it. It is perhaps to avoid such critical responses that support group members disclosed their insulin restriction in linguistically vague terms.

Finally, our close analysis of the keyword *diabetes* began by exploring the discursive connection between diabetes and eating disorders (including diabulimia). By constructing people with diabetes (who were often themselves) as experiencing heightened susceptibility to diabulimia and other eating disorders, we could argue that many of the contributors were able to avert some of the potential stigma and blame that regularly attends to eating disorders and, in this case, the perceived mismanagement of diabetes. We then focused on the word *control*, both as a collocate of *diabetes* and as a keyword in its own right. This turned out to be a topic for discursive contest, with contributors to the diabetes support groups construing diabulimia variously as something that signalled a lack of control on the part of the sufferer, but also as something that could, quite conversely, actually grant sufferers some degree of control, both over their pre-existing diabetes as well as over their lives more generally.

An overall finding emerging from this analysis, then, is that diabulimia is subject to a range of contesting discourses in the context of online diabetes support groups. Furthermore, it is also clear from this chapter that representations of diabulimia in this context do not focus just on concerns around body weight and body image but are shaped by ideas and discourses around autonomous diabetes management. In recent times, Western societies have witnessed an increased orientation towards a neoliberal model of public health (Lupton 1995), according to which individuals are responsibilized into accessing relevant expert health information, proactively managing their health risks and practising self-care, all to reduce the demands that ill health places on the state (Brown and Baker 2012). The neoliberal imperatives that imbue notions of health have profound implications for people who live with chronic diseases like diabetes, who are accordingly implored to take responsibility for and actively self-manage their condition in accordance with medical advice (Naemiratch and Manderson 2006). The discourses unpacked in this chapter signal a range of (sometimes conflicting) conceptions of, and relationships with, such neoliberal frameworks. For the majority of the contributors, diabulimia constitutes a deviation from this neoliberal imperative. On the other hand, other posts actually represented insulin restriction as a normal part of responsible diabetes management, signalling a potential overlap between the meaning of so-called normal and pathological diabetes-related practices. In a small minority of cases, the forum users construed insulin restriction as a means of relinquishing the demands and feelings of powerlessness associated with diabetes self-management. We will return to this variability in the discourse, and consider its possible implications for diabulimia and diabetes care, in the next chapter.

Discussion

Telling the right story; being the right self

7.1 Introduction

The foregoing chapters have examined three unique, specialized corpora of online support group interactions using a corpus-based discourse analytic approach. In doing so, they have offered original insights into the language used by large numbers of people suffering from anorexia nervosa, depression and diabulimia. In line with the aims outlined at the start of the book, the analysis has placed particular emphasis on the ways in which users of online support groups represent these conditions, as well as themselves in relation to them. Each chapter has also explored how participants in each corpus discuss issues that are more particular to their respective conditions. Specifically, we have considered the ways in which individuals with anorexia describe their weight loss practices, their compulsions to eat and efforts to 'eat more', including their use of dietary meal plans, which are constructed as a metaphorical guide to recovery. The analysis of the depression forum has considered some of the ways in which its members discuss antidepressant medication, and particularly their repeated emphasis on finding the 'right medication'. This chapter also illustrated ways in which participants discuss self-harming behaviour as both a source of emotional control and a practice over which they have lost control. Similarly, forum users described their suicidal ideation as beyond their control and sought to focus on the effects of suicide on their friends and family as a means of counteracting suicidal impulses. Finally, our analysis of diabulimia-related messages in three diabetes support groups demonstrated the ways in which individuals' conceptions of and relationships with their pre-existing diabetes intersect with their representations of diabulimia. For example, for the majority of the support group members, insulin restriction constituted deviance from prescribed diabetes self-management regimen. However, for others it provided a means of rejecting the burdensome obligation of managing their diabetes, while for some, under the right conditions, insulin restriction actually constituted a way to manage their chronic condition effectively.

This chapter synthesizes the findings from the three corpus analyses and identifies points of commonality and divergence between them. Given that we originally anticipated the discourses in each of the three corpora to be quite different (and, indeed, this was part of the rationale for analysing each corpus separately), the extent of the similarities between the three datasets, which we discuss in Sections 7.2 and 7.2.1 below, is quite striking. These similarities are not without exception, however, and our findings also point towards a discourse of individual responsibility that is more particular to the interactions related to diabulimia. We address this in Section 7.2.2 on responsibility and neoliberalism.

In discussing these findings, we are mindful of the need for corpus studies to produce findings that are 'both descriptive and explanatory' (Thornbury 2010: 271) and, as such, have sought to orient consistently to the question of 'why do participants represent their experience of mental illness in these ways?' Responding to this question over the following pages involves moving away from the discussion of language in and of itself to consider the social and cultural norms with which sufferers' linguistic choices are enmeshed. However, it is worth reiterating that the foregoing analysis did not set out to establish whether the similarities and differences in the discourse of each corpus reflect parallels and contrasts in the underlying psychopathologies of anorexia, depression and diabulimia. We have explained our reservations about research that uses decontextualized language data to make such claims in Chapter 1 and have no evidence to argue that overlaps in the discourse of the three corpora signify shared cognitive characteristics among their respective participants. Instead, in what follows, we focus on the way that representations of mental illness emerge at the interface of several factors: the participants' experiences themselves, the norms of the online community in which they are interacting, publically available discourses (such as the discourse of medicine), and how participants use these as resources for achieving interactional goals. As we have attempted to illustrate in the preceding chapters, these factors are imbricated with each other (Giles 2006). Consequently, the prevailing ways in which each of these conditions is represented articulate sufferers' experiences while also drawing upon broader discursive domains, orienting to the supportive aims of each forum and achieving more immediate communicative goals such as offering sympathy, disagreeing with another user, assessing others' problems and providing advice. The potential for representations of mental illness to serve these multiple functions simultaneously in turn explains their predominance in each corpus (Hunt and Harvey 2015); they allow users to construct the 'right' representation of anorexia, depression or diabulimia for the group and specific thread in which they are posting.

7.2 Talking about the condition and talking about the self

Although anorexia, depression and diabulimia are distinctive conditions with different core characteristics and treatments, the respective users of the fora studied throughout this book display a number of consistent linguistic practices. Chief among these is a tendency for the contributors to present their conditions nominally (i.e. as 'ED', 'depression' or 'diabulimia') rather than as personal attributes (i.e. 'I'm anorexic' and 'I'm diabulimic') or affective states (e.g. 'feeling depressed'). This pattern coheres with the more general tendency for diseases to be referred to nominally (Fleischman 1999). Frequency data indicates the relative dominance of these different representations in each corpus. In the *anorexia.net* corpus, *ED* occurs 623 times and *anorexic* occurs 29 times. In the *depression.net* data, *depression* features 442 times and *depressed* occurs 126 times, while *diabulimia* occurs 202 times and *diabulimic* 23 times in the *diabulimia.net* corpus. In each case, the data point towards a preference for objectifying nominal constructions of the respective condition in the forum users' discourse, with this preference being strongest among the *anorexia.net* users. Similarly, the construction *the*+[condition], which we argue is the most objectifying and distancing way of representing the illness, is most common in the anorexia data, with *the ED* accounting for 25 per cent of L1 collocates of *ED*, while *the depression* and *the diabulimia* account for 10.86 per cent and 3.43 per cent of L1 collocates of *depression* and *diabulimia*, respectively. This stronger preference for objectifying anorexia is also exemplified by its consistent representation as *the ED voice* on *anorexia.net*, a more specific personification than is apparent in the other two corpora, where users also opt for *suffering from* and *suffered with* constructions.

Closer analysis of each online corpus indicates that these collocational patterns are not simply accidental. For instance, newer users of *depression.net* tended to use *suffered with depression*, while more established forum members use *suffering from depression*. Although it was by no means an exclusive association, there is a shared tendency across all three corpora for grammatical constructions that align the sufferer with their condition to be used by individuals claiming to be recovering or to have recovered from their illness. That is, the aligning constructions *my+ED/depression/diabulimia* and *I am diabulimic* appear to correlate with users who talk about their conditions in a more positive light and typically from a perspective of recovery. This grammatical parallel between the separate fora suggests that those who claim to be experiencing relief from mental illness are also willing to represent it as a personal possession or attribute rather than distinct entity, perhaps indicating that these individuals are coming to terms with their condition (Schreiber 1996; Ridgway 2001) and are more able to claim responsibility for and ownership of it (Pierce et al. 2003). More generally, the variation in grammatical representations of each condition demonstrates that verbal representations of mental illnesses are not static, but vary depending on the sufferers' current experiences – especially in relation to recovery – as well as their socialization into a particular online community.

In each corpus, nominalizing references to conditions correlate with instances of illness personification, in which verbal and material processes characteristic of human agents are attributed to anorexia, depression or diabulimia. For example, *the ED* is presented as persuading, speaking and 'getting scared'; *the depression* is described as 'talking' and 'hitting'; *diabulimia* is said to 'strip' the sufferer of control, 'take control of your life' and to not 'stop at anything'. Members of *depression.net* also tended to distance themselves from depression's actions. This was typically achieved by contributors using intransitive verbs to present depression as 'starting' or 'lifting' independently of the sufferer or by avoiding explicitly presenting themselves as the grammatical objects of the transitive processes they attributed to their depression, such as by saying 'that's the way depression makes my mind work' rather than 'that's how depression makes me think'.

That comparable linguistic choices are made consistently across each corpus suggests that these choices are likely to play an important role for sufferers in conveying their experiences of mental illness. More specifically, we argue that the grammatical objectification and personification of psychological difficulty in each corpus serves two salient functions across the different fora. First, these tropes construct a separation between the identity of sufferer and their condition. Secondly, they construe mental health problems as beyond the control of individual sufferers, who present themselves as passive in the onset and continuation of their conditions. As a consequence, these two functions also act to nullify two corresponding forms of illness stigma: firstly, the 'negative evaluation' of a mentally ill identity and, secondly, the volitional stigma which attends the belief that illness (particularly an eating disorder like anorexia and diabulimia) is self-inflicted or endured voluntarily (Goffman 1963; Easter 2012: 1411). While previous research has interpreted this kind of distancing language as a means of managing gendered – and specifically masculine – identities (Galasiński 2008), the fact that such constructions were evident across posts ostensibly authored by both men and women (and especially in the overwhelmingly female *anorexia.net* forum) suggests that their function is likely to transcend gender boundaries (although gender may of course still play a role). When deployed in illness narratives and supportive messages in each forum, these linguistic strategies appear to enable sufferers to affirm an acceptable identity as someone living with a mental illness and to 'patch up the moral rupture' of an illness diagnosed on the basis of an individual's seemingly deliberate conduct (Kangas 2001: 77). As well as conveying their experiences of powerlessness and distress, therefore, the discursive naturalization and personification of mental illness apparent across each of the three preceding chapters may thus constitute cross-condition linguistic signatures of stigma management.

Additional evidence for this argument comes from Knapton's (2016, 2018) recent work on sufferers' narratives of obsessive-compulsive disorder. Knapton highlights the salience of personification in these accounts, noting that

> thoughts and other mental activities are often described as entities that are autonomous from the self and that have vast amounts of agency. Mental activities are therefore often externalized from the self and presented as outside of the person's control.
>
> (Knapton 2016: 2017)

Knapton's interpretation of this linguistic feature also matches those we have proffered in this study, namely that personification allows individuals to distance themselves from aspects of psychological distress that they regard as undesirable:

> By placing the mind and thoughts (and for some people, the disorder more broadly) as the grammatical subject of active voice constructions, these mental activities become agentive entities whose actions are constructed as relatively autonomous from the self. The responsibility for the content of the thoughts is thus potentially transferred from the real self to these agentive mental entities.
>
> (Knapton 2018: 19)

Although not explicitly phrased in terms of stigma, there are clear consistencies here with the ways in which participants in the present study seek to linguistically construct a sense of self that is distinct from each of the three stigmatized conditions. This discursive separation in turn permits sufferers to represent themselves as knowledgeable and rational in relation to their condition

(Galasiński 2008; Knapton 2018: 11), even while recounting seemingly irrational acts such as drastic weight loss, self-harm and severe insulin restriction.

Our qualitative discourse analysis of individual message threads further explains the quantitative evidence that objectifying constructions represent dominant discourses in each forum. In particular, Sections 4.6, 5.3.3 and 6.3 each illustrate the ways in which forum members use personified representations of anorexia, depression and diabulimia in order to construct mental illness as beyond individual control and to attribute unfavourable actions to their and others' conditions. In this regard, personifying mental illness is a potent discursive practice in these fora; not only does it function to distance sufferers from the stigma of their own conditions but it also serves as a resource for negotiating sensitive interactional tasks such as displaying solidarity and shared experience, accounting for others' non-recovery and resolving conflicting points of view between members (see Section 4.6, in particular). To put this another way, constructing anorexia, depression and diabulimia as independent entities rather than just diagnostic labels or sets of behaviours not only allows individuals to tell an acceptable story about their own illness, but also serves as the right model of mental illness for members of online communities looking to offer mutual, sympathetic support for one another.

Beyond the similar ways in which participants construct their respective illnesses, interactions in each of the fora demonstrate a number of other consistent rhetorical features. In particular, the foregoing analysis identified the use of extreme case formulations (Pomerantz 1986; Edwards 2000) to account for activities such as dietary restriction and self-injurious thinking. In each case, forum members used these formulations to situate their actions within extreme scenarios and thereby legitimize contentious practices as responses to acute psychological distress. For example, one *depression.net* user claims that they '[c]annot deal with stress at all and any type of pressure just makes me have suicidal thoughts'. The presence of such 'defensive detailing' (Drew 2006) in sufferers' posts serves as a reminder that accounts of mental illness cannot simply be regarded as reflections of an individual's psychology, but rather should be understood as having been designed to achieve particular interactional effects (Guise et al. 2007). Like the personification of each condition, one such effect is to mollify claims that they desire to engage in seemingly deleterious behaviours or are irrational for performing them. That is, members' messages appear to be designed, at least in part, to respond to the possibility that these are sanctionable acts by constructing an internal logic to their actions and demonstrating an awareness of their implications (Harris 2000; Drew 2006).

It is perhaps surprising to find that discursive strategies which serve to counteract stigma appear so consistently in forum users' messages, given that they are communicating in groups populated by fellow sufferers who are well placed to respond empathically to accounts of events that are embarrassing, degrading or socially maligned. A long-standing and repeated claim about the sorts of anonymous, spatially distal and asynchronous discussion fora examined in this book is that they enable participants to make face-threatening disclosures with a level of candour that would be unlikely – or which would result in censure – in face-to-face contexts (Wright and Bell 2003; Suler 2004). Indeed, members of the online communities represented in each of our corpora do attest to a range of profoundly painful experiences and stigmatized practices, not least deliberate self-harm. At the same time, as the foregoing discussion attests, sufferers in each forum design their contributions in order to provide socially preferred representations of themselves (as rational, as seeking to control their diabetes, as forced into harmful behaviours and so on). However, even in these anonymous and highly specific online illness communities, communication is clearly not disconnected from the values, norms and social expectations that are likely to infuse participants' offline lives. Seen in this light, a further benefit of online support groups is that they afford sufferers the opportunities to learn from others and practice narrating their own experiences in order to establish a sense that they are dealing with a debilitating condition in a legitimate manner (Bamberg 2012; Ziebland and Wyke 2012).

The interactional norms of each forum, visible in the form of the quantitatively dominant linguistic signatures of each corpus, are similarly interwoven with larger, culturally available discourses. Our discussion so far has focused particularly on participants' uptake of discourses of psychiatric medicine and neoliberal imperatives of personal responsibility, and the ways in which these discourses function to define the nature of sufferers' illness and their roles and responsibilities. We do not doubt that there are other important social forces at work in shaping the discourses surrounding anorexia, depression and diabulimia, both in the messages analysed in this study and more broadly (see Musolino et al. 2015). However, these discourses merit a more sustained examination because we believe that they play a particularly significant role in the forum messages we have analysed. Accordingly, the following two subsections address these two discourses, of psychiatric medicine and personal responsibility, in greater detail, considering their implications both for users of online support groups and healthcare professionals. The first subsection focuses on medicalization as a process that we perceive across all three corpora. However, the second, on neoliberalism and personal responsibility, focuses more exclusively on the diabulimia corpus since this theme emerged as particularly salient in the accounts of this condition (likely a corollary of its centrality to the management and experience of diabetes more generally (Peel et al. 2005)).

7.2.1 The self as patient: Illness and medicalization

The recurrent use of medical discourses was apparent across all of the online support fora making up the three corpora analysed in this study. To some extent, this should not be surprising; as discussed in the opening chapter, medicalization is a pervasive trend across developed nations, and, indeed, medical discourses are now very much the dominant means of understanding anorexia nervosa and depression (Hepworth 1999; Pilgrim and Bentall 1999). It is unsurprising, therefore, that medical discourses are available to lay members of the public to communicate about mental distress, even when they are discussing a condition such as diabulimia, which currently exists outside the boundaries of official psychiatric diagnosis (Williams et al. 2009; Brookes 2018).

What is more surprising, however, is the extent of the medicalized discourse in each corpus and its realization at numerous levels of linguistic granularity for the three conditions. At an orthographic and lexical level, the word 'diabulimia' is itself a blend of two established diagnostic categories, diabetes and bulimia, and the use of this label constitutes an attempt by sufferers to situate their experiences and behaviours within a medical framework. Users of the diabetes support groups also variously refer to diabulimia as a 'disorder', 'mental disorder' and 'eating disorder', thereby drawing on the language of medical pathology when discussing deliberate insulin restriction. Discussions of diabulimia regularly mention the condition alongside – and in some cases in conflation with – medically recognized eating disorders such as anorexia and bulimia, an association that confers medical legitimacy on diabulimia itself. Depression, too, is directly equated with physical conditions ('a broken bone' and 'fever') in order to construct it as worthy of medical intervention. As discussed above, the pervasive reference to these conditions using their (pseudo)medical diagnostic names means that sufferers verbally depict their conditions as distinct objects and, in doing so, align with the ontology of diseases discernible in medical discourse (Cassell 1976; Nijhof 1998; Fleischman 1999).

Rather more explicitly, all three conditions are at times expressly defined in accordance with key concepts of biomedicine so as to frame them as a form of biological malfunction: anorexia is described in terms of 'genes' and 'brain chemistry' (Section 4.6), depression is said to be a 'chemical imbalance' and to result from 'brain chemicals' not working normally (Section 5.3.2–5.3.3), and diabulimia is attributed to 'psychogenic causes' (Section 6.3). Although these are not the only definitions of diabulimia, depression and anorexia provided in the corpora, such biomedical descriptions routinely appear at interactively delicate points, such as disagreements, and are used to facilitate contextually relevant interactional tasks, such as offering sympathy and legitimizing advice.

A number of these longer interactional sequences themselves attest to medicalization insofar as sufferers' experiences are assessed and formulated as symptoms before being resolved into a diagnosis in a manner that emulates a clinical consultation. In the depression forum, for instance, a narrative in which a new member recounts having an 'ache in [her] head and heart' and claims 'there's only me that can help myself' is categorized by a forum moderator as indicating 'most of the classic symptoms of depression'. That an experience such as heart ache is used as a candidate reason for inferring the presence of a medical pathology suggests that forum participants exercise liberal criteria for diagnosing depression, with a diagnosis – however credible – offering members a means of responding sympathetically to others seeking help (Dowrick 2004).

Similarly, as described elsewhere (Brookes 2018: 8), discussions of diabulimia recurrently illustrate the contributors' propensity for specifying diagnostic criteria for diabulimia, assessing the magnitude of others' attested symptoms and determining whether that person could be categorized – 'diagnosed' – as having diabulimia (Section 6.3). Much like *depression.net*, therefore, not only do *diabulimia.net* members categorize each other's experiences as medical pathologies but this process of categorization itself imitates the genre of the primary care consultation, with individual contributors drawing on medical terminology to support their diagnostic interpretations. Given its relatively scarce psychiatric recognition, this diagnostic practice is particularly ironic in the case of diabulimia, since whether or not a forum contributor 'has diabulimia' reflects the extent to which the symptoms they describe match the forum's internal standards rather than any official diagnostic criteria. These diagnostic interactions therefore serve to reify the integrity of diabulimia as a genuine condition, shoring up its diagnostic boundaries rather than contesting its status as a real disease.

These types of diagnostic sequences regularly involve recommendations that the member being 'diagnosed' seek contact with healthcare professionals and professional forms of treatment. A preference for medical interventions was particularly strident in the recurrent discussion of antidepressant medication in *depression.net*, and its members' repeated recommendation to find the 'right medication'. One user in particular is advised to leave a general practitioner who is unwilling to prescribe antidepressants so that she can find another doctor who is willing to help her get the 'right meds' (Section 5.4). In this instance, depicting one member's psychological distress as amenable to medical treatment simultaneously (and paradoxically) overrules the opinion of a medical professional. In keeping with this preference for professional forms of treatment, there is little explicit discussion of treating depression, anorexia or diabulimia through non-professional means. It is, however, important to regard the forum members' participation in their respective electronic support groups as a proactive effort to manage their emotional difficulties outside of clinical settings.

Taken together, these interactional features consistently fulfil Conrad's defining criteria for medicalization, introduced in Chapter 1 as 'defining a problem in medical terms, using medical language to describe a problem, adopting a medical framework to understand a problem, or using a medical intervention to "treat" it' (1992: 211). Extending these criteria somewhat, we also see medicalization realized in lay individuals' simulation of communicative genres associated with professional healthcare, not least the diagnostic consultation. Medicalization, then, is not just defining a problem in medical terms, but enacting that definition as part of a broader emulation of institutional discourse with corresponding roles of patient and expert.

The preference for medicalizing experiences of psychological difficulty evident in our data stands somewhat in contrast to previous studies. Cornford et al. (2007) and Karasz (2005), for example, attest to lay individuals' preference for non-medical explanations that emphasize situational rather than biological causes of mental illness, while work with primary care clinicians has revealed their tendency to de-medicalize aspects of depression, anorexia and their treatments (McPherson and Armstrong 2009; Hunt and Churchill 2013; Hunt forthcoming).

There are, however, some exceptions to this medicalizing discourse. Testament, perhaps, to its controversial and contested medical status, a considerable minority of the diabetes forum contributors drew upon alternative discourses which conceived of diabulimia variously as deviant, as a normative part of diabetes management and as an active form of resistance to the neoliberal, responsibilizing imperative of diabetes self-management. In addition, on *anorexia.net*, eating in accordance with a professional meal plan is presented as a moral issue that warrants guilt, pride or feelings of 'fidelity'. This suggests that the dominance of medical discourses over alternative understandings of eating disorders is neither total nor one way on the fora. Instead, health-related behaviours and clinical technologies can equally be imbued with normative and emotional meanings. Likewise, the continuing (and by no means settled) negotiation of the medical status of diabulimia in our data provides further evidence of the capacity for so-called lay individuals to play a significant role in both the promotion and challenging of medicalizing ways of understanding and communicating about health and illness, with the context of peer-to-peer health fora acting as a prime site for the negotiation and re-negotiation of such meanings (Miah and Rich 2008). These features also blur the boundaries between nominally 'lay' and 'professional' or 'medical' understandings of these conditions; although the fora's interactions are concerned with personal narratives and emotional difficulties, these accounts of distress are interwoven with 'proto-professional' descriptions of anorexia, depression and diabulimia laced with biomedical concepts (de Swaan 1990; Stoppard 2000), with forum users presenting these conditions as issues of personal and moral significance while also drawing on scientific and medical concepts.

Although medicalization has tended to be regarded critically in the research literature on this topic, the process can carry significant advantages for those who are affected by the health concern in question (Miah and Rich 2008: 70). As we have discussed above, one such benefit for online forum users is neutralizing forms of stigma associated with illness. In addition, one highly feasible explanation for the abundance of medicalizing discourses across our corpora is that medical frameworks for understanding the body and its ailments afford an accessible means through which the different support group members can articulate their health-related experiences. Faced with the challenge of conveying complex and frequently painful thoughts to others, the language of medicine might simply offer individuals the most effective – or at least most accessible – set of linguistic and conceptual resources with which to articulate, comprehend and generally render more cohesive their otherwise ineffable experiences (Harvey 2012; Brookes 2018). Sufferers who learn to employ this medicalizing discourse as a result of their use of online fora will not only have learnt the preferred way of representing illness in that online community but may also find themselves better equipped to discuss their experiences with others offline.

An appealing potential outcome of medicalizing distress in this way is that challenging and debilitating experiences might then be treated with greater gravity by healthcare providers, practitioners and policy-makers (Moynihan et al. 2002). This is a consequence that is particularly pertinent for individuals with diabulimia and other conditions at the contested borders of medicine, where lay-driven medicalization provides a means of advocating for increased professional recognition and treatment (Barker 2008).

Medicalization can also effectively account for instances of non-adherent health behaviours. Given that patients with diabulimia can already feel stigmatized for failing to adhere to medically prescribed insulin regimens, medicalizing diabulimic practices can serve an important legitimizing function by providing an explanation for their non-adherence. As we have argued throughout Chapters 4 and 5, the same is true for people with anorexia and depression; constructing their experiences as one of medical pathology serves to countermand the contention that their behaviours were entered into voluntarily or that they had the ability to simply 'snap out' of them; as one member of *anorexia.net* claims, anorexia 'is no different than cancer. It is something that takes [sufferers] over', and over which they have little control.

However, the lack of agency associated with adopting medical understandings of anorexia, depression and diabulimia in turn reveals the pitfalls of medicalization for users of these fora. A feeling of lost control is common in experiences of long-term mental illness (Karp 1996) and throughout the preceding analysis we have noted the tendency for forum contributors to present themselves as passive sufferers of biological impairments that, while beyond their own control, are within the ambit of professional medical intervention. Although this position of passivity is not an inherent aspect of a medical model of illness, it is a role cued by framing psychological distress in medical terms. That is, presenting anorexia, depression and diabulimia as the result of factors beyond lay individuals' control corresponds with a position of limited power for the sufferer and a dependence upon professional intervention; in short, a position of patienthood.

Adopting this patient identity may lead sufferers to underestimate their capacity to make effective, non-medical changes to improve their well-being, as well as underestimating the value of non-medical changes themselves. Where access to professional interventions is limited or where medical treatments are ineffective, sufferers may also feel that their condition is not only beyond their control but also beyond hope. As we highlight in Chapter 4, the discursive separation of sufferer from condition and the representation of the sufferer as controlled by their disease is also a strategy employed by psychiatric professionals in order to undermine patients' resistance to particular treatments and day-to-day routines. As well as increasing sufferers' exposure to medical interventions, then, this same discourse may be harnessed to warrant the use of interventions that the sufferer ultimately experiences as oppressive (Malson et al. 2004). Again, this is an issue with particular relevance for eating disorders, where feelings of lost control feature prominently in sufferers' accounts of both the onset of illness and motivations for discontinuing treatment (Eivors et al. 2003). Similarly, some of the contributors to the diabetes support fora in this study expressed distress at their lack of self-determination over the management of their diabetes and lives more generally, in some cases citing this as a cause of their developing diabulimia in the first place. For these individuals, the increase in professional insulin monitoring that is likely to attend medical treatment for diabulimia may therefore be particularly distressing and will require careful management.

The emphasis on medical explanations of anorexia, depression and diabulimia in these fora may also foreclose alternative interpretations of these conditions and health beliefs more generally. In this respect, even while they involve contributors of different genders, the preference for medical models of psychological distress among the online communities in this study mirrors Stoppard's (2000) account of women's consciousness-raising support groups. Stoppard argues that discussions in women's consciousness-raising groups in the mid-twentieth century provided an opportunity to foreground the pervasive cultural and structural inequalities that give rise to women's mutual psychological distress. However, in a departure from their 1960s origins, Stoppard claims that contemporary feminist therapies for depression typically fail to integrate this contextualizing perspective and instead represent mental illness as an individualized pathology. In parallel with this, while clearly a venue in which women offer profound mutual support to each other, *anorexia. net* contains little discussion of gendered discourses of female body shape and physical regulation that might situate anorexia in relation to oppressive cultural norms. Instead, discussions tend to focus on individual therapies and personal meal plans (though this does, of course, also reflect the forms of professional treatment these sufferers are more likely to receive). Likewise, in the *diabulimia. net* corpus, insulin-induced weight gain was consistently imbued with a negative evaluative prosody and construed as unwanted and undesirable. Weight *loss*, on the other hand, tended to be framed positively, including being presented as a key component for managing diabetes, a representation which draws – harmfully – on the pervasive assumption that thinness equates to healthiness (Tischner and Malson 2012). However, there was little evidence of the contributors questioning the types of (gendered) cultural norms which position weight gain as negative and the desire to lose weight as not only positive but also natural and normal. Indeed, even contributors who were disparaging of others' insulin restriction frequently responded by recommending other, more 'normative' methods of weight loss, including diet and exercise, rather than questioning or even discussing the attested desire to lose weight which had led the original poster to those disordered practices in the first place.

Consequently, rather than fostering explanations of mental illness that critically examine the cultural and environmental causes of psychological distress, anorexia, depression, diabulimia and their respective aetiologies are largely depoliticized in these online interactions (Barker 2008). On *anorexia.net* in particular, forum members strongly disaffiliate from accounts that constitute anorexia as a choice rather than an 'illness', even if those accounts posit a more empowered role for the individual in managing their anorexia (Giordano 2005). Similarly, the discussion of diabulimia focused on its status as a medical problem to the extent that there was comparatively limited explicit exploration of the broader environmental and sociocultural forces potentially underlying this health phenomenon. Although discussion of such forces was not elided completely – some of the contributors openly proposed the demands of diabetes management and strained relationships with practitioners and family members as causes of diabulimia – such explanations were considerably less pervasive compared to the medicalizing discourses identified elsewhere in the corpus. Even while the equivalent details in *depression.net* discussions are somewhat more nuanced, the overall picture is much the same; although forum users typically attributed the onset of their unhappiness to a combination of traumatic experiences and environmental and interpersonal factors, the group's discussion of treatments was nevertheless focused on individualized medical interventions.

The persistent emphasis on locating the causes or treatment of distress at an individualized level means that online support groups that focus on medicalized understandings of suffering may thus be ineffective in establishing collective resistance to cultural practices that produce and oppress sufferers of mental health problems (Stoppard 2000). Therefore, although mutual peer support is the raison d'être of the support groups we have analysed, in practice this support involves the elision of politicized explanations of personal distress in favour of narrowly biomedical ones.

7.2.2 The responsible self: Illness and neoliberalism

The neoliberal imperatives that imbue notions of health have quite profound implications for people experiencing chronic illnesses, not least diabetes. These individuals are implored to take responsibility for and to actively self-manage their condition in accordance with medical advice (Broom and Whittaker 2004). The influence of neoliberal frameworks on diabetes management is surmised by Naemiratch and Manderson (2006: 1148) thus: 'from a clinical perspective, control of diabetes is relatively unproblematic: patients are advised to modify their diet, exercise regularly, lose weight if overweight, and if indicated, take medication orally or insulin by injection to ensure glycaemic control (that is, blood glucose levels are maintained at an acceptable level)' (see also Galvin 2002; Broom and Whittaker 2004). In what follows, we consider the ways that we interpret this responsibilizing, neoliberal imperative to have shaped how diabulimia is discursively constructed in the forum messages analysed in this study, while also touching briefly on the *anorexia.net* data.

As a condition characterized by the deliberate reduction of insulin, diabulimia tended, rather unsurprisingly, to be construed by the forum contributors as constituting a violation of the neoliberal imperative of diabetes self-management. We observed such representations to have a strong moral component, with those experiencing diabulimia frequently rendered in negative and potentially stigmatizing terms as deviant, irresponsible and out of control, not only of their diabetes but also of their lives more generally (Naemiratch and Manderson 2006: 1153). We interpret this feature of the forum posts as reflecting the broader penchant for diabetes control to be framed as a moral duty (Balfe 2007), whereby failure to control one's diabetes can elicit judgements of being 'bad' or deviant (Gomersall et al. 2011: 13). However, it is also important to bear in mind that such negative evaluations were not the sole preserve of those who claimed to manage their diabetes 'properly'; occasionally this discourse was also drawn upon by contributors who ostensibly identified as having diabulimia in order to negatively evaluate themselves and their own diabetes management. We would argue that the presence of such negative moral self-appraisals provides yet further evidence of the extent and influence of the neoliberal imperative over the ways that both diabulimia and diabetes are conceptualized and discussed in these online contexts.

The next implication of this neoliberal ideology is something of a consequence of the first. Specifically, our corpus analysis has elucidated the tendency for the majority of the *diabulimia.net* contributors to attest the ways in which they actually fulfilled this neoliberal expectation respecting the management of their diabetes, even when they also identified as experiencing diabulimia. This positive self-presentation was a two-part process. First, it involved constructing the self as experiencing diabulimia against one's volition by casting themselves as non-agentive with respect to the onset of the condition. Secondly, the forum contributors also constructed themselves as more agentive in regard to what might be perceived as more positive and less stigmatizing aspects of the diabulimia illness experience, for example attempts at recovery and being knowledgeable about their pre-existing and co-occurring diabetes. Presenting themselves as actually fulfilling the responsibilities of diabetes self-management *in spite of* their experiencing diabulimia might constitute a strategy for these forum members to guard against their attested emotions, experiences and concerns being conflated with, or simply dismissed as, 'bad' diabetes management (Balfe 2007). Such a strategy could thus, in turn, help the forum members to avert the attendant threat of stigma and to stave off accusations of moral failure (Galvin 2002: 112).

Other forum contributors, though still seeming to align with the neoliberal ideal of the diabetic who effectively and autonomously manages their condition, did so quite differently – by actually constructing diabulimia and its associated practices as constituting a part of effective and even normative diabetes self-management. Such constructions imply there to be some (perceived) overlap between 'pathologizsed' and therapeutically intended regimes of diabetes and weight self-management (Burns and Gavey 2008). As highlighted in Chapter 2, this conflation of disordered and normative weight practices is also true of individuals with anorexia, who enact the neoliberal ideals of bodily control through a hyper-disciplined micro-management of the body (and body weight in particular) (Malson 2008).

This argument might be extendable to the case of diabulimia, given that intense concerns about, and attempts to manage, body weight, which often sit at the heart of the diabulimia experience, might be interpreted as enacting 'par excellence' – to borrow Malson's (2008: 35–6) formulation – the kind of bodily control that is necessitated by the imperative of responsible diabetes self-management. Such overlap has been observed elsewhere, for instance by Paterson et al. (1998), who argue that accomplishing or at least performing autonomy and expertise in the context of diabetes self-management can involve active experimentation with diet, activity and medication. It would seem, therefore, that the practices associated with diabulimia constitute a series of culturally available techniques not only, or simply, for body weight management but also, in some cases, for autonomously managing one's diabetes. In other words, although the practices associated with diabulimia (namely, insulin restriction) are frequently distanced from and can be subjected to stigmatizing constructions in the forum messages we have examined, they also have the potential to be drawn upon in the discursive production of healthy and responsible diabetic selves.

This shared emphasis on the importance of individual bodily control is another point of significant overlap between the *anorexia.net* and *diabulimia.net* fora, with the relationship between disorder and personal control constituting a focal point for disagreement between the fora's respective users. Several messages posted to *anorexia.net* explicitly equate food restriction with personal control, while another forum member in response claims that 'EDs take all the control', leaving the sufferer with just 'the illusion of control' (Section 4.4). In a comparable exchange in the *diabulimia.net* corpus, one contributor writes that 'You start by thinking that you are in control [...] but before you realise what has happened you have been stripped of all control' (Section 6.5). Both responses acknowledge the sense of control afforded by disordered behaviours but seek to formulate this control as either temporary or illusory, with the ceding of control to anorexia or diabulimia identified as a defining characteristic in the classification of these conditions as pathologies. It seems telling that in neither forum is the ideal of personal control ever questioned; the primacy of the neoliberal demands of self-control is such that the imperative to recover from anorexia or diabulimia is one of regaining a position of unhindered autonomy.

Just as medicalizing perspectives on mental illness were occasionally challenged throughout each corpus in this study, neoliberal discourses of diabulimia were not universally accepted, since some of the forum contributors expressed openly negative experiences of, and attitudes towards, the neoliberal frameworks of diabetes self-management. In some cases, this involved establishing a direct causal link between the demands of diabetes self-management and the development of diabulimia, while in others diabulimia was constructed as a means through which individuals were able to actively resist and break from the burden of managing diabetes (see Chapter 6, Section 6.5). This finding is consistent with studies which report individuals with chronic diseases to experience their illness as interrupting or even taking over the routines of their normal lives (Charmaz 1991; Paterson et al. 1998). Indeed, it is in view of this that Goldman and Maclean (1998: 747) characterize diabetes as an 'assault on one's self'.

The foregoing discussion has underscored the complex and multifaceted ways in which ideas about diabetes, and more specifically the neoliberal imperatives of diabetes self-management, interact with and even shape the discourses that surround diabulimia in the context of online diabetes support groups. Indeed, individuals experiencing diabulimia could be discursively constructed as suffering from an eating disorder to which their diabetes makes them particularly susceptible; as being bad or deviant for failing their responsibilities to effectively manage their diabetes; as actually fulfilling such obligations despite suffering with diabulimia (but in some cases actually *through* their insulin restriction); or as restricting their insulin as a way of relinquishing their diabetes and the negative feelings they associate with it and the demands it places on them to closely monitor and control almost all aspects of their lives. Taken together, the diverse and conflicting ways in which the diabulimia accounts analysed in this study interact with neoliberal discourses of diabetes self-management suggest that people with diabetes can experience such responsibilizing demands in varying ways, and that both positive and negative experiences alike can feed into the development and discursive representation of diabulimia (Ingadottir and Halldorsdottir 2008). Thus, we would argue that people with diabulimia are subjected to a kind of double bind by the demands of the neoliberal imperative of diabetes self-management, by which such demands can at once be the cause of diabulimia, yet at the same time give rise to the stigma and censure that surround the condition and which contribute to understandings of it as a form of deviance.

7.3 Chapter summary

As the foregoing discussion attests, the discourses of mental health circulating within the fora of *anorexia.net*, *depression.net* and *diabulimia.net* are diverse; they testify to a plurality of experiences of illness and draw upon broader institutional and political discourses in complex ways. These accounts themselves can also be analysed from multiple perspectives so as to foreground the intra- and interpersonal functions of forum users' linguistic choices and their refraction of larger discourses of medicalization and neoliberalism. At the same time, the interactions across each forum also exhibit a number of consistencies, not least sufferers' attempts to distinguish their own sense of self from their mental health condition and to represent themselves as having the capacity to reflect rationally upon the history and implications of their illness. These consistent features, we argue, testify to the enduring stigma against mental illness and sufferers' need to exculpate themselves from the perceived taint of mental ill health.

Across the three corpora, it is clear that discourses which construct anorexia, depression and diabulimia as discrete, uncontrollable medical pathologies play a prominent role in forum users' negotiation of the stigma of mental illness. Medicalized representations of illness are both empowering in the sense that they can alleviate the perceptions that individuals are to blame for their suffering yet also limiting insofar as they offer only a diminished role for the sufferer in alleviating their distress. A similar dissonance is apparent in diabulimia sufferers' discourses of self-control and personal responsibility, with the imperative of responsible diabetes self-management being presented as both a justification for pursuing diabulimic weight loss practices and a means of condemning them. The multifaceted nature of these discourses and their heterogeneous use in online support groups have complex effects and implications for both sufferers and healthcare professionals. We address these in the next and final chapter of the book.

Beyond the forum
Implications and reflections

8.1 Introduction

This chapter considers the implications of the study's findings both for users and moderators of online health support platforms and for health professionals. Moving on from the discussion of anorexia, depression, diabulimia and online support groups, it also reflects upon the limitations and strengths of the study, using the former to identify avenues along which this study could be extended and enriched.

The conduct of the study – and particularly the corpus-based discourse analysis approach through which we have analysed the data – has also prompted methodological reflections on corpus-aided studies of discourse generally and on the use of corpus methods in the study of personal accounts of illness in particular. In looking ahead, we close this chapter by offering some critical and more programmatic comments on the potential of corpus-aided health communication research.

8.2 Implications for online health support and healthcare professionals

Much like other online contexts (Ziebland and Wyke 2012), the number of members registered to each forum in this study, the frequency with which they post messages and their sustained participation over the time periods sampled in each corpus indicate that the online support groups included in this study provide a valued facility for their respective users. All of the corpora contain instances in which forum participants report having difficulty discussing their conditions in offline settings, suggesting that online communication enables disclosure of concerns that would otherwise be left unsaid. Nowhere was this more profoundly evident than in those messages in which contributors expressed fears of sharing the information they were disclosing online with family members and practitioners. These disclosures frequently engender supportive responses and further discussion that sufferers may not receive during their offline interactions. In addition, the opportunities for narration afforded by each online support group allow users to reflect individually and collectively upon the effects of illness on their lives and to discursively construct positive self-identities. These findings corroborate extensive existing research that emphasizes the function of online communication in managing perceived stigma for illness (Bell 2007) and satisfying emotional needs that are not met elsewhere (Joinson 2003; Moorhead et al. 2013).

Given that both the interactions on *depression.net* and existing literature present self-injurious behaviour as a form of maladaptive expression (Harris 2000; Boynton and Auerbach 2004), it is worth highlighting the particular value of depression and self-harm support groups as venues for expressing distressing emotions. The orthodox understanding of suicide as an irrational behaviour hampers individuals' ability to seek help for fear of being labelled as mentally ill (Bennett et al. 2003), leading to limited disclosure to clinicians (Coggan et al. 1997). Negative experiences with healthcare providers can be a direct precursor of additional self-harm (Harris 2000) and potentiate suicidal behaviour by increasing an individual's sense of isolation and hopelessness of receiving help (Williams and Pollock 2000). While never encouraging suicide, the interactions on *depression.net* largely avoid this stigma and there are no identified instances of forum members explicitly describing others' suicidal ideation as irrational or pathological.

Non-critical discussions of suicide and the public nature of the medium also provide contributors with accessible, continuous and non-judgemental emotional support that has previously been identified as a factor protecting against suicide (Michel 2000). Indeed, given that users associate suicide with thwarted self-expression and loneliness (Section 5.5), the availability of an accessible venue in which to communicate with others and express emotions is likely to be beneficial. Furthermore, the ethos of mutual peer support evident in each forum included in this study provides users with the opportunity to adopt positive roles as listeners, advice givers and helpers that may otherwise be unavailable for those deemed mentally ill. Therefore, while the public reaction to websites permitting discussion of self-injurious behaviours has been largely condemnatory, expressing distress and stigmatized beliefs in a non-injurious manner may offer some users an alternative to suicidal ideation, rather than promoting it (Baker and Fortune 2008; Wiggins et al. 2016; Coulson et al. 2017). Similarly, users expressing difficult emotions through *anorexia.net* may find immediate relief from psychological distress that could otherwise lead them to restrict their diets or exercise excessively. The same could be said for users of *diabulimia.net* contemplating restricting their insulin either to control their weight or as a way of liberating themselves from the demands of, and negative feelings towards, their diabetes. However, we also accept that discussing self-harm with others who also engage in self-injurious behaviour, including insulin restriction, can serve to normalize and reinforce these practices and, where self-harm is constructed as inexorable, impede others from seeking help (Lewis et al. 2012). Indeed, it is for this reason that moderators of *anorexia.net* proscribe detailed descriptions of weight loss practices. In contrast, the supportive and accepting culture of *depression.net* means that users rarely responded to others' descriptions of self-harm by suggesting it was ultimately a maladaptive behaviour. However, our data do not afford the chance to assess the implications of this.

The analysis indicates that participation in the support groups' discussions will encourage new users to make contact with healthcare professionals (Section 6.3) and adhere to professional interventions such as meal plans (Section 4.4) and antidepressant medication (Section 5.4). Eivors et al. (2003) note that regarding anorexic practices as an index of lost control is a common precursor to anorexics seeking professional help. This view is of 'behaviours' and 'restricting' is expressed by several high-posting users of *anorexia.net* and, as a result, individuals who are initially reluctant to seek treatment for anorexia may be motivated to reinterpret their own 'behaviours' as pathological through encountering this framing in the forum. A remarkably similar framing of diabulimia is also apparent in the diabetes support fora, where the condition and its associated practices were explicitly described as constituting an 'eating disorder' that 'take[s] control of your life'.

There is also some evidence that forum interactions affect users' healthcare behaviours. For example, a member of *depression.net* who describes discontinuing taking antidepressants later acknowledges that he was wrong to do so (data not shown). Similarly, a new member who is told she has 'most of the classic symptoms of depression' (Section 5.3.3) subsequently posts a message describing an appointment with her GP which resulted in a prescription of Citalopram and claims, 'i probably would not have bothered going if i hadn't had such encouraging replies.' Participation on *depression.net* is also likely to increase users' exposure to psychologizing explanations of difficult experiences which, if reiterated in consultations, increase the likelihood of undiagnosed users receiving a diagnosis of depression (Kessler et al. 1999).

Healthcare professionals may look favourably on such online interactions as a means of encouraging contact with services and adherence to professional treatments. However, the promotion of medical diagnosis and treatment online may also be a source of tension between internet users and healthcare providers. Most obviously, individuals who are encouraged by their online activities to begin a 'moral career' (Rose 2006) as a person suffering from a treatable illness increase the demands on healthcare services that, in the UK at least, are increasingly stretched. Individuals convinced by the sophisticated proto-professional diagnoses of their internet peers might also experience a sense of conflict with clinicians who are unwilling to accommodate the recommendations and understandings of mental illness that sufferers have accrued through their participation in online support (Sosnowy 2014). In the case of diabulimia in particular, sufferers may attend primary care seeking recognition and treatment for a diagnosis that is only vaguely accounted for in diagnostic manuals. Similarly, users of *depression.net* who are urged to find the 'right meds' may pursue a prescription of antidepressants even when doctors are reluctant to prescribe and favour non-medical forms of treatment (Hunt forthcoming). This may lead forum users into confusion over the appropriate way to manage their distress and perhaps to discontinue consultations with practitioners who do not prescribe medication.

These predictions do not undermine the positive effects the fora have on the lives of sufferers. However, online group users and moderators should be aware that their electronic communities may emphasize professional diagnosis and clinical interventions at the expense of identifying wider material and cultural factors that may contribute to their members' distress (Schreiber and Hartrick 2002; Pilgrim and Dowrick 2006) and, as documented elsewhere, may raise members' expectations for forms of professional care that are not forthcoming (Bartlett and Coulson 2011; Mazanderani et al. 2013). This implication applies equally to healthcare professionals, who may well need to manage patients' expectations about the availability and suitability of particular treatments. Nevertheless, health professionals should be aware that a medicalizing perspective can be usefully de-stigmatizing for patients, even if they would not themselves adopt this perspective nor pursue the medical treatments their patients request.

The findings from the foregoing chapters carry several other implications relevant to the work of healthcare professionals. Chapter 4 demonstrated that externalization and personification of anorexia was a prevalent feature of messages on *anorexia.net*. As noted in Section 4.3.1, externalizing anorexia is advocated in both popular and CBT-based self-help literature as well as the leading Maudsley Methods for treating anorexia (see Rhodes 2003). However, for the users of *anorexia.net*, objectifying anorexia as 'the ED' or 'the ED voice' correlates with an expressed powerlessness over anorexia rather than signalling recovery. It also contrasts with forum users in recovery, who are more willing to represent anorexia as something they possess. Encouraging patients to personify their eating disorder may therefore inadvertently also promote a linguistic resource well suited to constructing themselves as passive and not responsible for their condition. At the very least, the findings signal a need to thoroughly investigate the therapeutic implications of encouraging patients to externalize and personify anorexia (Pugh 2016).

This study also found that the daily demands of self-care were interpreted and drawn upon by the forum contributors in nuanced and paradoxical ways. At the very least, the double bind of diabulimia, in which the norms of diabetes self-management can give rise to both diabulimia and its attendant stigma means that potentially scathing and value-laden judgements about people with diabulimia as 'lacking control' or being 'non-adherent' (Ingadottir and Halldorsdottir 2008: 615) are likely to be at best overly simplistic and at worst deeply stigmatizing.

Moreover, the inconsistent (and often negative) ways in which the *diabulimia.net* forum users were observed to interact with the neoliberal notion of individualized chronic illness management gives cause to question the usefulness of such a framework for promoting healthy and contented attitudes in people with diabetes towards their condition, as well as their bodies and health more generally. It falls beyond the scope of this study to motivate change on such broad a scale and, as linguists, we are neither qualified to recommend an alternative, nor even certain of what the best solution to this challenge is. Interesting discussions in this area are emergent and ongoing, with several authors proposing a promising notion of partnership between patient and practitioner in diabetes care (in contrast to a wholly individualizing or paternalistic model, which are likely to imply 'ownership' of care (and even condition) by either patient or practitioner, respectively) (Anderson and Funnell 2000; Gallant et al. 2002; Ingadottir and Halldorsdottir 2008; Mol 2008). Accordingly, the present study adds to calls for healthcare practitioners to develop diabetes care and management plans more collaboratively with their patients, with the aim of ensuring that patients are comfortable with and able to meet the disease management demands that are placed on them (Callaghan and Williams 1994; Paterson et al. 1998). However, we also acknowledge that such a bespoke level of diabetes care is likely to pose a significant challenge to increasingly over-burdened practitioners working within evermore rationalized healthcare systems.

Patients experiencing either anorexia or diabulimia present relatively infrequently in key healthcare contexts such as primary care, and general practitioners claim to have little training or clinical experience of patients with eating disorders (Reid et al. 2010). One way in which clinicians could be exposed to the discourse of those suffering from anorexia and diabulimia (as well as other eating disorders) is through examination of electronic support groups such as those included in this study. Medical education that includes exposure to online support communities would facilitate understanding of the interactions of sufferers, their diverse experiences and expectations of healthcare services, and their overarching concerns in relation to each condition. Through exploring interactions among online peers, clinicians could also be sensitized to the manner in which their patients articulate their concerns and the concepts that they co-develop online which may influence their beliefs about treatment. The study of online depression support groups may be similarly beneficial, particularly in light of patients' attested difficulties in discussing suicidality with clinicians (Michel 2000). Much like the learning of a foreign language, corpus linguistic methods would provide a strong evidence base on which to design such training and also permit trainee clinicians to study large volumes of naturally occurring patient data. In particular, corpus methods could demonstrate salient areas of patients' communication as well as the consistent linguistic choices through which they encode their understandings of illness and express beliefs about clinical interventions (Crawford and Brown 2010). In line with our arguments in the previous chapter, however, this training would need to emphasize that such linguistic choices can reflect the norms of online networks to which individual patients belong as well as their experiences of psychological distress themselves.

8.3 Methodological reflections

Online health fora constitute popular, accessible sources of support and, for patients in sparing contact with healthcare professionals, can represent a key source of healthcare information. As well as proving expedient to the compilation of corpora, the collection of data from such groups has therefore enabled analysis of a mode of interaction – computer-mediated communication

(CMC) – that serves as a principal means of communicating about mental health and illness. The use of web fora has also allowed for the study of non-elicited interactions that occur without the input of a researcher or healthcare professional. As such, the messages making up the three corpora analysed in this book have permitted us access to an otherwise unavailable context of sufferer-led health communication. To this end, the study has contributed to knowledge of the linguistic choices made by sufferers when articulating experiences of three contested conditions, the salient aspects of sufferers' experiences of psychological distress, the function of medicalized models of mental illness in the dynamics of support group interactions and the influence of neoliberal imperatives of diabetes self-management on experiences of diabulimia. Analysis of multiple illness communities has also enabled identification of consistent linguistic signatures and rhetorical strategies – illness objectification, personification and extreme case formulations – that feature across different fora, as well as accounts of group-specific concerns such as 'behaviours', antidepressant medication and diabetes management.

As all worthwhile findings should do, these insights inevitably encourage further questions. For example, the 'causal indeterminacy' inherent in the study of online behaviour (Herring 2004: 350) raises the question of whether the objectification and medicalization of illness illustrated in Chapters 4 to 6 are specifically encouraged by features of CMC. Similarly, the present data do not conclusively indicate whether the prevalence of the 'ED voice' concept originates from sufferers' own experiences, their exposure to professional and self-help therapies, their communication with other sufferers or from some combination of these and other factors. The unobtrusive nature of the study's data collection prevented such questions being posed directly to the discourse participants. However, they could be fruitfully investigated through interviews with online forum participants and comparisons between online fora and interactions in face-to-face support groups. The latter option would provide contrasting sufferer-led supportive talk that could be examined for verbal indications of illness reification and its function within the groups' interactions. The study of face-to-face support groups would also allow future research to account for sociolinguistic variables such as age, gender and ethnicity that are difficult to reliably ascertain from online profiles, but which correlate with particular linguistic styles.

Investigation of face-to-face groups would also help to capture the discourses of individuals with mental health difficulties who do not participate in online support groups. Like other internet-based health communication research, this study has been unable to capture the views of those experiencing mental health problems who are not computer literate or who are otherwise unwilling or unable to contribute to online platforms because they do not have regular or private internet access. Similarly, those sufferers who do not perceive a need for ongoing peer support or for whom psychological distress is short-lived are less likely to be represented in this study or research online support (Houston et al. 2002). This does not, however, detract from the valuable insights that are gained from online research, and the large number of individuals whose interactions can be examined. In addition, while this study has only investigated a small number of online communities, a preliminary analysis highlights the presence of similarly objectifying and medicalizing constructions in several other mental illness fora. Detailed examination of additional web communities – including those with non-Western users – would reveal the extent of the prevalence of the linguistic signatures identified here, as well as alternative discursive strategies.

A perennial issue for researchers interested in examining contemporary forms of online communication is keeping pace with the advent of new digital platforms to which the public migrate. Researchers must adapt to the increasingly diverse ecology of digital communication as well as augmenting existing methods in order to elucidate the forms of interaction afforded by individual platforms. In our own case, we are conscious that online health communication increasingly takes place on social media platforms that support a richer and more complex interaction of semiotic modes than those afforded by the largely text-based discussion fora examined in this study (see Ging and Garvey 2018; Koteyko and Atanasova 2018). While the extent of mental health communication on social media platforms makes them well suited to computer-assisted discourse analysis, traditional corpus linguistic methods require significant modification and integration with methods of multimodal discourse analysis in order to account for the full 'modal ensemble' of social media texts (Kress 2010; Caple 2018).

Regardless of the modal composition of a corpus and the methods used to interrogate it, individual corpus-aided discourse analyses will struggle to comprehensively explore all of the analytical possibilities of large datasets. While corpus methods offer principled and effective means for isolating the most frequent and statistically salient features of the data for closer, more fine-grained analysis, the extent of these features may still be too great for them to be examined exhaustively (Baker 2006; Harvey 2013a). In the case of this study, despite the rigorous insights that the corpus approach has offered into the expression of anorexia-, depression- and diabulimia-related concerns, the analysis has inevitably been restricted to a selection of keywords and only a minority of the messages in each corpus has been presented for scrutiny. Each of the three corpora therefore contains a number of under- and unexplored areas that warrant further interrogation. A useful starting point would be to examine the titles of healthcare practitioners that constitute keywords in each corpus. Analysis of these roles would supply further insights into sufferers' experiences of clinical diagnosis and intervention and their perceptions of the patient–professional relationship. In a similar vein, space constraints have also meant that discussions of medication 'side effects' in the *depression.net* corpus have not been presented here. Exploration of this collocation could help to illuminate sufferers' experiences of an aspect of taking antidepressants often cited as a reason for non-adherence (McMullen and Herman 2009), perhaps also offering a contrasting perspective to the more favourable representation of the 'right medication'. Participants in each corpus also consistently refer to the titles of family members and close social relations who occupy significant roles in their lives, whether as informal carers or possible antagonists (words such as *family* and *friend* typically have keyness values just below the threshold for our keyword analyses). Given the substantial role that family and friends can play in providing support for those experiencing mental health problems, analysis of these lexical items would shed light on a central – but frequently unheeded – facet of contemporary mental health care.

Despite these limitations, the choice of data and the analytical approach employed in this study also have a number of strengths. This study is one of the first to interrogate discourses of diabulimia and the linguistic practices of sufferers who disclose and discuss their experiences of this emerging condition online. The analytical focus on forum users' subjective constructions of diabulimia has allowed this study to provide a rich and novel illustration of the social and lived dynamics of this contested condition. The extended qualitative analysis in the preceding chapters also offers a counterpoise to the preponderance of quantitative, positivist paradigms in research on not only diabulimia, but also anorexia and depression.

At the same time, this study has clearly benefitted from the synthesis of qualitative discourse analysis with the quantitative methods of corpus linguistics. Most obviously, corpus techniques have been integral in identifying recurrent lexical items and multiword collocations throughout the three corpora. In doing so, they have contributed to illuminating discursive signatures used to express experiences of psychological distress and its management that are otherwise likely to have been overlooked. For example, Chapters 4 to 6 each identify the tendency for sufferers to use aligning constructions of illness – *my*+[condition] – in the broader context of discussing ongoing or previous successful treatments. It seems improbable that this highly granular but consistent grammatical distinction would be observed without software that enables researchers to attend closely to fine-grained linguistic patterns dispersed across large volumes of data and to easily examine such patterns in their contexts of use.

Corpus-driven methods of keyword and collocation analysis have also delivered summary information for large amounts of language and provided quantitative data that enabled insights into the relative dominance of different constructions of anorexia, depression and diabulimia at a corpus level. This degree of quantitative precision remains largely elusive in non-corpus discourse studies (Baker et al. 2008). In these respects, computer-assisted corpus tools constitute both expedient methods for interrogating our data and means of deriving findings on the basis of more robust volumes of data.

For researchers from a more traditional qualitative background, we have suggested that keyword analysis can offer a rapid, data-driven analogue to thematic coding for identifying overarching topics of discussion in large amounts of language data. Keyness analysis also has the advantage of being relatively free from researcher bias (though the choice of reference corpus, statistical measure and thematic categorization of keywords certainly are researcher driven). In this study, keyword analysis has highlighted lexical items – and corresponding discursive features – that had certainly escaped detection during manual reading of the data.

However, thematic coding is, of course, only one aspect of thematic analysis (Braun and Clarke 2006), and while we have sought to identify areas of consistency within and across each corpus, using automated keyness calculations as an entry point into each corpus somewhat militates against the construction of broader, more interpretive thematic categories that would arise from a manual, 'bottom-up' approach to coding. For example, when the original proposal and sample chapter for this book were submitted to the publishers, one reviewer suggested structuring Chapter 5 along broader themes of seeking help, getting help and overcoming the condition (i.e. in terms of themes that more closely encompass a potential illness trajectory). Organizing the chapter in this way would, we believe, have lent itself more readily to the construction of the sort of coherent overarching themes or theory that characterizes more conventional qualitative health research (though we accept that labels such as 'thematic analysis' refer to a range of different approaches – see Braun et al. 2019). However, clearly – and with the utmost respect for the reviewer's suggestion – we have not organized the analytical chapters in this manner and readers who anticipated overarching narratives that account for the 'what' and 'why' of the forum discussions as a whole may be duly disappointed. In response, we argue that there is no such discernible trajectory for the users of the fora in this study; even though stages of initial recognition, help-seeking and recovery are apparent across each corpus as a whole, for many participants, experiences of chronic mental illness appear to be characterized by painful stasis or repeated cycles of improving and declining well-being. The discourses in each corpus are also heterogeneous, with participants offering contrasting accounts of each condition as well as specific facets such as anorexic behaviours, antidepressants and diabetic 'control'. This diversity, we contend, defies – or at least hampers – attempts to abstract the data into 'a coherent and internally consistent account, with accompanying narrative' (Braun and Clarke 2006: 92). Instead, we offer a survey of specific discursive signatures while drawing attention to the situatedness and contingency of participants' discourse, illustrating how it is dependent on a range of broader discursive and local interactional factors that do not fit so neatly into decontextualized theories. It is for this reason, too, that we are cautious about claiming our findings would extrapolate to other eating disorder, depression and diabulimia support groups. The trade-off for the predictive power of a theory, then, is far greater attention to 'how' participants communicate their experiences, the interactional functions of how community members convey themselves, and what the implications of these discursive signatures are.

8.4 Corpus linguistics and health communication: Evidence-based or person-centred?

The quantitative and qualitative analysis of large amounts of language supports corpus linguistics' claim to be a 'data-driven' enterprise (Johns 1991). As well noted in Chapter 3, Adolphs et al. (2004) and Crawford and colleagues (2014; Brown et al. 2006; Crawford and Brown 2010) have repeatedly argued that this 'data-driven' approach confers upon corpus linguistics an 'evidence-based' philosophy that resonates with the (presumably positivist) epistemological proclivities of the healthcare professionals whose practices they seek to enhance. For instance, in contrast to traditional discourse analytic approaches, corpus linguistics can render evidentially robust results in a readily interpretable quantitative format. Wanting to enhance the uptake and disciplinary standing of corpus linguistics among non-linguists is certainly a laudable aim, as is these scholars' commitment to data-driven learning in professionals' health communication training. However, we argue that the label of 'evidence-based' rests uneasily on corpus linguistic studies of health communication. That is, it represents a questionable descriptive characterization of existing studies and engenders a number of challenges if used as a prescriptive template for how future research should be conducted.

From a descriptive perspective, it is not clear that foregoing corpus studies always provide robust results of the sort that characterizes 'gold standard' randomized control trials and meta-analyses (Bensing 2000). Corpus studies of health communication such as those of Adolphs et al. (2004) and Crawford et al. (2014) use small corpora comprised of relatively few individual texts and involving few participants. These corpora are less likely to be representative of the full breadth and diversity of language practices in the contexts under study and their interrogation is also more likely to be skewed towards individual longer texts or participants who simply speak more. Using online data allows for the creation of corpora whose size and participant numbers are greater by several orders of magnitude. However, corpora of online interactions – including those in this study – are frequently opportunistic datasets that lack reliable data on participants' demographic features, diagnoses and treatments of the sort that might allow for the correlation of linguistic style and clinical outcomes (though see Rude et al. 2004). To our knowledge, corpus methods are also yet to be integrated into clinical trials so as to correlate, say, the language used in therapeutic interactions with subsequent clinical outcomes. In light of this, the nature of the data and the manner of its collection mean that many corpus studies lack central components of reliable 'evidence' as it is construed in more conventional clinical research.

Even if the data used in existing corpus studies of health communication fall someway short, perhaps a stronger claim to the label of 'evidence-based' research lies in the analytical methods of corpus studies. Myriad studies illustrate that the data-driven – and nominally 'evidence-based' – aspect of corpus analysis is primarily operationalized through the presentation of frequency data and keyword and collocation analyses based on lexical frequencies. The provision of frequency information has been a core aspect of corpus linguistics and has contributed to the discipline's self-definition as offering a rationalized approach to language data. Starcke, for instance, claims that 'analysis of the frequency of linguistic items is the only available objective evidence for the significance of this item [sic] in the text' (2006: 88). As we note in Chapter 1, the focus on frequent items in critically oriented corpus studies has also helped researchers to counter accusations that critical discourse analyses are compromised by researchers' pre-analytical priorities (Widdowson 2004).

It should be obvious, however, that frequency information offers only one way to prioritize what is closely examined in a corpus. Accordingly, it should be noted that, by focusing primarily on linguistic features that are quantitatively dominant, corpus analyses may occlude statistical outliers – that is, the accounts of those speakers who express themselves idiosyncratically (Seale et al. 2006). For example, Section 5.5 examines the keywords *life* and *self* along with instances of *suicidal* and *suicide*, which both appear with significantly high frequencies in the *depression.net* corpus when compared to the Spoken BNC2014. Close consideration of these keywords provided insights into the discourse of those forum members who use these lexical items when discussing self-injurious behaviour. As elsewhere, this more granular examination of the data drew in part on collocation analysis that quantified collocational strength using MI³, a statistical measure that favours higher frequency collocations. But what of the forum user who claims that they wish to 'drive somewhere remote and never come home' or who gnomically refers to being 'sorely tempted' after alluding to the volume of medication they have stockpiled? While couched in more euphemistic terms (itself an interesting linguistic finding), these expressions are substantial, poignant disclosures for their respective authors and, from a researcher's perspective, signal the possibility of examining additional disclosures of suicidal ideation. However, these variable and oblique references to suicide are individually infrequent in the corpus and so will not be identified using keyword analysis. Their idiomatic form also means that even sophisticated, semantically sensitive corpus platforms such as *Wmatrix* (Rayson 2008) would not identify them as references to dying. As a result, they are unlikely to feature in any analysis driven primarily by computer-derived frequency counts; the views of these sufferers are discounted from further study because their expressions are lexically *atypical* rather than empirically irrelevant. Researchers should therefore remember that prioritizing corpus frequency in the pursuit of 'evidence-based' research not only shapes analysis but inadvertently warrants the marginalization or exclusion of potentially relevant data. Further, this exclusion occurs not because of the value of the data as a record of a sufferer's experience or example of suicide-related discourse, but because corpus analysis programmes have limited facilities for identifying complex discursive phenomena. While the impetus to be mindful of idiosyncratic expressions and resistant discourses is axiomatic in corpus-based discourse analysis (Baker 2006; Marchi and Taylor

2018), this obligation should be felt all the more keenly when dealing with data in which people are talking about ending their own lives. In cases such as these, overlooking idiosyncrasies and focusing solely on the aspects of the data for which there is the most – or most *visible* – evidence is not just partial analysis. Rather, it feels at odds with the fundamental commitment to the humane and empathetic treatment of participants that undergirds qualitative health inquiry (Morse 2016). As a prescription for conducting corpus-based health communication research, then, the focus on 'evidence-based' methods is clearly insufficient. Indeed, if we have reservations about the manner in which we have analysed and presented the data in this study, they stem from a feeling that we have underrepresented the extent of the suffering expressed by members of the fora we have studied. By abstracting their messages into collocation scores and thematically coherent but truncated extracts, we are aware that we risk overlooking the desperate and frequently heart-breaking crises that the participants describe.

There are parallels between corpus linguistics and quantitative healthcare research more generally here. Bensing (2000) notes that randomized control trials are often limited to homogenous patient groups who meet strict recruitment criteria and bear little resemblance to the individuals with diverse symptoms, comorbidities and coping strategies that physicians meet in practice. Similarly, we might claim that corpus frequency and keyword analyses narrow the population who are reflected in subsequent qualitative findings to those who choose contextually common lexical items. Additionally, corpus tools tend to efface individual speakers by abstracting their discourse into statistical representations and presenting their language use as a numbered line on a concordance that foregrounds linguistic consistencies over idiosyncratic utterances. Bensing (2000) goes on to argue that decisions based on evidence derived from meta-analyses of randomized control trials do not necessarily result in optimal, 'patient-centred' care for individual patients, and particularly those who would not fulfil the inclusion criteria of the clinical studies. What is needed, he argues, is care that integrates external scientific evidence into the specific context, needs and capacities of the individual patient (Bensing 2000; Byng 2012); care that is both 'evidence-based' and 'patient-centred'. As Mol (2008: 68) avers, 'good care depends on specification', and just as evidence from randomized control trials requires interpretation against particular patients (Sackett et al. 1996), quantitative corpus-driven findings must be viewed as only a partial heuristic of the data that must be interpreted to be meaningful in specific cases (Skelton and Hobbs 1999a). In light of this, throughout the analysis we have endeavoured to integrate the interrogation of frequent keywords with examination of less frequent lexical items and strings identified through intuition and manual reading of the corpora. In doing so, we have sought to bring together overarching trends with one-off expressions, exceptions and moments of resistance that would have been overlooked by a more stringent corpus-driven methodology.

In this vein, the foregoing analysis also underscores that fully apprehending the situated use of a linguistic feature requires the scope of the corpus analyst's lens to move beyond not just individual concordance lines but also larger stretches of discourse involving multiple participants (Mahlberg 2006). In this regard, across Chapters 4 to 6 we have attempted to contextualize findings derived from corpus analysis within the dynamics of each forum community. In particular, we have sought to evince how the dominant discourses of each forum are deployed strategically during interactions and that the use of these discourses results in new identities for those who come to define themselves as suffering from anorexia, depression or diabulimia. In contrast to previous studies that have examined corpora comprised of isolated texts (e.g. Harvey 2013a; Baker et al. 2019), this approach is particularly important when dealing with dialogic data such as discussion fora, where meanings emerge through sequences of messages involving multiple participants. We would argue that these aspects of the analysis, which have been entirely qualitative in orientation, have offered the most detailed insights into the three corpora by illustrating how the content of a text – representations of mental illness in this case – functions both within that utterance and interactively as part of a longer sequence of utterances.

More generally, regardless of whether corpora are composed of monologic or dialogic texts, it is essential that researchers employ an approach to discourse analysis that is conceptually and methodologically flexible to the nature of the data at hand and sensitive to the multiple contingent factors in which meaning is situated. In this regard, we are heartened by the willingness of corpus linguistic researchers to combine corpus methods with other forms of analysis (see Baker and Egbert 2016) in order to illuminate the 'blind spots' of their data (Marchi and Taylor 2018). Researchers should consider the size and composition of their corpora, too. The analysis in this study has been enriched by pre-analytical investigation of the organization, membership and moderation practices of each online community. This enabled our data to be interpreted in light of the – often unspoken – norms of each forum and offered a richer picture of participants' communicative practices. Researchers dealing with much larger corpora or those that have been compiled from multiple online communities and social networking platforms should thus be aware that these tacit contextual influences will be harder to discern and accommodate during analysis (Collins 2019), leading to a trade-off between the scope of the data and the granularity of its interpretation.

This more flexible approach has also extended to the way in which we have presented data. While in Chapter 4 we have discussed the grammatical and lexical collocates of *ED* separately, in Chapter 6 it was more appropriate to present the lexical and grammatical collocates of *diabulimia* together. The risk of this approach, inevitably, is the appearance of methodological inconsistency, particularly when analyses of different corpora appear in close proximity to each other. However, rather than a fixed (though consistent) model of reporting data, we recommend presenting the analysis in a way that is responsive to the contingencies of each corpus and which best allows its intricacies to be explicated and interpreted for the reader.

While corpus-aided discourse studies have come to be defined by methodological bricolage and appreciation of the various co-textual and contextual factors that shape language use, these characteristics contrast with alternative methods of quantitative linguistic analysis from computational linguistics and psychology (Blei et al. 2003; Pennebaker et al. 2007). In treating texts as 'bags of words', approaches such as topic modelling and Linguistic Inquiry and Word Count (*LIWC*) are more liable to draw researchers into offering haphazard summaries of the thematic content of a dataset, misinterpreting the meaning of words considered in isolation (or attributing them to pre-set psychological categories) and overlooking the manifold contingent factors from which discourses emerge (Brookes and McEnery 2019). They are, in short, characteristic of the perils of a purely 'evidence-based' approach to communication. In contrast to the contextualized qualitative analysis presented in the preceding chapters, a further shortcoming of these alternative approaches is the way in which they construe the data as homogenous and static. For example, the profiles emerging from a *LIWC* analysis render the data as the aggregate of psychological traits of its participants. If we accept the validity of such results, then they have a clear diagnostic value. Yet this aggregation effaces the heterogeneity in the data and masks the fact that its linguistic signatures emerge during interactions in which they are not just reiterated but also contested and undermined. It can appear that participants talk this way due to stable psychological dispositions, not that they talk in a variety of ways according to a host of contingent factors. For researchers or clinicians wishing to intervene in the context under study, then, the diagnostic potential of *LIWC* seems to outweigh its practical valence; that is, it can offer less insight into questions such as what form do dominant and resistant linguistic practices take in this context, what intrapersonal and interpersonal functions do they have for participants, and, for practices that are deemed problematic, what does the data itself suggest about how they could be challenged? Consequently, compared to alternative methods employed in other disciplines, we see corpus linguistics' combination of principled quantitative and theory-sensitive qualitative analysis as offering not only greater insight into the data at hand, but findings that have clearer implications for research users.

But where, then, does this leave corpus linguistics' status as a means of conducting 'evidence-based' health communication research? While some previous studies (Crawford and Brown 2010; Crawford et al. 2014) have been evangelical about the potential for the statistical elements of corpus linguistics to win over clinicians and quantitative health researchers, we offer a somewhat more tempered position. Like all interdisciplinary work, engaging in collaborative research with quantitative health researchers and convincing them of the merits of corpus-based discourse analysis present a number of challenges for corpus linguists to collectively overcome. These include the need to find common ground between different disciplinary perspectives on research ethics, the primacy of particular research questions, the way to value and assess outcomes and the implications of specific analytical findings. In addition, the particular mixed methods nature of corpus study and its ostensible 'evidence-based' approach present two unique demands. The first of these will arise as a consequence of promoting corpus linguistics on the basis of its 'data-driven', quantitative elements; on the one hand, clinicians are not simply number crunchers who care only for results that are presented in the form of p-values and effect sizes. On the other, clinical researchers who work with quantitative data already have established, successful research methods. It is our view that corpus linguists will need to work hard in the long term to persuade researchers who are already heavily invested in such methods that there is comparable value in the rather messier picture that emerges from the sort of corpus-based discourse analysis that we are advocating.

A second challenge for corpus linguists who aim to work with clinical researchers from quantitative backgrounds is the need to stand firm on the value and potential of qualitative research. Qualitative methodologies have unique strengths in facilitating rich, nuanced and complex interpretations of data. These methods are of undeniable benefit for the study of health communication and to health research more generally, and corpus-based discourse analysts seeking to foster interdisciplinary work on the basis of their own quantitative methods should ensure they do not implicitly devalue qualitative research by glossing its qualitative elements with a quantitative veneer.

Finally, appealing to clinicians from quantitative backgrounds is not the only way in which to expand the horizons of corpus research into health communication. We believe there is also significant value to be gained by promoting central corpus analysis methods to researchers who already operate in a primarily qualitative tradition. In particular, corpus linguistics furnishes qualitative researchers with a set of principled analytical methods with which to 'scale up' their analyses to larger datasets, with keyness analysis, in particular, offering a cognate method to thematic coding. Likewise, concordancing software and collocation analysis offer systematic means of identifying, scrutinizing and visualizing patterns of association in language data (Anthony 2018). Indeed, tools that approximate the frequency analysis and concordancing functions of *WordSmith Tools*, *Wmatrix*, *SketchEngine* and *AntConc* now feature in well-known qualitative analysis platforms such as *NVivo* and *ATLAS.ti*. Employing the more sophisticated versions of these applications along with the range of other tools that are offered by eminent corpus analysis interfaces would enable qualitative researchers to enhance their existing analytical practices. Crucially, this could be achieved without compromising the use of other, complementary forms of analysis or the overarching commitment of qualitative researchers to engage sensitively and carefully with the intricacies of their data.

In a society in which forms of mental distress are prevalent and increasingly visible, the need for research which addresses the topic of mental health has never been clearer. Although we are less sceptical than others about the capacity of psychiatric interventions to alleviate people's mental anguish, we are also certain of the need for more linguistic research which sheds further light on individuals' lived experiences of mental distress. Rather than providing an elusive 'evidence-based' gloss, we would argue that the virtue of corpus methods in this endeavour, as in the study of health communication generally, is that they enable multiple forms of investigation that are sensitive to both commonalities and idiosyncrasies in the data; they support analyses that are both statistically informed and fundamentally 'person-centred'.

Notes

Chapter 3

1 One duplicate message had to be removed from the *diabulimia.net* corpus. The post and word counts given in this table were obtained following the removal of this post.

2 We should note that the *diabulimia.net* corpus is imbalanced in terms of the degree to which each of its constituent support groups is represented; one website accounts for 56 per cent of the words in this corpus, another 29 per cent and then the final one 15 per cent. While this means that the norms of some of one online community are likely to influence the data more than the others, the support groups are all comparable in terms of their register features, the topic of the interactions and the rules and layouts of the websites.

3 Although note that recent research suggests this ought not to be a cause for concern in the kind of keyword-driven discourse analysis we are undertaking here. Smith et al. (2014) examined the effect of spelling variation on keywords generated from Harvey's (2013a) corpus of adolescent health emails in order to establish the extent to which misspellings and non-standard formulations skewed the keywords generated by the corpus software. In this study, keywords produced from a version of the corpus in which the spelling errors were corrected were compared against keywords generated from the original, unedited version of the same corpus. Interestingly, the researchers found each keyword's respective ranks to be very similar in both lists. This study therefore suggests that, depending on the research goals, keywords can be generated reliably without the need for spelling standardization (in electronic health communication data at least).

4 When conducting analyses of collocational strength using *WordSmith*, we used separate wordlist files in cases where the spellings of the node word had been standardized in the original data. This ensured that word lists and resultant MI^3 scores accurately reflected the corpus data.

5 As Collins observes, future studies undertaken in Europe will not be able to employ a post-hoc 'opt out' approach to consent, in which non-responses to consent requests are taken as implied consent, as the GDRP requires consent to be provided explicitly.

6 Although there is often overlap between computational keywords and the types of cultural keywords that a human analyst may intuitively regard as being salient in the texts they are analysing (Scott and Tribble 2006). A recent example is Jeffries and

Walker's (2019) study which combined measures of computational keyness with Williams's concept of 'cultural keywords' to examine keywords in the British press at the time of the New Labour Government in the UK.

Chapter 4

1 As noted in Chapter 3, *behaviours* is an example of a keyword in which the frequencies of US and UK spelling variants were manually combined for the purposes of keyword and collocation analyses. As a result, seven instances of *behaviors* from the original data are presented with the UK spelling in this chapter.

Chapter 5

1 The size and informal register of the spoken BNC2014 mean that the frequency of *depression* is relatively low ($n = 90$), and although it collocates significantly with *suffer*, *suffering* and *suffered*, these collocations are infrequent (three co-occurrences each). The frequency with which *depression* co-occurs with these collocates are much higher in the original, 100 million-word BNC, with a corresponding increase in MI^3 values.

Chapter 6

1 As noted in Chapter 3, these orthographic variations were standardized to ensure that our analysis captured the fullest possible range of discourses surrounding diabulimia. The frequency and keyness values given here reflect the corpus post-standardization.

References

Adolphs, S., Brown, B., Carter, R., Crawford, P. and Sahota, O. (2004), 'Applying corpus linguistics in a health care context', *Journal of Applied Linguistics*, 1(1): 9–28.

Affenito, S, G. and Adams, C. H. (2001), 'Are eating disorders more prevalent in females with type 1 diabetes mellitus when the impact of insulin omission is considered?', *Nutrition Reviews*, 59(6): 179–82.

Allan, K. and Burridge, K. (2006), *Forbidden Words*, Cambridge: Cambridge University Press.

Allen, G. (2011), *Intertextuality*, London and New York: Routledge.

Al-Mosaiwi, M. and Johnstone, T. (2018), 'In an absolute state: Elevated use of absolutist words is a marker specific to anxiety, depression, and suicidal ideation', *Clinical Psychological Science*, 6(4): 529–42.

American Psychiatric Association (1994), *Diagnostic and Statistical Manual of Mental Disorders*, 4th edn, Arlington, VA: APA.

American Psychiatric Association (2013), *Diagnostic and Statistical Manual of Mental Disorders*, 5th edn, Washington, DC: APA.

Anderson, R. M. and Funnell, M. M. (2000), 'Compliance and adherence are dysfunctional concepts in diabetes care', *The Diabetes Educator*, 26(4): 597–604.

Antaki, C. (1994), *Explaining and Arguing: The Social Organisation of Accounts*, London: Sage.

Antaki, C., Barnes, R. and Leudar, I. (2005), 'Diagnostic formulations in psychotherapy', *Discourse Studies*, 7(6): 627–47.

Antaki, C., Ardévol, E., Núñez, F. and Vayreda, A. (2005), '"For she knows who she is": Managing accountability in online forum messages', *Journal of Computer Mediated Communication*, 11(1): 114–32.

Anthony, L. (2018), 'Visualisation in corpus-based discourse studies', in C. Taylor and A. Marchi (eds), *Corpus Approaches to Discourse: A Critical Review*, 197–224, London and New York: Routledge.

Archer, M., Decoteau, C., Gorski, P., Little, D. Porpora, D., Rutzou, T., Smith, C., Steinmetz, G. and Vandenberghe, F. (2016), *What Is Critical Realism?* [online]. Available at http://www.asatheory.org/current-newsletter-online/what-is-critical-realism (accessed 14 March 2017).

Armstrong, N., Koteyko N. and Powell, J. (2011), '"Oh dear, should I really be saying that on here?" Issues of identity and authority in an online diabetes community', *Health*, 16(4): 347–65.

Aston, G. and Burnard, L. (1998), *The BNC Handbook: Exploring the British National Corpus with SARA*, Edinburgh: Edinburgh University Press.

Atanasova, D. (2018), '"Keep moving forward. LEFT RIGHT LEFT": A critical metaphor analysis and addressivity analysis of personal and professional obesity blogs', *Discourse, Context & Media*, 25: 5–12.

Attard, A. and Coulson, N. S. (2012), 'A thematic analysis of patient communication in Parkinson's disease online support group forums', *Computers in Human Behavior*, 28: 500–506.

Baker, D. and Fortune, S. (2008), 'Understanding self-harm and suicide websites: A qualitative interview study of young adult website users', *Crisis*, 29(3): 118–22.

Baker, P. (2004), 'Querying keywords: Questions of difference, frequency, and sense in keyword analysis', *Journal of English Linguistics*, 32(4): 346–59.

Baker, P. (2006), *Using Corpora in Discourse Analysis*, London: Continuum.

Baker, P. (2010), *Sociolinguistics and Corpus Linguistics*, Edinburgh: Edinburgh University Press.

Baker, P. and Egbert, J., eds (2016), *Triangulating Methodological Approaches in Corpus Linguistic Research*, London and New York: Routledge.

Baker, P. and McEnery, T. (2005), 'A corpus-based approach to discourses of refugees and asylum seekers in UN and newspaper texts', *Language and Politics*, 4(2): 197–226.

Baker, P. and McEnery, T. (2015), 'Introduction', in P. Baker and T. McEnery (eds), *Corpora and Discourse Studies: Integrating Discourse and Corpora*, 1–19, Basingstoke: Palgrave Macmillan.

Baker, P., Gabrielatos, C. and McEnery, T. (2013), *Discourse Analysis and Media Attitudes: The Representation of Islam in the British Press*, Cambridge: Cambridge University Press.

Baker, P., Brookes, G. and Evans, C. (2019), *The Language of Patient Feedback: A Corpus Linguistic Study of Online Health Communication*, London and New York: Routledge.

Baker, P., Gabrielatos, C., KhosraviNik, M., Krzyżanowski, M., McEnery, T. and Wodak, R. (2008), 'A useful methodological synergy? Combining critical discourse analysis and corpus linguistics to examine discourses of refugees and asylum seekers in the UK press', *Discourse & Society*, 19(3): 273–306.

Balfe, M. (2007), 'Diets and discipline: The narratives of practice of university students with Type 1 diabetes', *Sociology of Health & Illness*, 29: 136–53.

Bamberg, M. (2012), 'Narrative practice and identity navigation', in J. A. Holstein and J. F. Gubrium (eds), *Varieties of Narrative Analysis*, 99–124, Los Angeles: Sage.

Barak, A. (2007), 'Phantom emotions: Psychological determinants of emotional experiences on the Internet', in A. Joinson, K. Y. A. McKenna, T. Postmes and U. D. Reips (eds), *Oxford Handbook of Internet Psychology*, 303–29. Oxford: Oxford University Press.

Barker, K. (2008), 'Electronic support groups, patient consumers, and medicalization: The case of contested illness', *Journal of Health and Social Behavior*, 49(1): 20–36.

Baron, N. S. (1998), 'Letters by phone or speech by some other means: The linguistics of email', *Language and Communication*, 18(2): 133–70.

Baron, N. S. (2000), *Alphabet to E-mail: How Written English Evolved and Where It's Heading*, London and New York: Routledge.

Baron, N. S. (2008), *Always On: Language in an Online and Mobile World*, Oxford: Oxford University Press.

Bartlett, Y. K. and Coulson, N. (2011), 'An investigation into the empowerment effects of using online support groups and how this affects health professional/patient communication', *Patient Education and Counselling*, 83(1): 113–19.

Barton, D. and Lee, C. (2013), *Language Online: Investigating Digital Texts and Practices*, London and New York: Routledge.

Battaglia, M. R., Alemzadeh, R., Katte, H., Hall, P. and Perlmuter, L. (2006), 'Brief report: Disordered eating and psychosocial factors in adolescent females with type 1 diabetes mellitus', *Journal of Paediatric Psychology*, 31(6): 552–6.

Baym, N. K. and boyd, d. (2012), 'Socially mediated publicness: An introduction', *Journal of Broadcasting & Electronic Media*, 56(3): 320–29.

Beautrais, A. L. (2000), 'Risk factors for suicide and attempted suicide among young people', *Australian & New Zealand Journal of Psychiatry*, 34(3): 420–36.

Beck, A. T., Rush, A. J., Shaw, B. F. and Emery, G. (1979), *Cognitive Therapy of Depression*, New York: Guildford Press.

Becker, G. and Nachtigall, R. D. (1992), 'Eager for medicalisation: The social production of infertility as a disease', *Sociology of Health & Illness*, 14(4): 456–71.

Belica, C. (1996), 'Analysis of temporal changes in corpora', *International Journal of Corpus Linguistics*, 1(1): 61–73.

Bell, V. (2007), 'Online information, extreme communities and internet therapy: Is the internet good for our mental health?', *Journal of Mental Health*, 16(4): 445–57.

Bennett, S., Coggan, C. and Adams, P. (2003), 'Problematising depression: Young people, mental health and suicidal behaviours', *Social Science & Medicine*, 57(2): 289–99.

Bensing, J. (2000), 'Bridging the gap: The separate worlds of evidence-based medicine and patient-centred medicine', *Patient Education and Counseling*, 39(1): 17–25.

Bentall, R. (2003), *Madness Explained: Psychosis and Human Nature*, London: Penguin Allen Lane.

Berg, K. M. (2002), 'The illness experience: Eating disorders from the patient's perspective', in K. M. Berg, D. J. Hurley, J. A. McSherry and N. E. Strange (eds), *Eating Disorders: A Patient-Centred Approach*, 73–97, Oxford: Radcliffe Medical Press.

Bernal, M., Haro, J. M., Bernert, S., Brugha, T., de Graaf, R., Bruffaerts, R., Lépine, J. P., de Girolamo, G., Vilagut, G., Gasquet, I. and Torres, J. V. (2007), 'Risk factors for suicidality in Europe: Results from the ESEMED study', *Journal of Affective Disorders*, 101(1–3): 27–34.

Beumont, P. J. (2002), 'Clinical presentation of anorexia nervosa and bulimia nervosa', in C. G. Fairburn and K. D. Brownell (eds), *Eating Disorders and Obesity: A Comprehensive Handbook*, 2nd edn, 162–70, London: Guildford Press.

Bhaskar, R. (1975), *A Realist Theory of Science*, London: Verso.

Bhaskar, R. (1979), *The Possibility of Naturalism*, Atlantic Highlands, NJ: Humanities Press.

Bhaskar, R. (1990), *Reclaiming Reality*, London: Verso.

Biber, D. (1993), 'Representativeness in corpus design', *Literary and Linguistic Computing*, 8(4): 243–57.

Blei, D., Ng, A. Y., Jordan, M. I. (2003), 'Latent Dirichlet allocation', *Journal of Machine Learning Research*, 3(4–5): 993–1022.

Blommaert, J. (2005), *Discourse: A Critical Introduction*, Cambridge: Cambridge University Press.

Blommaert, J., Collins, J., Heller, M., Rampton, B., Slembrouck, S. and Verschueren, J. (2001), 'Discourse and critique: Part one', *Critique of Anthropology*, 21(1): 5–12.

Bordo, S. (2003), *Unbearable Weight: Feminism, Western Culture, and the Body*, Tenth anniversary edn, Berkeley: University of California Press.

Boughtwood, D. and Halse, C. (2010), 'Other than obedient: Girls' constructions of doctors and treatment regimes for anorexia nervosa', *Journal of Community and Applied Social Psychology*, 20(2): 83–94.

Boynton, P. and Auerbach, A. (2004), '"I cut because it helps": Narratives of self-injury in teenage girls', in B. Hurwitz, T. Greenhalgh and V. Skultans (eds), *Narrative Research in Health and Illness*, 95–114, London: BMJ Books.

Braun, V. and Clarke, V. (2006), 'Using thematic analysis in psychology', *Qualitative Research in Psychology*, 3(2), 77–101.

Braun, V., Clarke, V., Hayfield, N. and Terry, G. (2019), 'Thematic analysis', in P. Liamputtong (ed.), *Handbook of Research Methods in Health Social Sciences*, 843–60, Singapore: Springer.

Bray, A. and Colebrook, C. (1998), 'The haunted flesh: Corporeal feminism and the politics of (dis)embodiment', *Journal of Women in Culture and Society*, 24(1): 35–67.

Brezina, V., McEnery, T. and Wattam, S. (2015), 'Collocations in context: A new perspective on collocation networks', *International Journal of Corpus Linguistics*, 20(2): 139–73.

British Association for Applied Linguistics. (2016), *Recommendations on Good Practice in Applied Linguistics*, 3rd edn, British Association for Applied Linguistics. Available at https://www.baal.org.uk/wp-content/uploads/2016/10/goodpractice_full_2016.pdf.

Brodaty, H., Luscombe, G., Peisah, C., Anstey, K. and Andrews, G. (2001), 'A 25-year longitudinal, comparison study of the outcome of depression', *Psychological Medicine*, 31(8): 1347–59.

Brookes, G. (2018), 'Insulin restriction, medicalisation and the internet: A corpus-assisted study of diabulimia discourse in online support groups', *Communication & Medicine*, 15(1): 1–14.

Brookes, G. and McEnery, T. (2019), 'The utility of topic modelling for discourse studies: A critical evaluation', *Discourse Studies*, 21(1), 3–21.

Broom, A. and Tovey, P. (2008), *Therapeutic Pluralism: Exploring the Experiences of Cancer Patients and Professionals*, London and New York: London.

Broom, D. and Whittaker, A. (2004), 'Controlling diabetes, controlling diabetics: Moral language in the management of diabetes type 2', *Social Science & Medicine*, 58(11): 2371–82.

Brink, S. J. (1997), 'How to apply the diabetes control and complications trial experience to children and adolescents', *Annals of Medicine*, 29: 425–38.

Brown, B. J. and Baker, S. (2012), *Responsible Citizens: Individuals, Health and Policy Under Neoliberalism*, London: Anthem Press.

Brown, B. J., Crawford, P. and Carter, R. A. (2006), *Evidence-Based Health Communication*, Buckingham: Open University Press.

Brown, C. and Lloyd, K. (2001), 'Qualitative methods in psychiatric research', *Advances in Psychiatric Treatment*, 7(5): 350–6.

Brown, P. (1995), 'Naming and framing: The social construction of diagnosis and illness', *Journal of Health and Social Behaviour*, 1: 34–52.

Bruch, H. (1978), *The Golden Cage: The Enigma of Anorexia Nervosa*, Cambridge, MA: Harvard University Press.

Brumfit, C. (1995), 'Teacher professionalism and research', in G. Cook and B. Seidlhofer (eds), *Principles and Practice in Applied Linguistics*, 27–42, Oxford: Oxford University Press.

Bryden, K. S., Neil, A., Mayou, R. A., Peveler, R. C., Fairburn, C. G. and Dunger, D. B. (1999), 'Eating habits, body weight, and insulin misuse: A longitudinal study of teenagers and young adults with type 1 diabetes', *Diabetes Care*, 22(12): 1956–60.

Burchell, G. (1993), 'Liberal government and techniques of the self', *Economy and Society*, 22(3): 267–82.

Burns, M. and Gavey, N. (2008), 'Dis/orders of weight control: Bulimic and/or "healthy weight" practices', in S. Riley, M. Burns, H. Frith, S. Wiggins and P. Markula (eds), *Critical Bodies; Representations, Identities and Practices of Weight and Body Management*, 139–54, Basingstoke: Palgrave Macmillan.

Burr, V. (1995), *An Introduction to Social Constructionism*, London and New York: Routledge.

Burr, V. (2015), *Social Constructionism*, 3rd edn, London and New York: Routledge.

Burroughs, H., Lovell, K., Morley, M., Baldwin, R., Burns, A. and Chew-Graham, C. (2006), '"Justifiable depression": How primary care professionals and patients view late life depression? [*sic*] a qualitative study', *Family Practice*, 23(3): 369–77.

Burstow, B. (2015), *Psychiatry and the Business of Madness: An Ethical and Epistemological Accounting*, Basingstoke: Palgrave Macmillan.

Busfield, J. (2017), 'The concept of medicalisation reassessed', *Sociology of Health & Illness*, 39(5): 759–74.

Byng, R. (2012), 'Care for common mental health problems: Applying evidence beyond RCTs', *Family Practice*, 29(1): 3–7.

Callaghan, D. and Williams, A. (1994), 'Living with diabetes: Issues for nursing practice', *Journal of Advanced Nursing*, 20(1): 132–9.

Callum, A. and Lewis, L. (2014), 'Diabulimia among adolescents and young adults with type 1 diabetes', *Clinical Nursing Studies*, 2(4): 12–16.

Cameron, D. (2001), *Working with Spoken Discourse*, London: Sage.

Caple, H. (2018), 'Analysing the multimodal text', in. C. Taylor and A. Marchi (eds), *Corpus Approaches to Discourse: A Critical Review*, 85–109, London and New York: Routledge.

Carter, R. (2004), 'Introduction', in J. Sinclair (ed.), *Trust the Text: Language, Corpus and Discourse*, 1–6, London and New York: Routledge.

Carter, R. (2013), 'Preface', in K. Harvey (ed.), *Investigating Adolescent Health Communication: A Corpus Linguistics Approach*, xiii–xv, London: Bloomsbury.

Carter, R. and McCarthy, M. (2006), *Cambridge Grammar of English*, Cambridge: Cambridge University Press.

Cassell, E. J. (1976), 'Disease as an "it": Concepts of disease revealed by patients' presentation of symptoms', *Social Science & Medicine*, 10(3–4): 143–6.

Charmaz, K. (1991), *Good Days, Bad Days*, New Brunswick, NJ: Rutgers University Press.

Charteris-Black, J. (2012), 'Shattering the bell jar: Metaphor, gender, and depression', *Metaphor and Symbol*, 27(3): 199–216.

Charteris-Black, J. and Seale, C. (2010), *Gender and the Language of Illness*, Basingstoke: Palgrave Macmillan.

Chesley, K. and Loring-McNulty, N. E. (2003), 'Process of suicide: Perspective of the suicide attempter', *Journal of America Psychiatric Nurses Association*, 9(2): 41–5.

Chew-Graham, C. A., Mullin, S., May, C. R., Hedley, S. and Cole, H. (2002), 'Managing depression in primary care: Another example of the inverse care law?', *Family Practice*, 19(6): 632–7.

Chilvers, C., Dewey, M., Fielding, K., Gretton, V., Miller, P., Palmer, B., Weller, D., Churchill, R., Williams, I., Bedi, N., Duggan, C., Lee, A. and Harrison, G. (2001), 'Antidepressant drugs and generic counselling for treatment of major depression in primary care: Randomised trial with patient preference arms', *British Medical Journal*, 322: 1–5.

Chodoff, P. (2002), 'The medicalization of the human condition', *Psychiatric Services*, 53(5): 627–8.

Chomsky, N. (1957), *Syntactic Structures*, The Hague: Mouton.

Claridge, C. (2007), 'Constructing a corpus from the web: Message boards', in M. Hundt, N. Nesselhauf and C. Biewer (eds), *Corpus Linguistics and the Web*, 87–108, Amsterdam: Rodopi.

Clinard, M. B. and Meier, R. F. (2011), *Sociology of Deviant Behaviour*, 14th edn, Belmont, CA: Wadsworth Cengage Learning.

Coggan, C., Patterson, P. and Fill, J. (1997), 'Suicide: Qualitative data from focus group interviews with youth', *Social Science & Medicine*, 45(10): 1563–70.

Collins, L. C. (2019), *Corpus Linguistics for Online Communication: A Guide for Research*, London and New York: Routledge.

Collot, M. and Belmore, O. (1996), 'Electronic language: A new variety of English', in S. Herring (ed.), *Computer-Mediated Communication: Linguistics, Social and Cross-Cultural Perspectives*, 13–28, Amsterdam: John Benjamins.

Colton, P., Rodin, G., Bergenstal, R. and Parkin, C. (2009), 'Eating disorders and diabetes: Introduction and overview', *Diabetes Spectrum*, 22: 138–42.

Conrad, P. (1992), 'Medicalization and social control', *Annual Review of Sociology*, 18: 209–32.

Conrad, P. (2005), 'The shifting engines of medicalization', *Journal of Health and Social Behavior*, 46(1): 3–14.

Conrad, P. (2007), *The Medicalization of Society: On the Transformation of Health Conditions into Treatable Disorders*, Baltimore: The Johns Hopkins University Press.

Conrad, P. and Barker, K. K. (2010), 'The social constructions of illness: Key insights and policy implications', *Journal of Health and Social Behavior*, 51(1): S67–76.

Conrad, P. and Schneider, J. (1980), *Deviance and Its Medicalization: From Badness to Sickness*, St. Louis: Mosby.

Cook, G. (2003), *Applied Linguistics*, Oxford: Oxford University Press.

Corder, S. P. (1973), *Introducing Applied Linguistics*. Harmondsworth: Penguin Books.

Cornford, C. S., Hill, A. and Reilly, J. (2007), 'How patients with depressive symptoms view their condition: A qualitative study', *Family Practice*, 24(4): 358–64.

Coulson, N. S. and Knibb, R. C. (2007), 'Coping with food allergy: Exploring the role of the online support group', *CyberPsychology & Behavior*, 10(1): 145–8.

Coulson, N. S., Buchanan, H. and Aubeeluck, A. (2007), 'Social support in cyberspace: A content analysis of communication within a Huntington's disease online support group', Patient, *Education and Counseling*, 68(2): 173–8.

Coulson, N. S., Bullock, E. and Rodham, K. (2017), 'Exploring the therapeutic affordances of self-harm online support communities: An online survey of members', *JMIR Mental Health*, 4(4): e44.

Crawford, P. and Brown, B. (2010), 'Health communication: Corpus linguistics, data driven learning and education for health professionals', *Taiwan International ESP Journal*, 2(1): 1–26.

Crawford, P., Brown, B. and Harvey, K. (2014), 'Corpus linguistics and evidence-based health communication', in H. E. Hamilton and W. S. Chou (eds), *The Routledge Handbook of Language and Health Communication*, 75–90, London and New York: Routledge.

Crawford, P., Brown, B., Baker, C., Tischler, V. and Abrams, B. (2015), *Health Humanities*, Basingstoke: Palgrave Macmillan.

Crisafulli, M. A., Von Holle, A. and Bulik, C. M. (2008), 'Attitudes towards anorexia nervosa: The impact of framing on blame and stigma', *International Journal of Eating Disorders*, 41(4): 333–9.

Crookshank, F. G. (1923), 'The importance of a theory of signs and a critique of language in the theory of medicine', in C. Ogden and I. Richards (eds), *The Meaning of Meaning*, 5th edn, 327–55, New York: Harcourt Brace.

Crowe, M. (2000), 'Constructing normality: A discourse analysis of the DSM-IV', *Psychiatric and Mental Health Nursing*, 7(1): 69–77.

Crystal, D. (1995), *The English Language*, Cambridge: Cambridge University Press.

Crystal, D. (2001), *Language and the Internet*, 2nd edn, Cambridge: Cambridge University Press.

Crystal, D. (2011), *Internet Linguistics: A Student Guide*, London and New York: Routledge.

Darbar, N. and Mokha, M. (2008), 'Diabulimia: A body-image disorder in patients with type 1 diabetes mellitus', *Athletic Therapy Today*, 13: 31–3.

Das. T. K. (1984), 'Portmanteau ideas for organizational theorizing', *Organization Studies*, 5(3): 261–7.

Davies, C. E., Knol, L. L. and Turner, L. W. (2011), '"Training your taste buds": The language of success in diabetes "self-efficacy"', in P. McPherron and V. Ramanathan (eds), *Language, Body, and Health*, 171–90, Berlin: Mouton de Gruyter.

Day, K. and Keys, T. (2008), 'Starving in cyberspace: A discourse analysis of pro-eating disorder websites', *Journal of Gender Studies*, 17(1): 1–15.

de Swaan, A. (1990), *The Management of Normality*, London and New York: Routledge.

Deegan, P. (1996), 'Recovery as a journey of the heart', *Psychiatric Rehabilitation Journal*, 19(3): 91–7.

Demjén, Z., Marszalek, A., Semino, E. and Varese, F. (2019), 'Metaphor framing and distress in lived-experience accounts of voice-hearing', *Psychosis: Psychological, Social and Integrative Approaches*, 11(1): 16–27.

Demmen, J., Semino, E., Demjen, Z., Koller, V., Hardie, A., Rayson, P. and Payne, S. (2015), 'A computer-assisted study of the use of violence metaphors for cancer and end of life by patients, family carers and health professionals', *International Journal of Corpus Linguistics*, 20(2): 205–31.

Dowrick, C. (2004), *Beyond Depression: A New Approach to Understanding and Management*, Oxford: Oxford University Press.

Dowrick, C. (2009a), 'Reasons to be cheerful? Reflections on GPs' responses to depression', *British Journal of General Practice*, 59(566): 636–7.

Dowrick, C. (2009b), 'When diagnosis fails: A commentary on McPherson and Armstrong', *Social Science & Medicine*, 69(8): 1144–6.

Drake, R. E., Goldman, H., Leff, H. S., Lehman, A. F., Dixon, L., Mueser, K. T. and Torrey, W. C. (2001), 'Implementing evidence-based practices in routine mental health service settings', *Psychiatric Services*, 52(2): 179–82.

Dresner, E. and Herring, S. C. (2010), 'Functions of the nonverbal in CMC: Emoticons and illocutionary force', *Communication Theory*, 20(3): 249–68.

Drew, P. (2001), 'Spotlight on the patient', *Text and Talk*, 21(1–2): 261–8.

Drew, P. (2006), 'When documents "speak": Documents, language and interaction', in P. Drew, G. Raymond and D. Weinberg (eds), *Talk and Interaction in Social Research Methods*, 63–80, London: Sage.

Drew, P. and Sorjonen, M. (1997), 'Institutional dialogue', in T. A. van Dijk (ed.), *Discourse as Social Interaction*, 92–118, London: Sage.

Duncan, T. K., Sebar, B. and Lee, J. (2015), 'Reclamation of power and self: A meta-synthesis exploring the process of recovery from anorexia nervosa', *Advances in Eating Disorders: Theory, Research and Practice*, 3(2): 177–90.

Dunning, T. (1993), 'Accurate methods for the statistics of surprise and coincidence', *Computational Linguistics*, 19(1): 61–74.

Easter, M. M. (2012), '"Not all my fault": Genetics, stigma, and personal responsibility for women with eating disorders', *Social Science & Medicine*, 75(8): 1408–16.

Ebrahim, S. (2002), 'Editorial – The medicalisation of old age', *British Medical Journal*, 324: 861–3.

Edwards, D. (2000), 'Extreme case formulations: Softeners, investment and doing nonliteral', *Research on Language and Social Interaction*, 33(4): 347–73.

Edwards, D. and Potter, J. (1992), *Discursive Psychology*, London: Sage.

Eivors, A., Button, E., Warner, S. and Turner, K. (2003), 'Understanding the experience of drop-out from treatment for anorexia nervosa', *European Eating Disorders Review*, 11(2): 90–107.

Elgesem, D. (2015), 'Consent and information – Ethical considerations when conducting research on social media', in H. Fossheim and H. Ingierd (eds), *Internet Research Ethics*, 15–34, Oslo: Nordic Open Access Scholarly Publishing.

Epstein, R. M., Duberstein, P. R., Feldman, M. D., Rochlen, A. B., Bell, R. A., Kravitz, R. L., Cipri, C., Becker, J. D., Bamonti, P. M. and Paterniti, D. A. (2010), '"I didn't know what was wrong": How people with undiagnosed depression recognize, name and explain their distress', *Journal of General Internal Medicine*, 25(9): 954–61.

Evans, J., Rich, E., Davies, B. and Allwood, R. (2008), *Education, Disordered Eating and Obesity Discourse: Fat Fabrications*, London and New York: Routledge.

Evert, S. (2008), 'Corpora and collocations', in A. Lüdeling and M. Kytö (eds), *Corpus Linguistics: An International Handbook*, 1212–148, Berlin: Mouton de Gruyter.

Eysenbach, G. and Till, J. E. (2001), 'Ethical issues in qualitative research on internet communities', *British Medical Journal*, 323: 1103–5.

Fairburn, C. G. and Harrison, P. J. (2003), 'Eating disorders', *Lancet*, 361: 407–16.

Fairclough, N. (1989), *Language and Power*, London: Longman.

Fairclough, N. (2002), 'A reply to Henry Widdowson's "discourse analysis: A critical view"', in M. Toolan (ed.), *Critical Discourse Analysis: Critical Concepts in Linguistics, Vol. III*, 148–56, London and New York: Routledge.

Fairclough, N. (2003), *Analysing Discourse*, London and New York: Routledge.

Feldman, M. D., Franks, P., Duberstein, P. R., Vannoy, S., Epstein, R. and Kravitz, R. L. (2007), 'Let's not talk about it: Suicide inquiry in primary care', *Annals of Family Medicine*, 5(5): 412–8.

Firth, R. J. (1957), 'The technique of semantics', in R. J. Firth (ed.), *Papers in Linguistics 1934-1951*, 7–33, Oxford: Oxford University Press.

Fleischman, S. (1999), '*I am…, I have…, I suffer from…*: A linguist reflects on the language of illness and disease', *Journal of Medical Humanities*, 20(1): 3–32.

Fleischman, S. (2001), 'Language and medicine', in D. Schiffrin, D. Tannen and H. E. Hamilton (eds), *The Handbook of Discourse Analysis*, 470–502, Oxford: Blackwell.

Fleming, J. and Szmukler, G. I. (1992), 'Attitudes of medical professionals towards patients with eating disorders', *Australian and New Zealand Journal of Psychiatry*, 26(3): 436–43.

Flowerdew, L. (2004), 'The argument for using specialized corpora to understand academic and professional language', in U. Connor and T. Upton (eds), *Discourse in the Professions: Perspectives from Corpus Linguistics*, 11–13, Amsterdam: John Benjamins.

Foucault, M. (1969), *The Archaeology of Knowledge*, London and New York: Routledge.

Foucault, M. (1973), *The Birth of the Clinic: An Archaeology of Medical Perception*. London: Tavistock.

Foucault, M. (1979), *Discipline and Punish*. Harmondsworth: Penguin.

Fox Tree, J. E. and Schrock, J. C. (2002), 'Basic meanings of you know and I mean', *Journal of Pragmatics*, 34(6): 727–47.

Fox, N. and Ward, K. (2006), 'Health identities: From expert patient to resisting consumer', *Health*, 10(4): 461–79.

Fox, N., Ward, K. and O'Rourke, A. (2005), 'Pro-anorexia, weight-loss drugs and the internet: An "anti-recovery" explanatory model of anorexia', *Sociology of Health & Illness*, 27(7): 944–71.

Fox, S. and Duggan, M. (2013), 'Health online 2013', *Pew Internet and American Life Project Report*, Pew Research Centre.

Frankel, M. S. and Siang, S. (1999), *Ethical and Legal Aspects of Human Subjects Research on the Internet: A Report of an AAAS Workshop,* Washington, DC: American Association for the Advancement of Science.

Freeman, C. (2002), *Overcoming Anorexia Nervosa*, London: Robinson.

Fromm, E. (1976), *To Have or To Be?* London: Abacus.

Gabe, J. (2013), 'Medicalization', in J. Gabe and L. Monaghan (eds), *Key Concepts in Medical Sociology*, 2nd edn, 49–52, London: Sage.

Gablasova, D., Brezina, V., McEnery, T. (2017), 'Collocations in corpus-based language learning research: Identifying, comparing and interpreting the evidence', *Language Learning*, 67(1): 155–79.

Gabrielatos, C. (2018), 'Keyness analysis: Nature, metrics and techniques', in C. Taylor and A. Marchi (eds), *Corpus Approaches to Discourse: A Critical Review*, 225–58, London and New York: Routledge.

Galasiński, D. (2008), *Men's Discourses of Depression*, Basingstoke: Palgrave Macmillan.

Galasiński, D. (2013), *Fathers, Fatherhood and Mental Illness: A Discourse Analysis of Rejection*, Basingstoke: Palgrave Macmillan.

Galasiński, D. (2017), *Discourses of Men's Suicide Notes*, London: Bloomsbury.

Galasiński, D. (2018), 'Language of Depression?' [online], *Dariusz Galasiński*. Available at http://dariuszgalasinski.com/2018/02/04/language-of-depression/ (accessed 1 February 2019).

Gallant, M. H., Beaulieu, M. C. and Carnevale, F. A. (2002), 'Partnership: An analysis of the concept within the nurse-client relationship', *Journals of Advanced Nursing* 40(2): 149–57.

Galvin, R. (2002), 'Disturbing notions of chronic illness and individual responsibility: Towards a genealogy of morals', *Health*, 6(2): 107–37.

Georgaca, E. (2014), 'Discourse analytic research on mental distress: A critical overview', *Journal of Mental Health*, 23(2): 55–61.

Giaxoglou, K. (2017), 'Reflections on internet research ethics from language-focused research on web-based mourning: Revisiting the private/public distinction as a language ideology of differentiation', *Applied Linguistics Review*, 8(2–3): 229–50.

Gibson, J. M. E. and Kenrick, M. (1998), 'Pain and powerlessness: The experience of living with peripheral vascular disease', *Journal of Advanced Nursing*, 27(4): 737–45.

Giddens, A. (1991), *Modernity and Self-Identity*, Cambridge: Polity.

Giles, D. (2006), 'Constructing identities in cyberspace: The case of eating disorders', *British Journal of Social Psychology*, 45: 463–77.

Giles, D. C. and Newbold, J. (2011), 'Self-and other-diagnosis in user-led mental health online communities', *Qualitative Health Research*, 21(3): 419–28.

Gimlin, D. (1994), 'The anorexic as overconformist: Toward a reinterpretation of eating disorders', in K. A. Callaghan (ed.), *Ideals of Feminine Beauty: Philosophical, Social and Cultural Dimensions*, 99–112, Westport: Greenwood Press.

Ging, D. and Garvey, S. (2018), '"Written in these scars are the stories I can't explain": A content analysis of pro-ana and thinspiration image sharing on Instagram', *New Media & Society*, 20(3): 1181–200.

Giordano, S. (2005), *Understanding Eating Disorders*, Oxford: Oxford University Press.

Glasgow, S. M. (2012), 'The politics of self-craft: Expert patients and the public health management of chronic disease', *Sage Open*, 2(3): 1–11.

Goddard, A. and Geesin, B. (2011), *Language and Technology*, London and New York: Routledge.

Goebel-Fabbri, A., Fikkan, J., Franko, D., Pearson, K., Anderson, B. and Weinger, K. (2008), 'Insulin restriction and associated morbidity and mortality in women with type 1 diabetes', *Diabetes Care*, 31(3): 415–9.

Goffman, E. (1963), *Stigma*, Englewood Cliffs: Prentice-Hall.

Goldman, J. B. and Maclean, H. M. (1998), 'The significance of identity in the adjustment to diabetes among insulin users', *Diabetes Education*, 24(6): 741–8.

Gomersall, T., Madill, A. and Summers, L. K. M. (2011), 'A metasynthesis of the self-management of type 2 diabetes', *Qualitative Health Research*, 21(6): 853–71.

Grohol, J. M. (1998), 'Future clinical directions: Professional development, pathology and psychotherapy on-line', in J. Gackenbach (ed.), *Psychology and the Internet*,

Intrapersonal, Interpersonal and Transpersonal Implications, 111–40, San Diego, CA: Academic Press.

Guise, J., Widdicombe, S. and McKinlay, A. (2007), '"What is it like to have ME?": The discursive construction of ME in computer-mediated communication and face-to-face interaction', *Health*, 11(1): 87–108.

Gull, W. W. (1868), 'The address in medicine: Delivered before the annual meeting of the B.M.A. at Oxford', *The Lancet*, 2: 171–6.

Gull, W. W. (1874), 'Anorexia nervosa (apepsia hysterica, anorexia hysterica)', *Transactions of the Clinical Society*, 7: 22–8.

Gwyn, R. (2002), *Communicating Health and Illness*, London: Sage.

Halliday, M. A. K. (1994), *An Introduction to Functional Grammar*, 2nd edn, London: Edward Arnold.

Halliday, M. A. K. (2002), 'On the grammar of pain', in M. Toolan (ed.), *Critical Discourse Analysis: Critical Concepts in Linguistics, Vol. III*, 303–30, London and New York: Routledge.

Hamilton, H. E. (1996), 'Reported speech and survivor identity in on-line bone marrow transplantation narratives', *Journal of Sociolinguistics*, 2(1): 53–67.

Hardie, A. (2014), 'Log ratio – An informal introduction', *ESRC Centre for Corpus Approaches to Social Science*. Lancaster: Lancaster University [blog]. Available at http://cass.lancs.ac.uk/log-ratio-an-informal-introduction/.

Hardin, P. K. (2003), 'Shape-shifting discourses of anorexia nervosa: Reconstituting psychopathology', *Nursing Inquiry*, 10(4): 209–17.

Harper, D. J. (1995), 'Discourse analysis and "mental health"', *Journal of Mental Health*, 4(4): 347–58

Harris, J. (2000), 'Self-harm: Cutting the bad out of me', *Qualitative Health Research*, 10(2): 164–73.

Harvey, D. (2005), *A Brief History of Neoliberalism*, Oxford: Oxford University Press.

Harvey, K. (2008), *Adolescent Health Communication: A Corpus Linguistics Approach*. Unpublished doctoral thesis, University of Nottingham, UK.

Harvey, K. (2012), 'Disclosures of depression: Using corpus linguistics methods to interrogate young people's online health concerns', *International Journal of Corpus Linguistics*, 17(3): 349–79.

Harvey, K. (2013a), *Investigating Adolescent Health Communication: A Corpus Linguistics Approach*, London: Bloomsbury.

Harvey, K. (2013b), 'Medicalisation, pharmaceutical promotion and the Internet: A critical multimodal discourse analysis of hair loss websites', *Social Semiotics*, 23(5): 691–714.

Harvey, K. and Brown, B. (2012), 'Health communication and psychological distress: Exploring the language of self-harm', *Canadian Modern Language Review*, 68(3): 316–40.

Harvey, K., Brown, B., Crawford, P., Macfarlane, A. and McPherson, A. (2007), '"Am I normal?" Teenagers, sexual health and the internet', *Social Science & Medicine*, 65(4): 771–81.

Hasken, J., Kresl, L., Nydegger, T. and Temme, M. (2010), 'Diabulimia and the role of school health personnel', *Journal of School Health*, 80(10): 465–9.

Hastings, A., McNamara, N., Allan, J. and Marriott, M. (2016), 'The importance of social identities in the management of and recovery from 'Diabulimia': A qualitative exploration', *Addictive Behaviors Reports*, 4, 78–86.

Heartfield, J. (2002), *The 'Death of the Subject' Explained*, Sheffield: Sheffield Hallam University Press.

Hepworth, J. (1999), *The Social Construction of Anorexia Nervosa*, London: Sage.

Herring, S. (2004), 'Computer-mediated discourse analysis: An approach to researching online behaviour', in S. A. Barab, R. King and J. H. Gray (eds), *Designing for Virtual Communities in the Service of Learning*, 338–76, Cambridge: Cambridge University Press.

Herring, S. C. and Dainas, A. R. (2017), '"Nice picture comment!" Graphicons in Facebook comment threads', *Proceedings of the Fiftieth Hawai'i International Conference on System Sciences (HICSS-50)*, Los Alamitos, CA: IEEE.

Herzlich, C. (1973), *Health and Illness: A Social Psychological Analysis*, London: Academic Press.

Herzog, W., Deter, H. C., Fiehn, W. and Petzold, E. (1997), 'Medical findings and predictors of long-term physical outcome in anorexia nervosa: A prospective, 12-year follow-up study', *Psychological Medicine*, 27(2): 269–79.

Hoek, H. W. (2006), 'Incidence, prevalence and mortality of anorexia nervosa and other eating disorders', *Current Opinion in Psychiatry*, 19(4): 389–94.

Holmes, G. R., Offen, L. and Waller, G. (1997), 'See no evil, hear no evil, speak no evil: Why do relatively few male victims of childhood sexual abuse receive help for abuse-related issues in adulthood?', *Clinical Psychology Review*, 17(1): 69–88.

Hopton, J. (2006), 'The future of critical psychiatry', *Critical Social Policy*, 26(1): 57–73.

Horne, J. and Wiggins, S. (2009), 'Doing being "on the edge": Managing the dilemma of being authentically suicidal in an online forum', *Sociology of Health & Illness*, 31(2): 170–84.

Horne, O. and Csipke, E. (2009), 'From feeling too little and too much, to feeling more and less? A nonparadoxical theory of the functions of self-harm', *Qualitative Health Research*, 19(5): 655–67.

Horton-Salway, M. (2004), 'The local production of knowledge: Disease labels, identities and category entitlements in ME support group talk', *Health*, 8(3): 351–71.

Houston, T. K., Cooper, L. A. and Ford, D. E. (2002), 'Internet support groups for depression: A 1-year prospective cohort study', *American Journal of Psychiatry*, 159(12): 2062–8.

Hughes, J. (2010), 'Addressing the new teen trend of "diabulimia": Moral quandaries of a pediatric endocrinologist', *University of Western Ontario Medical Journal*, 79(1): 11–13.

Hughner, R. S. and Kleine, S. S. (2004), 'Views of health in the lay sector: A compilation and review of how individuals think about health', *Health*, 8(4): 395–422.

Hunston, S. (2002), *Corpora in Applied Linguistics*, Cambridge: Cambridge University Press.

Hunston, S. (2007), 'Semantic prosody revisited', *International Journal of Corpus Linguistics*, 12(2): 249–68.

Hunt, D. (forthcoming), 'Corpus linguistics: Examining tensions in general practitioners' views about diagnosing and treating depression', in G. Brookes and D. Hunt (eds), *Analysing Health Communication: Discourse Approaches*, Basingstoke: Palgrave.

Hunt, D. and Churchill, R. (2013), 'Diagnosing and managing anorexia nervosa in UK primary care: A focus group study', *Family Practice*, 30: 459–65.

Hunt, D. and Harvey, K. (2015), 'Health communication and corpus linguistics: Using corpus tools to analyse eating disorder discourse online', in P. Baker and T. McEnery (eds), *Corpora and Discourse Studies: Integrating Discourse and Corpora*, 134–54, Basingstoke: Palgrave Macmillan.

Hutchby, I. and Wooffitt, R. (1998), *Conversation Analysis*, Cambridge: Polity Press.

Hutchins, W. J. (1978), 'The concept of "aboutness" in subject indexing', *Aslib Proceedings*, 30(5): 172–81.

Ingadottir, B. and Halldorsdottir, S. (2008), 'To discipline a "dog": The essential structure of mastering diabetes', *Qualitative Health Research*, 18(5): 606–19.

Jammal, A. (1988), 'Les vocabulaires des spécialités médicales: pourquoi et comment les fabrique-t-on? [The vocabularies of medical specialities: Why and how are they created?]', *Meta*, 33(4): 535–41.

Jaworska, S. and Kinloch, K. (2018), 'Using multiple data sets', in C. Taylor and A. Marchi (eds), *Corpus Approaches to Discourse*, 126–45, London and New York: Routledge.

Jeffries, L. and Walker, B. (2019), *Keywords in the Press: The New Labour Years*, London: Bloomsbury.

Johanson, R., Newburn, M. and Macfarlane, A. (2002), 'Has the medicalisation of childbirth gone too far?', *British Medical Journal*, 324(7342): 892–5.

Johns, T. F. (1991), 'Should you be persuaded: Two examples of data-driven learning', in T. F. Johns and P. King (eds), *Classroom Concordancing*, 1–13, Birmingham: Empirical Language Research.

Johnson, D. and Murray, J. F. (1985), 'Do doctors mean what they say?', in D. J. Enright (ed.), *Fair of Speech: The Uses of Euphemism*, 151–8, Oxford: Oxford University Press.

Joinson, A. N. (1999), 'Social desirability, anonymity and internet-based questionnaires', *Behavior Research Methods, Instruments and Computers*, 31(3): 433–8.

Joinson, A. N. (2001), 'Self-disclosure in computer-mediated communication: The role of self-awareness and visual anonymity', *European Journal of Social Psychology*, 31: 177–92.

Joinson, A. N. (2003), *Understanding the Psychology of Internet Behaviour: Virtual Worlds, Real Lives*, Basingstoke: Palgrave Macmillan.

Jones, R. (2012), *Discourse Analysis: A Resource Book for Students*, London and New York: Routledge.

Jones, R. (2013), *Health and Risk Communication: An Applied Linguistic Perspective*, London and New York: Routledge.

Kangas, I. (2001), 'Making sense of depression: Perceptions of melancholia in lay narratives', *Health*, 5(1): 76–92.

Karasz, A. (2005), 'Cultural differences in conceptual models of depression', *Social Science & Medicine*, 60(7): 1625–35.

Karp, D. A. (1996), *Speaking of Sadness*, Oxford: Oxford University Press.

Kessler, D., Lloyd, K., Lewis, G. and Gray, D. P. (1999), 'Cross sectional study of symptom attribution and recognition of depression and anxiety in primary care', *British Medical Journal*, 318: 436–9.

Kessler, R. C., Berglund, P., Borges, G., Nock, M. and Wang, P. S. (2005), 'Trends in suicide ideation, plans, gestures, and attempts in the United States, 1990–1992 to 2001–2003', *JAMA*, 293(20): 2487–95.

Kilgarriff, A. and Grefenstette, G. (2003), 'Introduction to the special issue on web as corpus', *Computational Linguistics*, 29(3): 1–15.

King, B. W. (2009), 'Building and analysing corpora of computer-mediated communication', in P. Baker (ed.), *Contemporary Corpus Linguistics*, 301–20, London: Continuum.

Kirsch, I., Deacon, B. J., Huedo-Medina, T. B., Scoboria, A., Moore, T. J. and Johnson, B. T. (2008), 'Initial severity and antidepressant benefits: A meta-analysis of data submitted to the food and drug administration', *PLoS Medicine*, 5(2): e45.

Kiyimba, N. (2016), 'Using discourse and conversation analysis to study clinical practice in adult mental health', in M. O'Reilly and J. N. Lester (eds), *The Palgrave Handbook of Adult Mental Health*, 45–63, Basingstoke: Palgrave Macmillan.

Kleinman, A. (1988), *The Illness Narratives: Suffering, Healing, and the Human Condition*, New York: Basic Books.

Klonsky, E. D. (2007), 'The functions of deliberate self-injury: A review of the evidence', *Clinical Psychology Review*, 27(2): 226–39.

Klonsky, E. D. (2009), 'The functions of self-injury in young adults who cut themselves: Clarifying the evidence for affect-regulation', *Psychiatry Research*, 166(2–3): 260–8.

Knapton, O. (2013), 'Pro-anorexia: Extensions of ingrained concepts', *Discourse & Society*, 24(4): 461–77.

Knapton, O. (2016), 'Experiences of obsessive-compulsive disorder: Activity, state, and object episodes', *Qualitative Health Research*, 26(14): 2009–23.

Knapton, O. (2018), 'The linguistic construction of the self in narratives of obsessive compulsive disorder', *Qualitative Research in Psychology* [online first]. Available at https://www.tandfonline.com/doi/abs/10.1080/14780887.2018.1499834?journalCode=uqrp20.

Knowles, G. M. and Moon, R. (2006), *Introducing Metaphor*, London and New York: Routledge.

Knudsen, P., Hansen, E. H., Traulsen, J. M. and Eskildsen, K. (2002), 'Changes in self-concept whilst using SSRI antidepressants', *Qualitative Health Research*, 12(7): 932–44.

Koller, V. and Mautner, G. (2004), 'Computer application in critical discourse analysis', in C. Coffin, A. Hewings and K. O'Halloran (eds), *Applying English Grammar: Functional and Corpus Approaches*, 216–28, London: Arnold.

Koteyko, N. and Atanasova, D. (2018), 'Mental health advocacy on Twitter: Positioning in Depression Awareness Week tweets', *Discourse, Context & Media*, 25: 52–9.

Kövecses, Z. (2005), *Metaphor in Culture: Universality and Variation*, Cambridge: Cambridge University Press.

Kress, G. (2010), *Multimodality: A Social Semiotic Approach to Contemporary Communication*, London and New York: Routledge.

Kwan, S. and Graves, J. (2013), *Framing Fat: Competing Constructions in Contemporary Culture*, New Brunswick, NJ: Rutgers University Press.

Lakoff, G. and Johnson, M. (1980), *Metaphors We Live By*, London: University of Chicago Press.

Lamerichs, J. (2003), 'Discourse of support: Exploring online discussions on depression'. PhD thesis, Wageningen University, The Netherlands.

Lamerichs, J. and te Molder, H. F. M. (2003), 'Computer-mediated communication: From a cognitive to a discursive model', *New Media & Society*, 5(4): 451–73.

Largier, C. (2002), 'Aspekte der Debatte in argumentationsorientierten Internet-Foren: die Abtreibungsebatte in Frankreich und Deutschland', *Deutsche Sprache*, 30: 287–306.

Lasègue, E. C. (1873), 'On Hysteria Anorexia', *Medical Times and Gazette*, 2: 265–6.

Lask, B. and Hage, T. W. (2013), 'Therapeutic engagement', in B. Lask and R. Bryant-Waugh (eds), *Eating Disorders in Childhood and Adolescence*, 4th edn, 197–221, New York: Routledge.

Lave, J. and Wenger, E. (1991), *Situated Learning: Legitimate Peripheral Participation*, Cambridge: Cambridge University Press.

Lavrova, N. (2010), 'Linguistic contamination: Word-building peculiarities and stylistic functions', *International Journal of Arts and Sciences*, 3(14): 223–30.

Laye-Gindhu, A. and Schonert-Reichl, K. A. (2005), 'Nonsuicidal self-harm among community adolescents: Understanding the "whats" and "whys" of self-harm', *Journal of Youth and Adolescence*, 34(5): 447–57.

Lee, S. (1995), 'Self-starvation in context: Towards a culturally sensitive understanding of anorexia nervosa', *Social Science & Medicine*, 41(1): 25–36.

Leech G. (2000), 'Grammars of spoken English: New outcomes of corpus-oriented research', *Language Learning*, 50(4): 675–724.

Leech, G. (1991), 'The state of the art in corpus linguistics', in K. Aijmer and B. Altenberg (eds), *English Corpus Linguistics: Studies in Honour of Jan Svartvik*, 8–29, London: Longman.

Lester, J. N. and O'Reilly, M. (2016), 'The history and landscape of conversation and discourse analysis', in M. O'Reilly and J. N. Lester (eds), *The Palgrave Handbook of Adult Mental Health Disorders*, 23–34, Basingstoke: Palgrave Macmillan.

Lewis, S. (1995), 'A search for meaning: Making sense of depression', *Journal of Mental Health*, 4(4): 369–82.

Lewis, S. E. (1996), *The Social Construction of Depression: Experience, Discourse and Subjectivity*. PhD thesis, University of Sheffield.

Lewis, S. P., Heath, N. L., Michal, N. J. and Duggan, J. M. (2012), 'Non-suicidal self-injury, youth, and the internet: What mental health professionals need to know', *Child and Adolescent Psychiatry and Mental Health*, 6(1): 13.

Lipták A. K. and Reintges, C. H. (2006), 'Have = be + Prep: New evidence for the preposition incorporation analysis', in M. Frascarelli (ed.), *Phases of Interpretation*, 112–28, Berlin: Mouton de Gruyter.

Littlefield, C. H., Craven, J. L., Rodin, G. M., Daneman, D., Murray, M. A. and Rydall, A. C. (1992), 'Relationship of self-efficacy and binging to adherence to diabetes regimen among adolescents', *Diabetes Care*, 15 (1): 90–4.

Locher, M. A. (2013), 'Internet advice', in. S Herring, D. Stein and T. Virtanen (eds), *Pragmatics of Computer-Mediated Communication*, 339–62, Berlin: De Gruyter.

Louw, B. (1993), 'Irony in the text or insincerity in the writer? The diagnostic potential of semantic prosodies', in M. Baker, G. Francis and E. Tognini-Bonelli (eds), *Text and Technology: In Honour of John M. Sinclair*, 157–76, Amsterdam: John Benjamins.

Louw, B. (2000), 'Contextual prosodic theory: Bringing semantic prosodies to life', in C. Heffer and H. Sauntson (eds), *Words in Context: A Tribute to John Sinclair on His Retirement*, 48–94, Birmingham: University of Birmingham.

Love, R., Dembry, C., Hardie, A., Brezina, V. and McEnery, T. (2017), 'The spoken BNC2014: Designing and building a spoken corpus of everyday conversations', *International Journal of Corpus Linguistics*, 22(3): 319–44.

Lupton, D. (1994), 'Food, memory and meaning: The symbolic and social nature of food events', *The Sociological Review*, 42(4): 664–85.

Lupton, D. (1995), *The Imperative of Health: Public Health and the Regulated Body*, London: Sage.

Lupton, D. (2016), *The Quantified Self*, London: Polity Press.

Lyons, E. J., Mehl, M. R. and Pennebaker, J. W. (2006), 'Pro-anorexics and recovering anorexics differ in their linguistic internet self-presentation', *Journal of Psychosomatic Research*, 60(3): 253–6.

Mackenzie, J. (2017), 'Identifying informational norms in Mumsnet Talk: A reflexive-linguistic approach to internet research ethics', *Applied Linguistics Review*, 8(2–3): 293–314.

Mahlberg, M. (2006), 'Lexical cohesion', *International Journal of Corpus Linguistics*, 11(3), 363–83.

Malik, S. H. and Coulson, N. S. (2008), 'The male experience of infertility: A thematic analysis of an online infertility support group bulletin board', *Journal of Reproductive and Infant Psychology*, 26(1): 18–30.

Malson, H. (1998), *The Thin Woman: Feminism, Post-Structuralism and the Social Psychology of Anorexia Nervosa*, London and New York: Routledge.

Malson, H. (2008), 'Deconstructing un/healthy body-weight and weight management', in S. Riley, M. Burns, H. Frith, S. Wiggins and P. Markula (eds), *Critical Bodies*, 27–42, Basingstoke: Palgrave.

Malson, H., Finn, D. M., Treasure, J., Clark, S. and Anderson, G. (2004), 'Constructing "the eating disordered patient": A discourse analysis of accounts of treatment experiences', *Journal of Community and Applied Social Psychology*, 14(6): 473–89.

Marchi, A. and Taylor, C. (2018), 'Introduction: Partiality and reflexivity', in C. Taylor and A. Marchi (eds), *Corpus Approaches to Discourse: A Critical Review*, 1–15, London and New York: Routledge.

Markham, A. N. and Buchanan, E. (2012), *Ethical Decision-Making and Internet Research: Recommendations from the AOIR Ethics Working Committee* (version 2.0). Available at http://www.aoir.org/reports/ethics2.pdf.

Markham, A. N. and Buchanan, E. (2015), 'Ethical considerations in digital research contexts', in J. Wright (ed.), *Encyclopedia for Social & Behavioral Sciences*, 2nd edn, 606–13, London: Elsevier Science.

Markula, P., Burns, M. and Riley, S. C. E. (2008), 'Introducing critical bodies: Representations, identities and practices of weight and body management', in S. C. E. Riley, M. Burns, H. Frith and P. Markula (eds), *Critical Bodies: Representations, Practices and Identities of Weight and Body Management*, 1–23, Basingstoke: Palgrave Macmillan.

Mathieu, J. (2008), 'What is diabulimia?', *Journal of the Academy of Nutrition and Dietetics*, 108(5): 769–70.

Mautner, G. (2005), 'Time to get wired: Using web-based corpora in critical discourse analysis', *Discourse & Society*, 16(6): 809–28.

Mautner, G. (2009), 'Corpora and critical discourse analysis', in P. Baker (ed), *Contemporary Approaches to Corpus Linguistics,* 32–46. London: Continuum.

Maxwell, M. (2005), 'Women's and doctors' accounts of their experiences of depression in primary care: The influence of social and moral reasoning on patients' and doctors' decisions', *Chronic Illness*, 1(1): 61–71.

Mazanderani, F., O'Neill, B. and Powell, J. (2013), '"People power" or "pester power"? YouTube as a forum for the generation of evidence and patient advocacy', *Patient Education and Counseling*, 93(3): 420–5.

McCarron, R. M. (2013), 'The DSM-5 and the art of medicine: Certainly uncertain', *Annals of Internal Medicine*, 159(5): 360–1.

McCaughey, M. (1999), 'Fleshing out the discomforts of femininity', in J. Sobal and D. Maurer (eds), *Weighty Issues*, 133–55, New York: Aldine De Gruyter.

McDonald, D. and Woodward-Kron, R. (2016), 'Member roles and identities in online support groups: Perspectives from corpus and systemic functional linguistics', *Discourse & Communication*, 10(2): 157–75.

McEnery, T. (2006), *Swearing in English: Bad Language, Purity and Power from 1586 to the Present*, London and New York: Routledge.

McEnery, T. and Gabrielatos, C. (2006), 'English corpus linguistics', in B. Aarts and A. McMahon (eds), *The Handbook of English Linguistics*, 33–71, Oxford: Blackwell.

McEnery, T. and Hardie, A. (2012), *Corpus Linguistics: Method, Theory and Practice*, Cambridge: Cambridge University Press.

McEnery, T. and Wilson, A. (2001), *Corpus Linguistics: An Introduction*, 2nd edn, Edinburgh: Edinburgh University Press.

McEnery, T., Xiao, R. and Tono, Y. (2006), *Corpus-Based Language Studies: An Advanced Resource Book*, London and New York: Routledge.

McKague, M. and Verhoef, M. (2003), 'Understandings of health and its determinants among clients and providers at an urban community health center', *Qualitative Health Research*, 13(5): 703–17.

McMullen, L. M. (1999), 'Metaphors in the talk of "depressed" women in psychotherapy', *Canadian Psychology*, 40(2): 102–11.

McMullen, L. M. and Herman, J. (2009), 'Women's accounts of their decision to quit taking antidepressants', *Qualitative Health Research*, 19(11): 1569–79.

McPherson, S. and Armstrong, D. (2009), 'Negotiating "depression", in primary care: A qualitative study', *Social Science & Medicine*, 69(8): 1137–43.

Miah, A. and Rich, E. (2008), *The Medicalization of Cyberspace*, London and New York: Routledge.

Micali, N., Hagberg, K. W., Petersen, I. and Treasure, J. L. (2013), 'The incidence of eating disorders in the UK in 2000–2009: Findings from the General Practice Research Database', *BMJ Open*, 3(5): e002646.

Michel, K. (2000), 'Suicide prevention in primary care', in K. Hawton and K. van Heeringen (eds), *The International Handbook of Suicide and Attempted Suicide*, 661–75, Chichester: Wiley.

Mills, S. (2005), *Discourse*, 2nd edn, London and New York: Routledge.

Mintz, D. (1992), 'What in a word: The distancing function of language in medicine', *The Journal of Medical Humanities*, 13(4): 223–33.

Mishler, E. (1984), *The Discourse of Medicine: Dialects of Medical Interviews*. Norwood, NJ: Ablex.

Mol, A. (2008), *The Logic of Care*, London and New York: Routledge.

Moorhead, S. A., Hazlett, D. E., Harrison, L., Carroll, J. K., Irwin, A. and Hoving, C. (2013), 'A new dimension of health care: Systematic review of the uses, benefits, and limitations of social media for health communication', *Journal of Medical Internet Research*, 15(4): e85.

Morley, J. and Partington, A. (2009), 'A few frequently asked questions about semantic – Or evaluative – Prosody', *International Journal of Corpus Linguistics*, 14(2): 139–58.

Morris, S and Twaddle, S. (2007), 'Anorexia nervosa', *British Medical Journal*, 334: 894–98.

Morrow, P. R. (2006), 'Telling about problems and giving advice in an internet discussion forum: Some discourse features', *Discourse Studies*, 8(4): 532–48.

Morse, J. M. (2016), *Qualitative Research: Creating a New Discipline*, Walnut Creek, CA: Left Coast Press.

Moynihan, R., Heath, I. and Henry, D. (2002), 'Selling sickness: The pharmaceutical industry and disease mongering', *British Medical Journal*, 324(7342): 886–91.

Mulderrig, J. (2018), 'Multimodal strategies of emotional governance: A critical analysis of "nudge" tactics in health policy', *Critical Discourse Studies*, 15(1): 39–67.

Mullany, L., Smith, C., Harvey, K. and Adolphs, S. (2015), '"Am I anorexic?": Weight, eating and discourses of the body in online adolescent health communication', *Communication and Medicine*, 12(2–3): 211–23.

Musolino, C., Warin, M., Wade, T. and Gilchrist, P. (2015), '"Healthy anorexia": The complexity of care in disordered eating', *Social Science & Medicine*, 139: 18–25.

Naemiratch, B. and Manderson, L. (2006), 'Control and adherence: Living with diabetes in Bangkok, Thailand', *Social Science & Medicine*, 63(5): 1147–57.

National Institute for Clinical Excellence (2004), *Eating Disorders: Core Interventions in the Treatment and Management of Anorexia Nervosa, Bulimia Nervosa and Related Eating Disorders*. Leicester: British Psychological Society and the Royal College of Psychiatrists.

National Institute for Health and Clinical Excellence. (2009), *Depression: The Treatment and Management of Depression in Adults*, Updated edn, Leicester: British Psychological Society and the Royal College of Psychiatrists.

Nettleton, S. (2013), *The Sociology of Health and Illness*, 3rd edn, London: Polity Press.

Neumark-Sztainer, D., Wall, M., Guo, J., Story, M., Haines, J. and Eisenberg, M. (2006), 'Obesity, disordered eating, and eating disorders in longitudinal study of adolescents: How do dieters fare 5 years later?', *Journal of the American Diet Association*, 106(4): 559–68.

Nijhof, G. (1998), 'Naming as naturalization in the medical encounter', *Journal of Pragmatics*, 30(6): 735–53.

Nissenbaum, H. (2010), *Privacy in Context: Technology, Policy, and the Integrity of Social Life*, Stanford: Stanford University Press.

Nosek, B. A., Banaji, M. R. and Greenwald, A. G. (2002), 'E-Research: Ethics, security, design, and control in psychological research on the internet', *Journal of Social Issues*, 58(1): 161–76.

O'Reilly, M. and Lester, J. N. (2016), 'Introduction: The social construction of normality and pathology', in M. O'Reilly and J. N. Lester (eds), *The Palgrave Handbook of Adult Mental Health Disorders*, 1–19, Basingstoke: Palgrave Macmillan.

O'Halloran, K. and Coffin, C. (2004), 'Checking over-interpretation and under-interpretation: Help from corpora in critical linguistics', in C. Coffin and A. Hewings (eds), *Applying English Grammar: Functional and Corpus Approaches*, 275–97, London: Hodder Arnold.

Orbach, S. (1986), *Hunger Strike: The Anorectic's Struggle as a Metaphor for Our Age*, New York: W. W. Norton.

Orpin, D. (2005), 'Corpus linguistics and critical discourse analysis: Examining the ideology of sleaze', *International Journal of Applied Linguistics*, 10(1): 37–61.

Page, R., Barton, D., Unger, J. and Zappavigna, M. (2014), *Researching Language and Social Media: A Student Guide*, London and New York: Routledge.

Parsons, T. (1951), *The Social System*, Glencoe, IL: The Free Press.

Paterson, B. L., Thorne, S. and Dewis, M. (1998), 'Adapting to and managing diabetes', *Journal of Nursing Scholarship*, 30(1): 57–62.

Peel, E., Parry, O., Douglas, M. and Lawton, J. (2005), 'Taking the biscuit? A discursive approach to managing diet in type 2 diabetes', *Journal of Health Psychology*, 10(6): 779–91.

Peeters, R. (2013), 'Responsibilisation on government's terms: New welfare and the governance of responsibility and solidarity', *Social Policy and Society*, 12(4): 583–95.

Pennebaker, J. W. and Lay, T. C. (2002), 'Language use and personality during crises: Analyses of Mayor Rudolph Giuliani's press conferences', *Journal of Research in Personality*, 36(3): 271–82.

Pennebaker, J. W., Booth, R. J. and Francis, M. E. (2007), *Linguistic Inquiry and Word Count: LIWC* [Computer software], Austin, TX: LIWC Net.

Pennebaker, J. W., Groom, C. J., Loew, D. and Dabbs, J. M. (2004), 'Testosterone as a social inhibitor: Two case studies of the effect of testosterone treatment on language', *Journal of Abnormal Psychology*, 113(1): 172–75.

Piccinelli, M. and Wilkinson, G. (1994), 'Outcome of depression in psychiatric settings', *British Journal of Psychiatry*, 164(3): 297–304.

Pierce, J. L., Kostova, T. and Dirks, K. T. (2003), 'The state of psychological ownership: Integrating and extending a century of research', *Review of General Psychology*, 7(1): 84–107.

Pilgrim, D. and Bentall, R. (1999), 'The medicalisation of misery: A critical realist analysis of the concept of depression', *Journal of Mental Health*, 8(3): 261–74.

Pilgrim, D. and Dowrick, C. (2006), 'From a diagnostic-therapeutic to a social-existential response to "depression"', *Journal of Public Mental Health*, 5(2): 6–12.

Pilling, S., Anderson, I., Goldberg, D., Meader, N. and Taylor, C. (2009), 'Depression in adults, including those with a chronic physical health problem: Summary of NICE guidance', *British Medical Journal*, 339: 1025–27.

Poirier, S. and Brauner, D. J. (1988), 'Ethics and the daily language of medical discourse', *Hastings Centre Report*, 18(4): 5–9.

Pomerantz, A. (1986), 'Extreme case formulations: A way of legitimizing claims', *Human Studies*, 9(2–3): 219–29.

Potter, J. (1996), *Representing Reality*, London: Sage.

Potter, J., Wetherell, M. and Chitty, A. (1991), 'Quantification rhetoric – Cancer on television', *Discourse & Society*, 2(3): 333–65.

Pounds, G., Hunt, D. and Koteyko, N. (2018), 'Expression of empathy in a Facebook-based diabetes support group', *Discourse, Context and Media*, 25: 34–43.

Powers, M., Richter, S., Ackard, D., Gerken, S., Meier, M. and Criego, A. (2012), 'Characteristics of persons with an eating disorder and type 1 diabetes and psychological comparisons with persons with an eating disorder and no diabetes', *International Journal of Eating Disorders*, 45: 252–6.

Pugh, M. (2016), 'The internal "anorexic voice": A feature or fallacy of eating disorders?', *Advances in Eating Disorders*, 4(1): 75–83.

Rayson, P. (2008), 'From key words to key semantic domains', *International Journal of Corpus Linguistics*, 13(4): 519–49.

Reaven, G. M. (1988), 'Banting lecture 1988: Role of insulin resistance in human disease', *Diabetes*, 37(12):1595–607.

Reeves, A., Bowl, R., Wheeler, S. and Guthrie, E. (2004), 'The hardest words: Exploring the dialogue of suicide in the counselling process—A discourse analysis', *Counselling and Psychotherapy Research*, 4(1): 62–71.

Reid, M., Williams, S. and Burr, J. (2010), 'Perspectives on eating disorders and service provision: A qualitative study of healthcare professionals', *European Eating Disorders Review*, 18(5): 390–8.

Rhodes, P. (2003), 'The Maudsley model of family therapy for children and adolescents with anorexia nervosa: Theory, clinical practice and empirical support', *American and New Zealand Journal of Family Therapy*, 24(4): 191–8.

Rich, E. (2006), 'Anorexic dis(connection): Managing anorexia as an illness and an identity', *Sociology of Health & Illness*, 28(3): 284–305.

Riddle, M. C. (2002), 'The underuse of insulin therapy in North America', *Diabetes Metabolism Research and Reviews*, 18(3): S42–S49.

Ridge, D. and Ziebland, S. (2006), '"The old me could never have done that": How people give meaning to recovery following depression', *Qualitative Health Research*, 16(8): 1038–53.

Ridgway, P. (2001), 'ReStorying psychiatric disability: Learning from first person recovery narratives', *Psychiatric Rehabilitation Journal*, 24(4): 335–43.

Rimmon-Kenan, S. (2002), 'The story of "I": Illness and narrative identity', *Narrative*, 19(1): 9–27.

Ringlstetter, C., Schulz, K. U. and Mihov, S. (2006), 'Orthographic errors in web pages: Toward cleaner web corpora', *Computational Linguistics*, 32(3): 295–340.

Robinson, J., Cox, G., Bailey, E., Hetrick, S., Rodrigues, M., Fisher, S. and Herrman, H. (2016), 'Social media and suicide prevention: A systematic review', *Early Intervention in Psychiatry*, 10(2): 103–21.

Roen, K., Scourfield, J. and McDermott, E. (2008), 'Making sense of suicide: A discourse analysis of young people's talk about suicidal subjecthood', *Social Science & Medicine*, 67(12): 2089–97.

Rogers, A. and Pilgrim, D. (1997), 'The contribution of lay knowledge to the understanding and promotion of mental health', *Journal of Mental Health*, 6(1): 23–35.

Rose, N. (2006), 'Diseases without borders? The expanding scope of psychiatric practice', *BioSocieties*, 1(4): 465–84.

Rose, N. (2007), 'Beyond medicalisation', *The Lancet*, 369(9562): 700–702.

Rothblum, E. D. (1994), '"I'll die for the revolution but don't ask me not to diet": Feminism and the continuing stigmatization of obesity', in P. Fallon, M. A. Katzman and S. Wooley (eds), *Feminist Perspectives on Eating Disorders*, 53–76, New York: Guildford Press.

Rude, S. S., Gortner, E. M. and Pennebaker, J. W. (2004), 'Language use of depressed and depression-vulnerable college students', *Cognition and Emotion*, 18: 1121–33.

Ruth-Sahd, L. A., Schneider, M. and Haagen, B. (2009), 'Diabulimia: What it is and how to recognize it in critical care', *Dimensions of Critical Care Nursing*, 28(4): 147–53.

Rydall, A. C., Rodin, G. M., Olmsted, M. P., Devenyi, R. G. and Daneman, D. (1997), 'Disordered eating behavior and microvascular complications in young women with insulin-dependent diabetes mellitus', *The New England Journal of Medicine*, 336: 1849–954.

Sackett, D. L., Rosenberg, W. M., Gray, J. M., Haynes, R. B. and Richardson, W. S. (1996), 'Evidence based medicine: What it is and what it isn't', *British Medical Journal*, 312(7023): 71–2.

Sacks, H. (1992), *Lectures on Conversation, Volumes I and II*, edited by G. Jefferson with Introduction by E. A. Schegloff, Oxford: Blackwell.

Sainsbury Centre for Mental Health. (2010), *The Economic and Social Costs of Mental Health Problems in 2009/10*, London: Sainsbury Centre.

Salem, D. A., Bogat, G. A. and Reid, C. (1997), 'Mutual help goes on-line', *Journal of Community Psychology*, 25: 189–207.

Sandaunet, A. G. (2008a), 'The challenge of fitting in: Non-participation and withdrawal from an online self-help group for breast cancer patients', *Sociology of Health & Illness*, 30(1): 131–44.

Sandaunet, A. G. (2008b), 'A space for suffering? Communicating breast cancer in an online self-help context', *Qualitative Health Research*, 18(12): 1631–41.

Sartorius, N. (2007), 'Stigma and mental health', *Lancet*, 370: 810–11.

Schaefer, J. (2004), *Life Without Ed*, New York: McGraw Hill.

Schaefer, J. (2009), *Goodbye Ed, Hello Me*, New York: McGraw Hill.

Schegloff, E. A. (1968), 'Sequencing in conversational openings', *American Anthropologist*, 70(6): 1075–95.

Schmidt, U. (2002), 'Risk factors for eating disorders', in C. G. Fairburn and K. D. Brownell (eds), *Eating Disorders and Obesity: A Comprehensive Handbook*, 2nd edn, 246–50, London: Guildford Press.

Schreiber, R. (1996), '(Re)Defining my self: Women's process of recovery from depression', *Qualitative Health Research*, 6(4): 469–91.

Schreiber, R. and G. Hartrick. (2002), 'Keeping it together: How women use the biomedical explanatory model to manage the stigma of depression', *Issues in Mental Health Nursing*, 23(2): 91–105.

Schuler, G., Petersen, K-G., Khalaf, A-N. and Kerp, L. (1989), 'Insulin abuse in long standing IDDM', *Diabetes Research and Clinical Practice*, 6(2): 145–8.

Scott, M. (1996), *WordSmith Tools*, Oxford: Oxford University Press.

Scott, M. (2016), *WordSmith Tools version 7*, Stroud: Lexical Analysis Software.

Scott, M. and Tribble, C. (2006), *Textual Patterns: Key Words and Corpus Analysis in Language Education*, Amsterdam: John Benjamins.

Scott, S. (2006), 'The medicalisation of shyness: From social misfits to social fitness', *Sociology of Health & Illness*, 28(2): 133–53.

Seale, C. (2001), 'Sporting cancer: Struggle language in news reports of people with cancer', *Sociology of Health & Illness*, 23(3): 308–29.

Seale, C., Charteris-Black, J., MacFarlane, A. and McPherson, A. (2010), 'Interviews and internet forums: A comparison of two sources of qualitative data', *Qualitative Health Research*, 20(5): 595–606.

Seale, C., Ziebland, S. and Charteris-Black, J. (2006), 'Gender, cancer experience and internet use: A comparative keyword analysis of interviews and online cancer support groups', *Social Science & Medicine*, 62(10): 2577–90.

Seligman, M. E. P. (1975), *Helplessness: On Depression, Development and Death*, San Francisco: Freeman.

Semino, E. (2008), *Metaphor in Discourse*, Cambridge: Cambridge University Press.

Serpell, L., Treasure, J., Teasdale, J. and Sullivan, V. (1999), 'Anorexia nervosa: Friend or foe?', *International Journal of Eating Disorders*, 25(2): 177–86.

Shaban, C. (2013), 'Diabulimia: Mental health condition or media hyperbole?', *Practical Diabetes*, 30(3): 104–5.

Sharma, A. E. (2013), *Diabulimia: Towards Understanding, Recognition, and Healing*, South Carolina: CreateSpace.

Shaw, A. and Favazza, A. (2010), 'Insulin under-dosing and omission should be included in DSM-V criteria for bulimia nervosa (letter to the editor)', *Journal of Neuropsychiatry and Clinical Neuroscience*, 22(3): 352.

Shih, G. H. (2011), *Diabulimia: What It Is and How to Treat It*, Lexington, KY: Grace Huifeng Shih.

Sinclair, J. (1991), *Corpus, Concordance, Collocation*, Oxford: Oxford University Press.

Sinclair, J. (2003), *Reading Concordances*, Harlow: Pearson.

Sinclair, J. (2004), *Trust the Text*, London and New York: Routledge.

Skårderud, F. (2007a), 'Eating one's words, Part I: "Concretised metaphors" and reflective function in anorexia nervosa—An interview study', *European Eating Disorders Review: The Professional Journal of the Eating Disorders Association*, 15(3): 163–74.

Skårderud, F. (2007b), 'Eating one's words, part II: The embodied mind and reflective function in anorexia nervosa—Theory', *European Eating Disorders Review: The Professional Journal of the Eating Disorders Association*, 15(4): 243–52.

Skelton, J. R. and Hobbs, F. D. R. (1999a), 'Concordancing: Use of language-based research in medical communication', *The Lancet*, 353(9147): 108–11.

Skelton, J. R. and Hobbs, F. D. R. (1999b), 'Descriptive study of cooperative language in primary care consultations by male and female doctors', *British Medical Journal*, 318: 576–9.

Skelton, J. R., Wearn, A. M. and Hobbs, F. D. R. (2002a), '"I" and "we": A concordancing analysis of how doctors and patients use first person pronouns in primary care consultations', *Family Practice*, 19(5): 484–8.

Skelton, J. R., Wearn, A. M. and Hobbs, F. D. R. (2002b), 'A concordance-based study of metaphoric expressions used by general practitioners and patients in consultation', *British Journal of General Practice*, 52(475): 114–18.

Smith, C. J., Adolphs, S., Harvey, K. and Mullany, L. (2014), 'Spelling errors and keywords in born-digital data: A case study using the Teenage Health Freak Corpus', *Corpora*, 9(2): 137–54.

Smithson, J., Sharkey, S., Hewis, E., Jones, R., Emmens, T., Ford, T. and Owens, C. (2011), 'Problem presentation and responses on an online forum for young people who self-harm', *Discourse Studies*, 13(4): 487–501.

Sneijder, P. and te Molder, H. F. M. (2004), 'Health should not have to be a problem: Talking health and accountability in an internet forum on veganism', *Journal of Health Psychology*, 9(4): 599–616.

Sontag, S. (1978), *Illness as Metaphor*, New York: Farrar, Straus & Giroux.

Sosnowy, C. (2014), 'Practicing patienthood online: Social media, chronic illness, and lay expertise', *Societies*, 4(2): 316–29.

Staiano, K. V. (1986), *Interpreting Signs of Illness*, Berlin: Mouton de Gruyter.

Starcke, B. (2006), 'The phraseology of Jane Austen's *Persuasion*: Phraseological units as carriers of meaning', *ICAME Journal*, 30: 87–104.

Steger, M and Roy, R. (2010), *Neoliberalism: A Very Short Introduction*, Oxford: Oxford University Press.

Steinhausen, H. (2002), 'The outcome of anorexia nervosa in the 20th century', *American Journal of Psychiatry*, 159(8): 1284–93.

Stephens, C., Carryer, J. and Budge, C. (2004), 'To have or to take: Discourse, positioning, and narrative identity in women's accounts of HRT', *Health*, 8(3): 329–50.

Stewart, C., Smith, B. and Sparkes, A. (2011), 'Sporting autobiographies of illness and the role of metaphor', *Sport in Society*, 14(5): 577–93.

Stewart, M. C., Keel, P. K. and Schiavo, R. S. (2006), 'Stigmatization of anorexia nervosa', *International Journal of Eating Disorders*, 39(4): 320–25.

Stommel, W. (2009), *Entering an Online Support Group on Eating Disorders: A Discourse Analysis*, Amsterdam: Rodopi.

Stommel, W. and Koole, T. (2010), 'The online support group as a community: A micro-analysis of the interaction with a new member', *Discourse Studies*, 12(3): 357–78.

Stommel, W. and Lamerichs, J. (2014), 'Communication in online support groups: Advice and beyond', in H. Hamilton and W.-Y. S. Chou (eds), *Routledge Handbook of Language and Health Communication*, 198–211, London and New York: Routledge.

Stoppard, J. (2000), *Understanding Depression: Feminist Social Constructionist Approaches*, London and New York: Routledge.

Strober, M. and Johnson, C. (2012), 'The need for complex ideas in anorexia nervosa: Why biology, environment, and psyche all matter, why therapists make mistakes, and why clinical benchmarks are needed for managing weight correction', *International Journal of Eating Disorders*, 45(2): 155–78.

Stubbs, M. (1983), *Discourse Analysis: The Sociolinguistic Analysis of Natural Language*, Chicago: University of Chicago Press.

Stubbs, M. (1994), 'Grammar, text, and ideology: Computer-assisted methods in the linguistics of representation', *Applied Linguistics*, 15(2): 201–23.

Stubbs, M. (1996), *Text and Corpus Analysis*, Oxford: Blackwell.

Stubbs, M. (2001), *Words and Phrases: Corpus Studies of Lexical Semantics*, London: Blackwell.

Stubbs, M. (2011), 'Sequence and order: The neo-Firthian tradition of corpus semantics', International Computer Archive of Modern and Medieval English (ICAME) 32. University of Oslo, 1–5 June 2011.

Suler, J. (2004), 'The online disinhibition effect', *CyberPsychology & Behaviour*, 7(3): 321–6.

Sunderland, J. (2004), *Gendered Discourses*, Basingstoke: Palgrave Macmillan.

Surtees, P. G. and Barkley, C. (1994), 'Future imperfect: The long-term outcome of depression', *British Journal of Psychiatry*, 164: 327–41.

Sveningsson Elm, M. (2009), 'How do various notions of privacy influence decisions in qualitative internet research?', in A. Markham and N. Baym (eds), *Internet Inquiry: Conversations about Method*, 69–87, Thousand Oaks, CA: Sage.

Swartz, L. (1987), 'Illness negotiation: The case of eating disorders', *Social Science & Medicine*, 24(7): 613–18.

Sweeting, H., Walker, L., MacLean, A., Patterson, C., Räisänen, U. and Hunt, K. (2015), 'Prevalence of eating disorders in males: A review of rates reported in academic research and UK mass media', *International Journal of Men's Health*, 14(2): 86–112.

Szasz, T. (1960), 'The myth of mental illness', *American Psychologist*, 15(2): 113–18.

Tausczik, Y. R. and Pennebaker, J. W. (2010), 'The psychological meaning of words: LIWC and computerized text analysis methods', *Journal of Language and Social Psychology*, 29(1): 24–54.

ten Have, P. (2002), 'Sequential structures and categorical implications in doctor-patient interaction: Ethnomethodology and history', *Paul Ten Have*. Available at http://www.paultenhave.nl/seqstruct.html.

Teubert, W. (1999), *Corpus Linguistics – A Partisan View*. Available at http://tractor.bham. ac.uk/ijcl/teubert_cl.html.

Teubert, W. (2005), 'My version of corpus linguistics', *International Journal of Corpus Linguistics*, 10(1): 1–13.

Thomas, G. and Wyatt, S. (1999), 'Shaping cyberspace – Interpreting and transforming the internet', *Research Policy*, 28: 681–98.

Thomas-MacLean, R. and Stoppard, J. M. (2004), 'Physicians' constructions of depression: Inside/outside the boundaries of medicalization', *Health*, 8(3): 275–93.

Thornbury, S. (2010), 'What can a corpus tell us about discourse?', in A. O'Keeffe and M. McCarthy (eds), *The Routledge Handbook of Corpus Linguistics*, 270–87, London and New York: Routledge.

Thorne, S. E. (1997), 'Phenomenological positivism and other problematic trends in health science research', *Qualitative Health Research*, 7(2): 287–93.

Tierney, S. and Fox, J. R. (2010), 'Living with the anorexic voice: A thematic analysis', *Psychology and Psychotherapy: Theory, Research and Practice*, 83(3): 243–54.

Tischner, I. and Malson, H. (2012), 'Deconstructing health and the un/healthy fat woman', *Journal of Community and Applied Social Psychology*, 22(1): 50–62.

Titscher, S., Meyer, M., Wodak, R. and Vetter, E. (2000), *Methods of Text and Discourse Analysis*, translated by Bryan Jenner, London: Sage.

Toolan, M. (2002), 'What is critical discourse analysis and why are people saying such terrible things about it', in M. Toolan (ed.), *Critical Discourse Analysis: Critical Concepts in Linguistics, Vol. III*, 218–41, London and New York: Routledge.

van der Geest, S. and Whyte, S. R. (1989), 'The charm of medicines: Metaphors and metonyms', *Medical Anthropology Quarterly*, 3(4): 345–67.

van Dijk, T. A. (1977), *Text and Context: Explorations in the Semantics and Pragmatics of Discourse*, London: Longman.

van Dijk, T. A. (2008), *Discourse & Power*, Basingstoke: Palgrave Macmillan.

van Leeuwen, T. (2008), *Discourse and Practice*, Oxford: Oxford University Press.

Vayreda, A. and Antaki, C. (2009), 'Social support and unsolicited advice in a bipolar disorder online forum', *Qualitative Health Research*, 19(7): 931–42.

Veen, M., te Molder, H. F. M., Gremmen, C. and van Woerkum, C. (2010), 'Quitting is not an option: An analysis of online talk between celiac disease patients', *Health*, 14(1): 23–40.

Victor, S. E., Scott, L. N., Stepp, S. D. and Goldstein, T. R. (2018), 'I want you to want me: Interpersonal stress and affective experiences as within-person predictors of nonsuicidal self-injury and suicide urges in daily life', *Suicide and Life-Threatening Behavior* [online first]. doi.org/10.1111/sltb.12513.

Warner, R. (1976), 'The relationship between language and disease concepts', *Journal of Psychiatry in Medicine*, 7(1): 57–68.

Weinger, K. and Beverly, E. A. (2010), 'Barriers to achieving glycemic targets: Who omits insulin and why?', *Diabetes Care*, 33(2): 450–2.

Wenger, E. (1998), *Communities of Practice: Learning, Meaning and Identity*, Cambridge: Cambridge University Press.

White, M. and Dorman, S. M. (2001), 'Receiving social support online: Implications for health education', *Health Education Research*, 16(6), 693–707.

Widdows, H. (2018), *Perfect Me: Beauty as an Ethical Ideal*, Princeton NJ: Princeton University Press.

Widdowson, H. (2002), 'Discourse analysis: A critical view', in M. Toolan (ed.), *Critical Discourse Analysis: Critical Concepts in Linguistics Vol. III,* 131–47. London: Routledge.

Widdowson, H. (2004), *Text, Context, Pretext: Critical Issues in Discourse Analysis*, Oxford: Blackwell.

Wiggins, S., McQuade, R. and Rasmussen, S. (2016), 'Stepping back from crisis points: The provision and acknowledgment of support in an online suicide discussion forum', *Qualitative Health Research*, 26(9): 1240–51.

Williams, J. M. G. and Pollock, L. R. (2000), 'The psychology of suicidal behaviour', in K. Hawton and K. van Heeringen (eds), *The International Handbook of Suicide and Attempted Suicide*, 79–93, Chichester: Wiley.

Williams, K., King, J. and Fox, J. R. (2016), 'Sense of self and anorexia nervosa: A grounded theory', *Psychology and Psychotherapy: Theory, Research and Practice*, 89(2): 211–28.

Williams, R. (1983), *Keywords: A Vocabulary of Culture and Society*, Revised edn, Oxford: Oxford University Press.

Williams, S. (2000), 'Chronic illness as biographical disruption or biographical disruption as chronic illness? Reflections on a core concept', *Sociology of Health & Illness*, 22(1): 40–67.

Williams, S. and Reid, M. (2010), 'Understanding the experience of ambivalence in anorexia nervosa: The maintainer's perspective', *Psychology and Health*, 25(5): 551–67.

Williams, S. J., Gabe, J. and Davis, P. (2009), *Pharmaceuticals and Society: Critical Discourses and Debates*, Chichester: John Wiley.

Willig, C. (2000), 'A discourse-dynamic approach to the study of subjectivity in health psychology', *Theory & Psychology*, 10(4): 547–70.

Willner, P. (1985), *Depression: A Psychobiological Synthesis*, New York: Wiley.

Winzelberg, A. (1997), 'The analysis of an electronic support group for individuals with eating disorders', *Computers in Human Behaviour*, 13(3): 393–407.

Wittink, M. N., Dahlberg, B., Biruk, C. and Barg, F. K. (2008), 'How older adults combine medical and experiential notions of depression', *Qualitative Health Research*, 18(9): 1174–83.

Wolf, M., Sedway, J., Bulik, C. M. and Kordy, H. (2007), 'Linguistic analyses of natural written language: Unobtrusive assessment of cognitive style in eating disorders', *International Journal of Eating Disorders*, 40(8): 711–17.

Wolf, N. (1991), *The Beauty Myth: How Images of Beauty Are Used Against Women*, New York: Morrow.

Wooffitt, R. (2005), *Conversation Analysis and Discourse Analysis: A Comparative and Critical Introduction*, London: Sage.

Woolrich, R. A., Cooper, M. J. and Turner, H. M. (2006), 'A preliminary study of negative self-beliefs in anorexia nervosa: A detailed exploration of their content, origins and functional links to "not eating enough" and other characteristic behaviours', *Cognitive Therapy and Research*, 30(6): 735–48.

World Health Organisation (1992), *The ICD-10 Classification of Mental and Behavioural Disorders: Clinical Descriptions and Diagnostic Guidelines*, New York: World Health Organisation.

World Health Organisation. (2017), *Depression and Other Common Mental Disorders: Global Health Estimates*, Geneva: World Health Organisation.

World Medical Association. (2013), 'World Medical Association Declaration of Helsinki: Ethical principles for medical research involving human subjects', *JAMA*, 310(20): 2191–94.

Wright, K. B. and Bell, S. B. (2003), 'Health-related support groups on the internet: Linking empirical findings to social support and computer-mediated communication theory', *Journal of Health Psychology*, 8(1): 39–54.

Zabka, C. (2011), 'The evolving price of perfection', *Journal of Renal Nutrition*, 21: e21–24.

Ziebland, S. and Wyke, S. (2012), 'Health and illness in a connected world: How might sharing experiences on the internet affect people's health?', *Milbank Quarterly*, 90(2): 219–49.

Ziółkowska, J. and Galasiński, D. (2017), 'Discursive construction of fatherly suicide', *Critical Discourse Studies*, 14(2): 150–66.

Zola, I. K. (1972), 'Medicine as an institution of social control', *Sociological Review*, 20: 487–504.

Index